Essential Atlas of
NEPHROLOGY

Essential Atlas of
NEPHROLOGY

Editor-in-Chief

Robert W. Schrier, MD
Professor and Chairman
Department of Medicine
University of Colorado School of Medicine
Denver, Colorado

Contributing Editors

William M. Bennett, MD
Professor (retired)
Department of Medicine
University of Oregon Health Sciences University;
Director
Department of Renal Transplantation
Legacy/Good Samaritan Hospital
Portland, Oregon

Tomas Berl, MD
Head, Division of Renal Diseases and Hypertension
University of Colorado School of Medicine
Denver, Colorado

Joseph V. Bonventre, MD, PhD
Massachusetts General Hospital
Charlestown, Massachusetts

Arthur H. Cohen, MD
Department of Pathology
Cedars-Sinai Medical Center
Los Angeles, California

Richard J. Glassock, MD
Department of Internal Medicine
University of Kentucky Chandler Medical Center
Lexington, Kentucky

Jean-Pierre Grünfeld, MD
Necker University Hospital
Paris, France

William L. Henrich, MD
Professor
Department of Medicine
University of Maryland School of Medicine;
Chairman
Department of Medicine
University of Maryland Medical Center
Baltimore, Maryland

Saulo Klahr, MD
Simon Professor of Medicine
Department of Internal Medicine
Washington University School of Medicine;
Seattle, Washington;
Physician
Barnes-Jewish Hospital
St. Louis, Missouri

Christopher S. Wilcox, MD, PhD
George E. Schreiner Professor of Nephrology
Department of Medicine
Georgetown University
Washington, DC

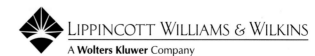
LIPPINCOTT WILLIAMS & WILKINS
A **Wolters Kluwer** Company
Philadelphia · Baltimore · New York · London
Buenos Aires · Hong Kong · Sydney · Tokyo

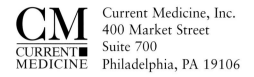 Current Medicine, Inc.
400 Market Street
Suite 700
Philadelphia, PA 19106

Developmental Editor: Elise M. Paxson
Editorial Assistant: Annmarie D'Ortona
Cover Design: William Whitman, Jr.
Design and Layout: Christine Keller-Quirk
Assistant Production Manager: Simon Dickey

Essential atlas of nephrology / editor-in-chief, Robert W. Schrier ;
contributing editors, William M Bennett ... [et al.] ; with 9
contributors
   p. ; cm.
  Includes bibliographical references and index.
  ISBN 0-7817-3530-0
  1. Kidneys--Diseases--Atlases. 2. Nephrology--Atlases.
  [DNLM: 1. Kidney Diseases--Atlases. WJ 17 E78 2001]   I.
Schrier, Robert W. II. Bennett, William M., 1938-
  RC903 .E85 2001
  616.6'1'00222---dc21
                 00-065629

ISBN 0-7817-3530-0

Printed in Hong Kong by Paramount

10 9 8 7 6 5 4 3 2

The publisher and editors acknowledge the contributions made by the many
authors, whose images appear in this volume, to the original series.

Distributed worldwide by Lippincott Williams & Wilkins

Preface

The *Essential Atlas of Nephrology* is a compilation of the most important images from the five-volume *Atlas of Diseases of the Kidney*. The images were chosen by all eight Section Editors of the latter series, all of whom are internationally prominent in their respective areas.

Tomas Berl is the Section Editor of the "Disorders of Water, Electrolytes, and Acid-Base" chapter. Joseph Bonventre is the Section Editor for the "Acute Renal Failure" chapter, which includes ischemic and nephrotoxic insults. Section Editors Arthur Cohen and Richard Glassock ("Glomerulonephritis and Vasculitis") focus on the most recent advances in immuno-pathology and treatments of the glomerulonephritides and vas-culitides. Jean-Pierre Grünfeld's chapter on "Tubulointerstitial Disease" focuses on interstitial nephritis and hereditary renal disease, including urinary tract infections, reflux, obstruction, cystic diseases, metabolic disorders, and the array of renal tubu-lar disorders. Christopher Wilcox is the Section Editor for "Hypertension and the Kidney." Treatment of end-stage renal disease is examined in two chapters: William Bennett covers "Transplantation as Treatment of End-stage Renal Disease," and William Henrich presents "Dialysis as Treatment of End-stage Renal Disease."

Saulo Klahr is the Section Editor for "Systemic Diseases and the Kidney."

The Section Editors and their authors from the *Atlas of Diseases of the Kidney* deserve the most credit for this *Essential Atlas of Nephrology*. I would like to thank Abe Krieger, President of Current Medicine, for initiating this aptly named "essential" reference tool. Thanks also to the develop-ment editor, Elise Paxson, and the excellent illustrators at Current Medicine, as well as for support from Jan Darling in my office.

Robert W. Schrier, MD

Contents

Disorders of Water, Electrolytes, and Acid-Base

Tomas Berl

CHAPTER

1

Horacio J. Androgué, Robert J. Anderson, Robert Bacallao, Kevin T. Bush, Marc E. De Broe, Wilfred Druml, Brian G. Dwinnel, David H. Ellison, Michael S. Goligorsky, Katrina J. Kelly, Rajiv Kumar, Sumit Kumar, Moshe Levi, Fernando Liaño, Wilfred Lieberthal, Stuart T. Linas, Nicolaos E. Madias, James T. McCarthy, Ravindra L. Mehta, Steven B. Miller, Bruce A. Molitoris, Cynthia C. Nast, Sanjay K. Nigam, Fredrick V. Osorio, Babu J. Padanilam, Julio Pascual, Mordecai Popovtzer, Lorraine C. Racusen, Hiroyuki Sakurai, Rick G. Schnellman, Kim Solez, Tatsuo Tsukamoto

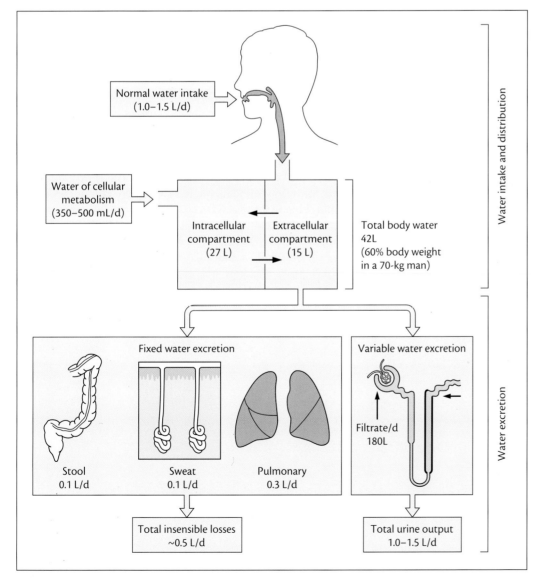

FIGURE 1-1

Principles of normal water balance. In most steady-state situations, human water intake matches water losses through all sources. Water intake is determined by thirst (*see* Fig. 1-2) and by cultural and social behaviors. Water intake is finely balanced by the need to maintain physiologic serum osmolality between 285 to 290 mOsm/kg. Both water that is drunk and that is generated through metabolism are distributed in the extracellular and intracellular compartments that are in constant equilibrium. Total body water equals approximately 60% of total body weight in young men, about 50% in young women, and less in older persons. Infants' total body water is between 65% and 75%. In a 70-kg man, in temperate conditions, total body water equals 42 L, 65% of which (22 L) is in the intracellular compartment and 35% (19 L) in the extracellular compartment.

Assuming normal glomerular filtration rate to be about 125 mL/min, the total volume of blood filtered by the kidney is about 180 L/d. Only about 1 to 1.5 L is excreted as urine, however, on account of the complex interplay of the urine concentrating and diluting mechanism and the effect of antidiuretic hormone to different segments of the nephron.

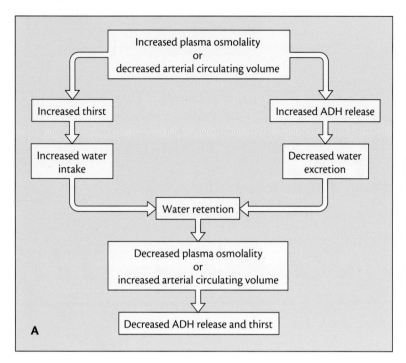

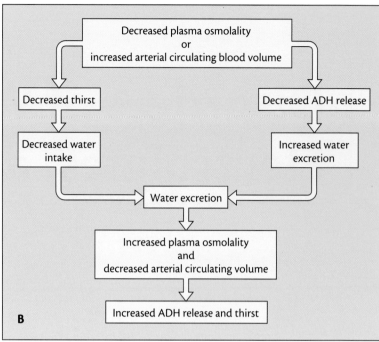

FIGURE 1-2

Pathways of water balance (conservation [**A**], and excretion [**B**]). In humans and other terrestrial animals, the thirst mechanism plays an important role in H_2O balance. Hypertonicity is the most potent stimulus for thirst: only 2% to 3 % changes in plasma osmolality produce a strong desire to drink water. This absolute level of osmolality at which the sensation of thirst arises in healthy persons, called the *osmotic threshold for thirst*, usually averages about 290 to 295 mOsm/kg H_2O (approximately 10 mOsm/kg H_2O above that of antidiuretic hormone [ADH] release). The so-called thirst center is located close to the osmoreceptors but is anatomically distinct. Between the limits imposed by the osmotic thresholds for thirst and ADH release, plasma osmolality may be regulated still more precisely by small osmoregulated adjustments in urine flow and water intake. The exact level at which balance occurs depends on various factors such as insensible losses through skin and lungs, and the gains incurred from eating, normal drinking, and fat metabolism. In general, overall intake and output come into balance at a plasma osmolality of 288 mOsm/kg, roughly halfway between the thresholds for ADH release and thirst [1].

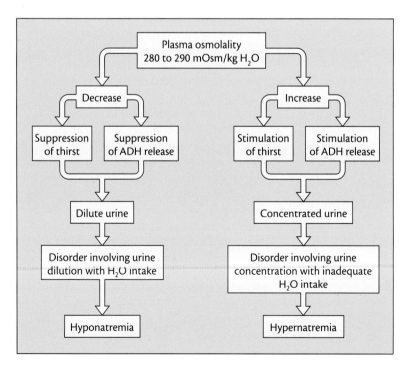

FIGURE 1-3

Pathogenesis of dysnatremias. The countercurrent mechanism of the kidneys in concert with the hypothalamic osmoreceptors via antidiuretic hormone (ADH) secretion maintain a very finely tuned balance of water (H_2O). A defect in the urine-diluting capacity with continued H_2O intake results in hyponatremia. Conversely, a defect in urine concentration with inadequate H_2O intake culminates in hypernatremia. Hyponatremia reflects a disturbance in homeostatic mechanisms characterized by excess total body H_2O relative to total body sodium, and hypernatremia reflects a deficiency of total body H_2O relative to total body sodium [2]. (*Adapted from* Halterman and Berl [3].)

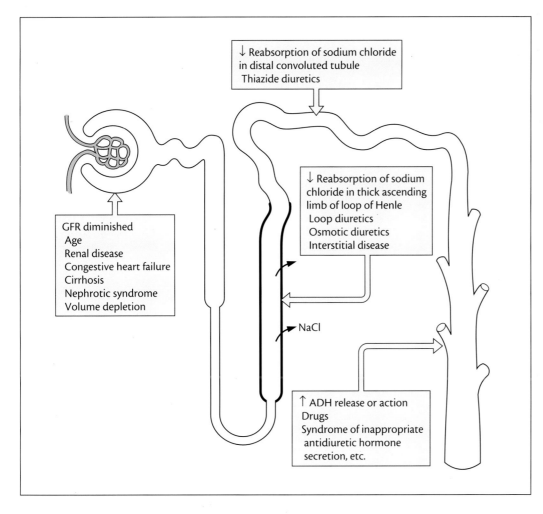

FIGURE 1-4

Pathogenesis of hyponatremia. Hyponatremia results from disorders of the diluting capacity of the kidney in the following situations:

1. *Intrarenal factors* such as a diminished glomerular filtration rate (GFR), or an increase in proximal tubule fluid and sodium reabsorption, or both, which decrease distal delivery to the diluting segments of the nephron, as in volume depletion, congestive heart failure, cirrhosis, or nephrotic syndrome.

2. *A defect in sodium chloride transport* out of the water-impermeable segments of the nephrons (*ie*, in the thick ascending limb of the loop of Henle). This may occur in patients with interstitial renal disease and administration of thiazide or loop diuretics.

3. *Continued secretion of antidiuretic hormone (ADH)* despite the presence of serum hypo-osmolality mostly stimulated by nonosmotic mechanisms [3].

NaCl—sodium chloride.

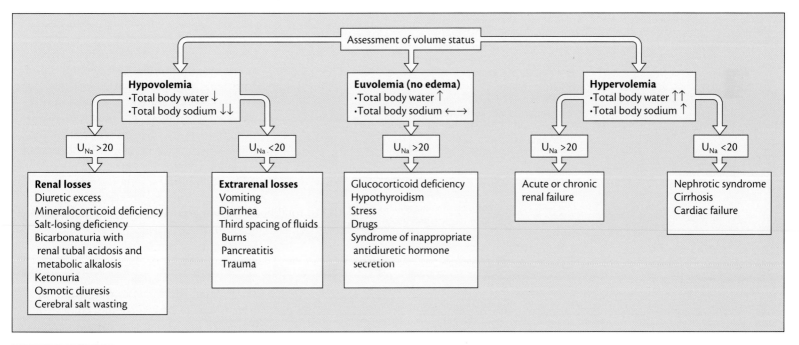

FIGURE 1-5

Diagnostic algorithm for hyponatremia. The next step in the evaluation of a hyponatremic patient is to assess volume status and identify it as hypovolemic, euvolemic or hypervolemic. The patient with hypovolemic hyponatremia has both total body sodium and water deficits, with the sodium deficit exceeding the water deficit. This occurs with large gastrointestinal and renal losses of water and solute when accompanied by free water or hypotonic fluid intake. In patients with hypervolemic hyponatremia, total body sodium is increased but total

body water is increased even more than sodium, causing hyponatremia. These syndromes include congestive heart failure, nephrotic syndrome, and cirrhosis. They are all associated with impaired water excretion. Euvolemic hyponatremia is the most common dysnatremia in hospitalized patients. In these patients, by definition, no physical signs of increased total body sodium are detected. They may have a slight excess of volume but no edema [3]. (*Adapted from* Halterman and Berl [3].)

HYPONATREMIC PATIENTS AT RISK FOR NEUROLOGIC COMPLICATIONS

Complication	Persons at Risk
Acute cerebral edema	Postoperative menstruant females
	Elderly women taking thiazides
	Children
	Psychiatric polydipsic patients
	Hypoxemic patients
Osmotic demyelination syndrome	Alcoholics
	Malnourished patients
	Hypokalemic patients
	Burn victims
	Elderly women taking thiazide diuretics

FIGURE 1-6

Hyponatremic patients at risk for neurologic complications. Those at risk for cerebral edema include postoperative menstruant women, elderly women taking thiazide diuretics, children, psychiatric patients with polydipsia, and hypoxic patients. In women, and, in particular, menstruant ones, the risk for developing neurologic complications is 25 times greater than that for nonmenstruant women or men. The increased risk was independent of the rate of development, or the magnitude of the hyponatremia [4]. The osmotic demyelination syndrome or central pontine myelinolysis seems to occur when there is rapid correction of low osmolality (hyponatremia) in a brain already chronically adapted (more than 72 to 96 hours). It is rarely seen in patients with a serum sodium value greater than 120 mEq/L or in those who have hyponatremia of less than 48 hours' duration [4,5]. (*Adapted from* Lauriat and Berl [5].)

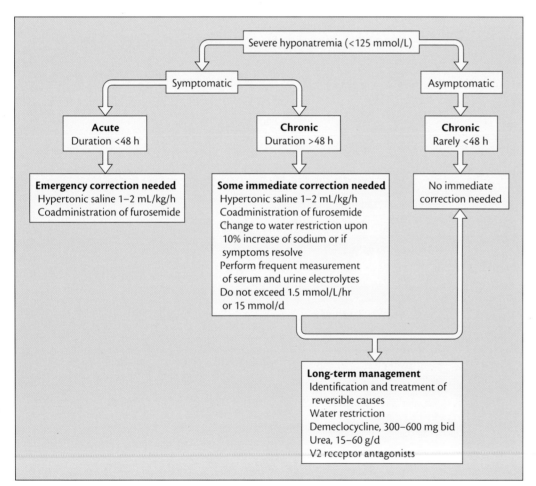

FIGURE 1-7

Treatment of severe euvolemic hyponatremia (<125 mmol/L). The evaluation of a hyponatremic patient involves an assessment of whether the patient is symptomatic, and if so, the duration of hyponatremia should be ascertained. The therapeutic approach to the hyponatremic patient is determined more by the presence or absence of symptoms than by the absolute level of serum sodium. Acutely hyponatremic patients are at great risk for permanent neurologic sequelae from cerebral edema if the hyponatremia is not promptly corrected. On the other hand, chronic hyponatremia carries the risk of osmotic demyelination syndrome if corrected too rapidly. The next step involves a determination of whether the patient has any risk factors for development of neurologic complications.

The commonest setting for acute, symptomatic hyponatremia is hospitalized, postoperative patients who are receiving hypotonic fluids. In these patients, the risk of cerebral edema outweighs the risk for osmotic demyelination. In the presence of seizures, obtundation, and coma, rapid infusion of 3% sodium chloride (4 to 6 mL/kg/h) or even 50 mL of 29.2% sodium chloride has been used safely. Ongoing careful neurologic monitoring is imperative [3].

A. GENERAL GUIDELINES FOR THE TREATMENT OF SYMPTOMATIC HYPONATREMIA*

Acute hyponatremia (duration < 48 hrs)

Increase serum sodium rapidly by approximately 2 mmol/L/h until symptoms resolve

Full correction probably safe but not necessary

Chronic hyponatremia (duration > 48 hrs)

Initial increase in serum sodium by 10% or 10 mmol/L

Perform frequent neurologic evaluations; correction rate may be reduced with improvement in symptoms

At no time should correction exceed rate of 1.5 mmol/L/h, or increments of 15 mmol/d

Measure serum and urine electrolytes every 1–2 h

*The sum of urinary cations (U_{Na} + U_K) should be less than the concentration of infused sodium, to ensure excretion of electrolyte-free water.

B. APPROACH TO INCREASING THE SERUM SODIUM CONCENTRATION

Calculate the net water loss needed to raise the serum sodium (S_{Na}) from 110 mEq/L to 120 mEq/L in a 50-kg person.

Example

Current S_{Na} × Total body water (TBW) = Desired S_{Na} × New TBW

Assume that TBW = 60% of body weight

Therefore TBW of patient = 50 × 0.6 = 30 L

$$New\ TBW = \frac{110\ mEq/L \times 30\ L}{120\ mEq/L} = 27.5\ L$$

Thus the electrolyte-free water loss needed to raise the S_{Na} to 120 mEq/L = Present TBW − New TBW = 2.5 L

Calculate the time course in which to achieve the desired correction (1 mEq/h)—in this case, 250 mL/h

Administer furosemide, monitor urine output, and replace sodium, potassium, and excess free water lost in the urine

Continue to monitor urine output and replace sodium, potassium, and excess free water lost in the urine

FIGURE 1-8

General guidelines for the treatment of symptomatic hyponatremia, **A**, Included herein are general guidelines for treatment of patients with acute and chronic symptomatic hyponatremia. In the treatment of chronic symptomatic hyponatremia, since cerebral water is increased by approximately 10%, a prompt increase in serum sodium by 10% or 10 mEq/L is permissible. Thereafter, the patient's fluids should be restricted. The total correction rate should not exceed 1.0 to 1.5 mEq/L/h, and the total increment in 24 hours should not exceed 15 mmol/d [3]. A specific example as to how to increase a patient's serum sodium is illustrated in *part B*.

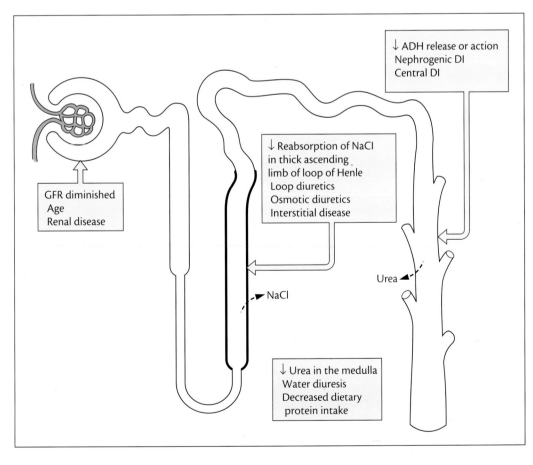

FIGURE 1-9

Pathogenesis of hypernatremia. The renal concentrating mechanism is the first line of defense against water depletion and hyperosmolality. When renal concentration is impaired, thirst becomes a very effective mechanism for preventing further increases in serum osmolality. Hypernatremia results from disturbances in the renal concentrating mechanism. This occurs in interstitial renal disease, with administration of loop and osmotic diuretics, and with protein malnutrition, in which less urea is available to generate the medullary interstitial tonicity.

Hypernatremia usually occurs only when hypotonic fluid losses occur in combination with a disturbance in water intake, typically in elders with altered consciousness, in infants with inadequate access to water, and, rarely, with primary disturbances of thirst [2]. ADH—antidiuretic hormone; DI—diabetes insipidus; GFR—glomerular filtration rate.

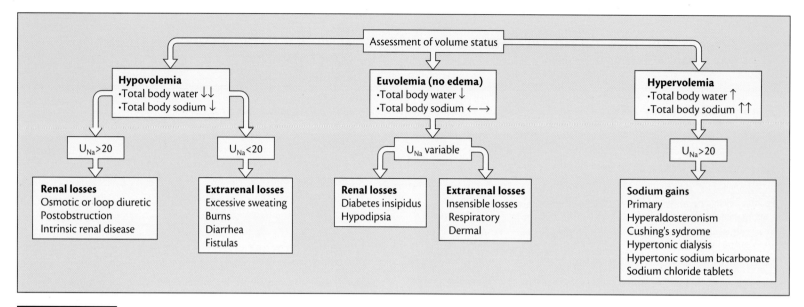

FIGURE 1-10

Diagnostic algorithm for hypernatremia. As for hyponatremia, the initial evaluation of the patient with hypernatremia involves assessment of volume status. Patients with hypovolemic hypernatremia lose both sodium and water, but relatively more water. On physical examination, they exhibit signs of hypovolemia. The causes listed reflect principally hypotonic water losses from the kidneys or the gastrointestinal tract.

Euvolemic hypernatremia reflects water losses accompanied by inadequate water intake. Since such hypodipsia is uncommon, hypernatremia usually supervenes in persons who have no access to water or who have a neurologic deficit that impairs thirst perception—the very young and the very old. Extrarenal water loss occurs from the skin and respiratory tract, in febrile or other hypermetabolic states. Very high urine osmolality reflects an intact osmoreceptor–antidiuretic hormone–renal response. Thus, the defense against the development of hyperosmolality requires appropriate stimulation of thirst and the ability to respond by drinking water. The urine sodium (U_{Na}) value varies with the sodium intake. The renal water losses that lead to euvolemic hypernatremia are a consequence of either a defect in vasopressin production or release (central diabetes insipidus) or failure of the collecting duct to respond to the hormone (nephrogenic diabetes insipidus) [6]. (*Adapted from Halterman and Berl [3].*)

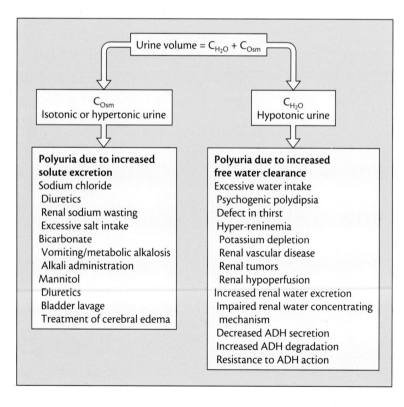

FIGURE 1-11

Physiologic approach to polyuric disorders. Among euvolemic hypernatremic patients, those affected by polyuric disorders are an important subcategory. Polyuria is arbitrarily defined as urine output of more than 3 L/d. Urine volume can be conceived of as having two components: the volume needed to excrete solutes at the concentration of solutes in plasma (called the *osmolar clearance*) and the other being the *free water clearance*, which is the volume of solute-free water that has been added to (positive free water clearance [C_{H_2O}]) or subtracted (negative C_{H_2O}) from the isotonic portion of the urine osmolar clearance (Cosm) to create either a hypotonic or hypertonic urine.

Consumption of an average American diet requires the kidneys to excrete 600 to 800 mOsm of solute each day. The urine volume in which this solute is excreted is determined by fluid intake. If the urine is maximally diluted to 60 mOsm/kg of water, the 600 mOsm will need 10 L of urine for effective osmotic clearance. If the concentrating mechanism is maximally stimulated to 1200 mOsm/kg of water, osmotic clearance will occur in a minimum of 500 mL of urine. This flexibility is affected when drugs or diseases alter the renal concentrating mechanism.

Polyuric disorders can be secondary to an increase in solute clearance, free water clearance, or a combination of both. ADH—antidiuretic hormone.

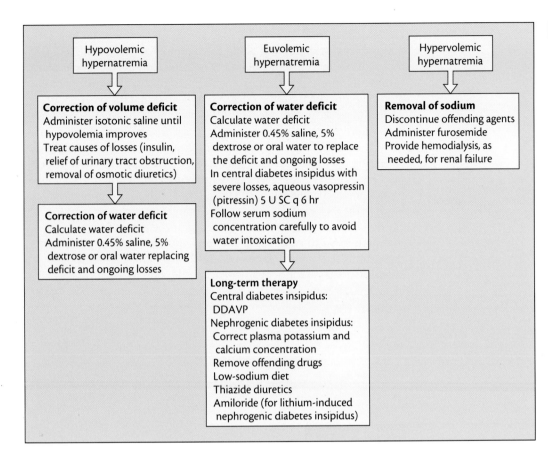

Hypovolemic hypernatremia	Euvolemic hypernatremia	Hypervolemic hypernatremia

Correction of volume deficit
Administer isotonic saline until hypovolemia improves
Treat causes of losses (insulin, relief of urinary tract obstruction, removal of osmotic diuretics)

Correction of water deficit
Calculate water deficit
Administer 0.45% saline, 5% dextrose or oral water replacing deficit and ongoing losses

Correction of water deficit
Calculate water deficit
Administer 0.45% saline, 5% dextrose or oral water to replace the deficit and ongoing losses
In central diabetes insipidus with severe losses, aqueous vasopressin (pitressin) 5 U SC q 6 hr
Follow serum sodium concentration carefully to avoid water intoxication

Long-term therapy
Central diabetes insipidus:
DDAVP
Nephrogenic diabetes insipidus:
Correct plasma potassium and calcium concentration
Remove offending drugs
Low-sodium diet
Thiazide diuretics
Amiloride (for lithium-induced nephrogenic diabetes insipidus)

Removal of sodium
Discontinue offending agents
Administer furosemide
Provide hemodialysis, as needed, for renal failure

FIGURE 1-12

Management options for patients with hypernatremia. The primary goal in the treatment of hypernatremia is restoration of serum tonicity. Hypovolemic hypernatremia in the context of low total body sodium and orthostatic blood pressure changes should be managed with isotonic saline until blood pressure normalizes. Thereafter, fluid management generally involves administration of 0.45% sodium chloride or 5% dextrose solution. The goal of therapy for hypervolemic hypernatremias is to remove the excess sodium, which is achieved with diuretics plus 5% dextrose. Patients who have renal impairment may need dialysis. In euvolemic hypernatremic patients, water losses far exceed solute losses, and the mainstay of therapy is 5% dextrose. To correct the hypernatremia, the total body water deficit must be estimated. This is based on the serum sodium concentration and on the assumption that 60% of the body weight is water [2]. (*Adapted from* Halterman and Berl [3].)

Disorders of Sodium Balance

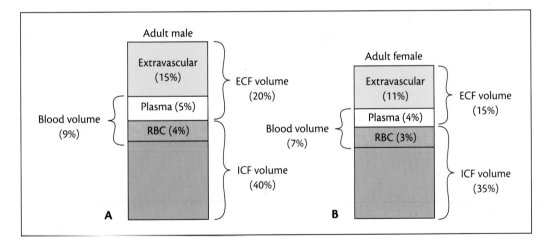

FIGURE 1-13

Fluid volumes in typical adult men and women, given as percentages of body weight. In men (**A**), total body water typically is 60% of body weight (total body water = Extracellular fluid [ECF] volume + intracellular fluid [ICF] volume). The ECF volume comprises the plasma volume and the extravascular volume. The ICF volume comprises the water inside erythrocytes (RBCs) and inside other cells. The blood volume comprises the plasma volume plus the RBC volume. Thus, the RBC volume is a unique component of ICF volume that contributes directly to cardiac output and blood pressure. Typically, water comprises a smaller percentage of the body weight in a woman (**B**) than in a man; thus, when expressed as a percentage of body weight, fluid volumes are smaller. Note, however, that the percentage of total body water that is intracellular is approximately 70% in both men and women.

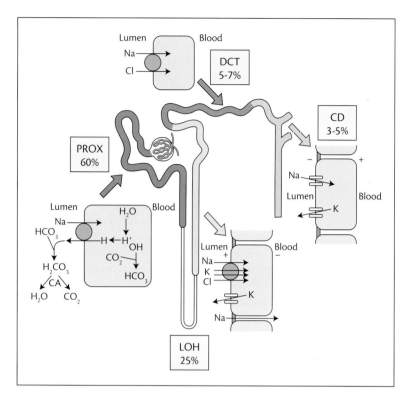

FIGURE 1-14

Sodium (Na) reabsorption along the mammalian nephron. About 25 moles of Na in 180 L of fluid daily is delivered into the glomerular filtrate of a normal person. About 60% of this load is reabsorbed along the proximal tubule (PROX), indicated in dark blue; about 25% along the loop of Henle (LOH), including the thick ascending limb indicated in light blue; about 5% to 7% along the distal convoluted tubule (DCT), indicated in dark gray; and 3% to 5% along the collecting duct (CD) system, indicated in light gray. All Na transporting cells along the nephron express the ouabain-inhibitable sodium-potassium adenosine triphosphatase (Na-K ATPase) pump at their basolateral (blood) cell surface. (The pump is not shown here for clarity.) Unique pathways are expressed at the luminal membrane that permit Na to enter cells. The most quantitatively important of these luminal Na entry pathways are shown here. CA—carbonic anhydrase; Cl—chloride; CO_2—carbon dioxide; H—hydrogen; H_2CO_3—carbonic acid; HCO_3—bicarbonate; K—potassium; OH—hydroxyl ion.

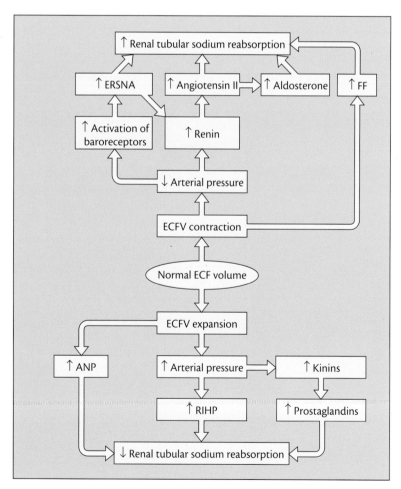

FIGURE 1-15

Integrated response of the kidneys to changes in extracellular fluid (ECF) volume. This composite figure illustrates natriuretic and anti-natriuretic mechanisms. For simplicity, the systems are shown operating only in one direction and not all pathways are shown. The major antinatriuretic systems are the renin-angiotensin-aldosterone axis and increased efferent renal sympathetic nerve activity (ERSNA). The most important natriuretic mechanism is pressure natriuresis, because the level of renal perfusion pressure (RPP) determines the magnitude of the response to all other natriuretic systems. Renal interstitial hydrostatic pressure (RIHP) is a link between the circulation and renal tubular sodium reabsorption. Atrial natriuretic peptide (ANP) is the major systemic natriuretic hormone. Within the kidney, kinins and renomedullary prostaglandins are important modulators of the natriuretic response of the kidney. AVP—arginine vasopressin; FF—filtration fraction. (*Adapted from* Gonzalez-Campoy and Knox [7].)

CAUSES OF VOLUME EXPANSION

Primary renal sodium retention (with hypertension but without edema)
  Hyperaldosteronism (Conn's syndrome)
  Cushing's syndrome
  Inherited hypertension (Liddle's syndrome, glucocorticoid remediable hyperaldo-
    steronism, pseudohypoaldosteronism type II, others)
  Renal failure
  Nephrotic syndrome (mixed disorder)

Secondary renal sodium retention
  Hypoproteinemia
    Nephrotic syndrome
    Protein-losing enteropathy
    Cirrhosis with ascites
  Low cardiac output
    Hemodynamically significant pericardial effusion
    Constrictive pericarditis
    Valvular heart disease with congestive heart failure
    Severe pulmonary disease
    Cardiomyopathies
  Peripheral vasodilation
    Pregnancy
    Gram-negative sepsis
    Anaphylaxis
    Arteriovenous fistula
    Trauma
    Cirrhosis
    Idiopathic edema (?)
    Drugs: minoxidil, diazoxide, calcium channel blockers (?)
  Increased capillary permeability
    Idiopathic edema (?)
    Burns
    Allergic reactions, including certain forms of angioedema
    Adult respiratory distress syndrome
    Interleukin-2 therapy
    Malignant ascites
  Sequestration of fluid ("3rd spacing," urine sodium concentration low)
    Peritonitis
    Pancreatitis
    Small bowel obstruction
    Rhabdomyolysis, crush injury
    Bleeding into tissues
    Venous occlusion

FIGURE 1-16

Causes of volume expansion. In volume expansion, total body sodi-um (Na) content is increased. In primary renal Na retention, volume expansion is modest and edema does not develop because blood pressure increases until Na excretion matches intake. In secondary Na retention, blood pressure may not increase sufficiently to increase urinary Na excretion until edema develops.

CAUSES OF VOLUME DEPLETION

Extrarenal losses (urine sodium concentration low)
  Gastrointestinal salt losses
    Vomiting
    Diarrhea
    Nasogastric or small bowel aspiration
    Intestinal fistulae or ostomies
    Gastrointestinal bleeding
  Skin and respiratory tract losses
    Burns
    Heat exposure
    Adrenal insufficiency
    Extensive dermatologic lesions
    Cystic fibrosis
    Pulmonary bronchorrhea
    Drainage of large pleural effusion

Renal losses (urine sodium concentration normal or elevated)
  Extrinsic
    Solute diuresis (glucose, bicarbonate, urea, mannitol, dextran, contrast dye)
    Diuretic agents
    Adrenal insufficiency
    Selective aldosterone deficiency
  Intrinsic
    Diuretic phase of oliguric acute renal failure
    Postobstructive diuresis
    Nonoliguric acute renal failure
    Salt-wasting nephropathy
      Medullary cystic disease
      Tubulointerstitial disease
      Nephrocalcinosis

FIGURE 1-17

Causes of volume depletion. In volume depletion, total body sodium is decreased.

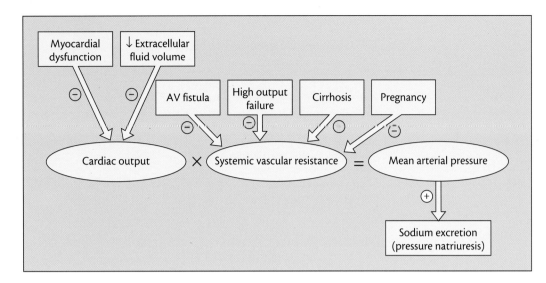

FIGURE 1-18

Summary of mechanisms of sodium (Na) retention in volume contraction and in depletion of the "effective" arterial volume. In secondary Na retention, Na retention results primarily from a reduction in mean arterial pressure (MAP). Some disorders decrease cardiac output, such as congestive heart failure owing to myocardial dysfunction; others decrease systemic vascular resistance, such as high-output cardiac failure, atriovenous fistulas, and cirrhosis. Because MAP is the product of systemic vascular resistance and cardiac output, all causes lead to the same result. Small changes in MAP lead to large changes in urinary Na excretion. Although edematous disorders usually are characterized as resulting from contraction of the effective arterial volume, the MAP, as a determinant of renal perfusion pressure, may be the crucial variable. The mechanisms of edema in nephrotic syndrome are more complex.

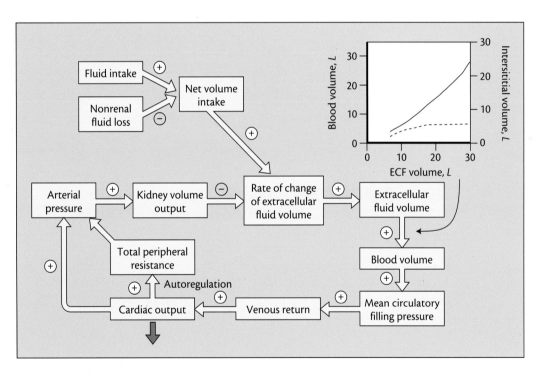

FIGURE 1-19

Mechanism of extracellular fluid (ECF) volume expansion in congestive heart failure. A primary decrease in cardiac output (indicated by dark blue arrow) leads to a decrease in arterial pressure, which decreases pressure natriuresis and volume excretion. These decreases expand the ECF volume. The inset graph shows that the ratio of interstitial volume (*solid line*) to plasma volume (*dotted line*) increases as the ECF volume expands because the interstitial compliance increases [8]. Thus, although expansion of the ECF volume increases blood volume and venous return, thereby restoring cardiac output toward normal, this occurs at the expense of a *disproportionate* expansion of interstitial volume, often manifested as edema.

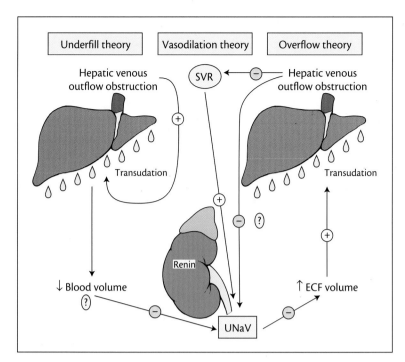

FIGURE 1-20

Three theories of ascites formation in hepatic cirrhosis. Hepatic venous outflow obstruction leads to portal hypertension. According to the *underfill theory*, transudation from the liver leads to reduction of the blood volume, thereby stimulating sodium (Na) retention by the kidney. As indicated by the question mark near the term *blood volume*, a low blood volume is rarely detected in clinical or experimental cirrhosis. Furthermore, this theory predicts that ascites would develop before renal Na retention, when the reverse generally occurs. According to the *overflow theory*, increased portal pressure stimulates renal Na retention through incompletely defined mechanisms. As indicated by the question mark near the arrow from hepatic venous outflow obstruction to $U_{Na}V$, the nature of the portal hypertension–induced signals for renal Na retention remains unclear. The *vasodilation theory* suggests that portal hypertension leads to vasodilation and relative arterial hypotension. Evidence for vasodilation in cirrhosis that precedes renal Na retention is now convincing [9].

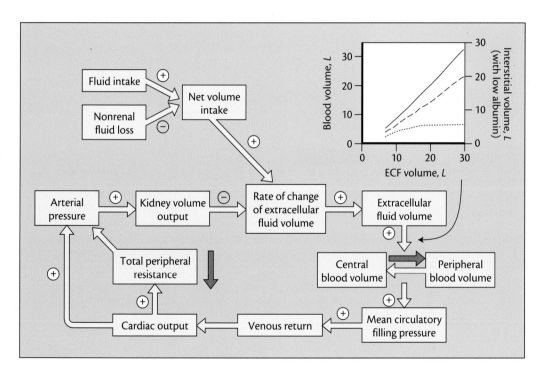

FIGURE 1-21

Mechanisms of sodium (Na) retention in cirrhosis. A primary decrease in systemic vascular resistance (indicated by dark arrow) leads to a decrease in arterial pressure. The reduction in systemic vascular resistance, however, is not uniform and favors movement of blood from the central ("effective") circulation into the peripheral circulation. Hypoalbuminemia shifts the interstitial to blood volume ratio upward (compare the interstitial volume with normal [*dashed line*], and low [*solid line*], protein levels in the inset graph). Because cardiac output increases and venous return must equal cardiac output, dramatic expansion of the extracellular fluid (ECF) volume occurs.

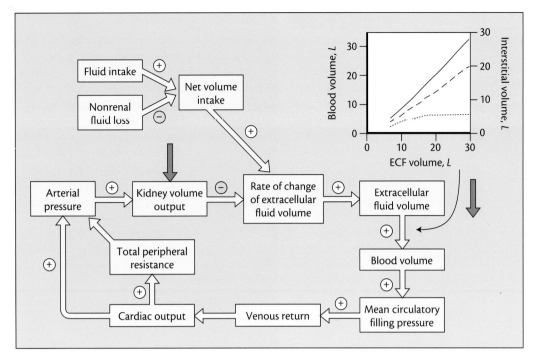

FIGURE 1-22

Mechanisms of extracellular fluid (ECF) volume expansion in nephrotic syndrome. Nephrotic syndrome is characterized by hypoalbuminemia, which shifts the relation between blood and interstitial volume upward (dashed to solid lines in inset). These effects of hypoalbuminemia are evident when serum albumin concentrations decrease by more than half. In addition, however, hypoalbuminemia may induce vasodilation and arterial hypotension that lead to sodium (Na) retention, independent of transudation of fluid into the interstitium. Unlike other states of hypoproteinemia and vasodilation, however, nephrotic syndrome usually is associated with normotension or hypertension. Natriuresis may take place before increases in serum albumin concentration in patients with nephrotic syndrome, implicating an important role for primary renal Na retention in this disorder (dark blue arrow). The decrease in urinary Na excretion may play a larger role in patients with acute glomerulonephritis than in patients with minimal change nephropathy.

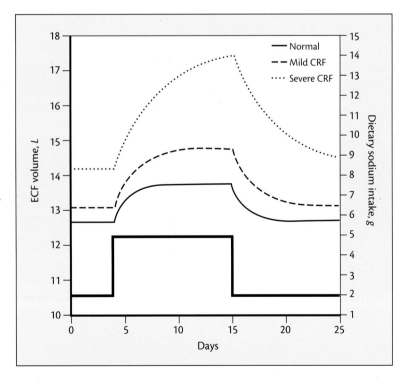

FIGURE 1-23

Effects of dietary sodium (Na) intake on extracellular fluid (ECF) volume in chronic renal failure (CRF) [10]. Compared with normal persons, patients with CRF have expanded ECF volume at normal Na intake. Furthermore, the time necessary to return to neutral balance on shifting from one to another level of Na intake is increased. Thus, whereas urinary Na excretion equals dietary intake of Na within 3 to 5 days in normal persons, this process may take up to 2 weeks in patients with CRF. This time delay means that not only are these patients susceptible to volume overload, but also to volume depletion.

Diseases of Potassium Metabolism

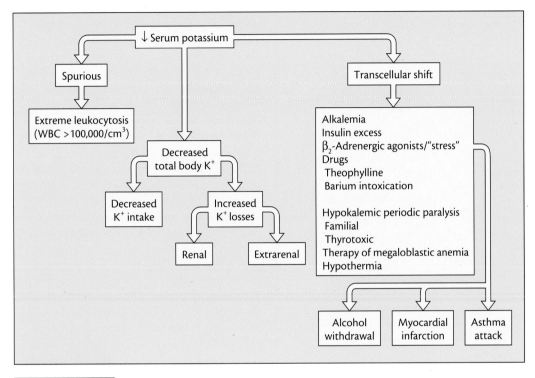

Overview of diagnostic approach to hypokalemia: hypokalemia without total body potassium depletion. Hypokalemia can result from transcellular shifts of potassium into cells without total body potassium depletion or from decreases in total body potassium. Perhaps the most dramatic examples occur in catecholamine excess states, as after administration of

$\beta_2$adreneric receptor (β_2AR) agonists or during "stress." It is important to note that, during some conditions (eg, ketoacidosis), transcellular shifts and potassium depletion exist simultaneously. Spurious hypokalemia results when blood specimens from leukemia patients are allowed to stand at room temperature; this results in leukocyte uptake of potassium from serum and artifactual hypokalemia. Patients with spurious hypokalemia do not have clinical manifestations of hypokalemia, as their in vivo serum potassium values are normal. Theophylline poisoning prevents cAMP breakdown. Barium poisoning from the ingestion of soluble barium salts results in severe hypokalemia by blocking channels for exit of potassium from cells. Episodes of hypokalemic periodic paralysis can be precipitated by rest after exercise, carbohydrate meal, stress, or administration of insulin. Hypokalemic periodic paralysis can be inherited as an autosomal-dominant disease or acquired by patients with thyrotoxicosis, especially Chinese males. Therapy of megaloblastic anemia is associated with potassium uptake by newly formed cells, which is occasionally of sufficient magnitude to cause hypokalemia [11].

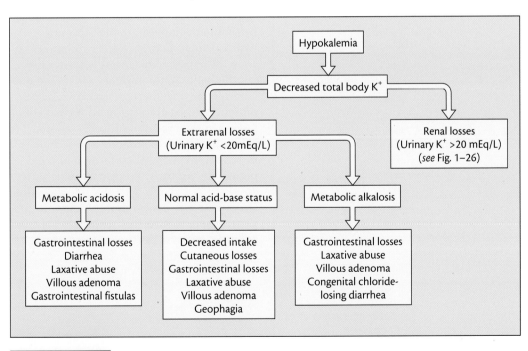

Diagnostic approach to hypokalemia: hypokalemia with total body potassium depletion secondary to extrarenal losses. In the absence of redistribution, measurement of urinary potassium is helpful in determining whether hypokalemia is due to renal or to extrarenal potassium losses. The normal kidney responds to several (3 to 5) days of potassium depletion with appropriate renal potassium conservation. In the absence of severe polyuria, a "spot"

urinary potassium concentration of less than 20 mEq/L indicates renal potassium conservation. In certain circumstances (eg, diuretics abuse), renal potassium losses may not be evident once the stimulus for renal potassium wasting is removed. In this circumstance, urinary potassium concentrations may be deceptively low despite renal potassium losses. Hypokalemia due to colonic villous adenoma or laxative abuse may be associated with metabolic acidosis, alkalosis, or no acid-base disturbance. Stool has a relatively high potassium content, and fecal potassium losses could exceed 100 mEq per day with severe diarrhea. Habitual ingestion of clay (pica), encountered in some parts of the rural southeastern United States, can result in potassium depletion by binding potassium in the gut, much as a cation exchange resin does. Inadequate dietary intake of potassium, like that associated with anorexia or a "tea and toast" diet, can lead to hypokalemia, owing to delayed renal conservation of potassium; however, progressive potassium depletion does not occur unless intake is well below 15 mEq of potassium per day.

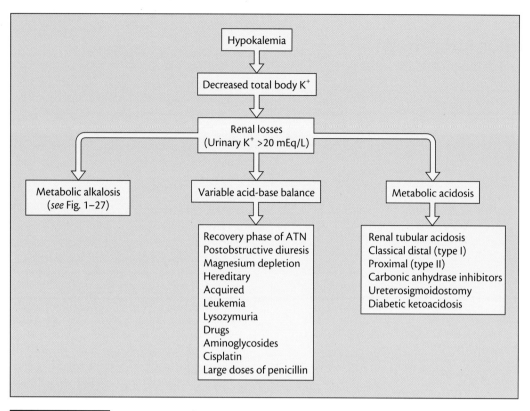

FIGURE 1-26

Diagnostic approach to hypokalemia: hypokalemia due to renal losses with normal acid-base status or metabolic acidosis. Hypokalemia is occasionally observed during the diuretic recovery phase of acute tubular necrosis (ATN) or after relief of acute obstructive uropathy, pre-

sumably secondary to increased delivery of sodium and water to the distal nephrons. Patients with acute monocytic and myelomonocytic leukemias occasionally excrete large amounts of lysozyme in their urine. Lysozyme appears to have a direct kaliuretic effect on the kidneys (by an undefined mechanism). Penicillin in large doses acts as a poorly reabsorbable anion, resulting in obligate renal potassium wasting. Mechanisms for renal potassium wasting associated with aminoglycosides and cisplatin are ill-defined. Hypokalemia in type I renal tubular acidosis is due in part to secondary hyperaldosteronism, whereas type II renal tubular acidosis can result in a defect in potassium reabsorption in the proximal nephrons. Carbonic anhydrase inhibitors result in an acquired form of renal tubular acidosis. Ureterosigmoidostomy results in hypokalemia in 10% to 35% of patients, owing to the sigmoid colon's capacity for net potassium secretion. The osmotic diuresis associated with diabetic ketoacidosis results in potassium depletion, although patients may initially present with a normal serum potassium value, owing to altered transcellular potassium distribution.

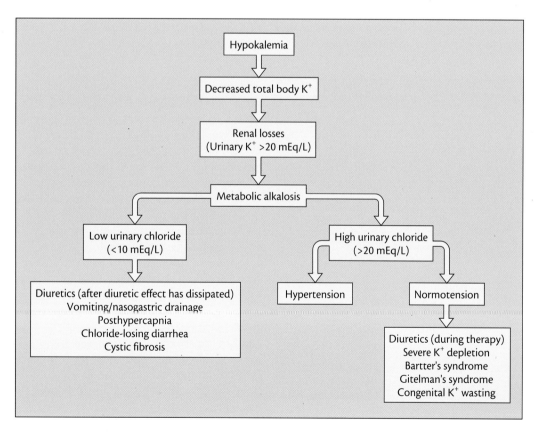

FIGURE 1-27

Diagnostic approach to hypokalemia: hypokalemia due to renal losses with metabolic alkalosis. The urine chloride value is helpful in distinguishing the causes of hypokalemia. Diuretics are a common cause of hypokalemia; however, after discontinuing diuretics, urinary potassium and chloride may be appropriately low. Urine diuretic screens are warranted for patients suspected of surreptious diuretic abuse. Vomiting results in chloride and sodium depletion, hyperaldosteronism, and renal potassium wasting. Posthypercapnic states are often associated with chloride depletion (from diuretics) and sodium avidity. If hypercapnia is corrected without replacing chloride, patients develop chloride-depletion alkalosis and hypokalemia.

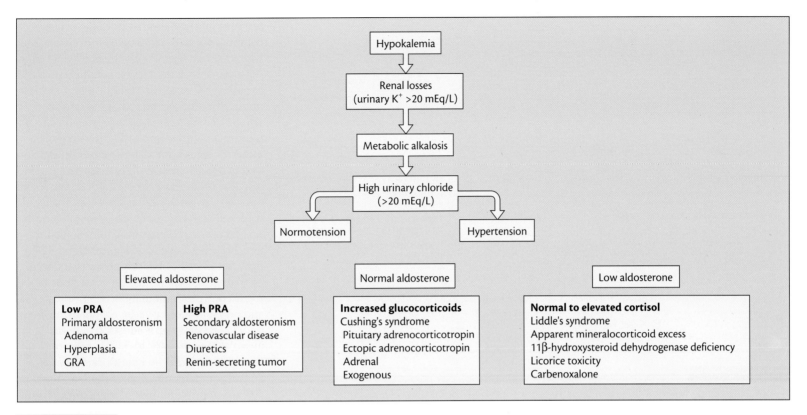

FIGURE 1-28

Diagnostic approach to hypokalemia: hypokalemia due to renal losses with hypertension and metabolic alkalosis.

FIGURE 1-29

Treatment of hypokalemia.

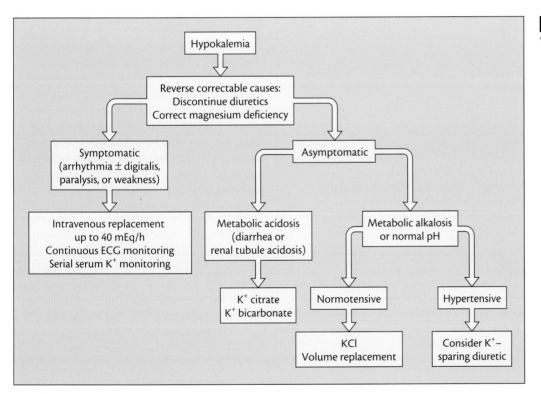

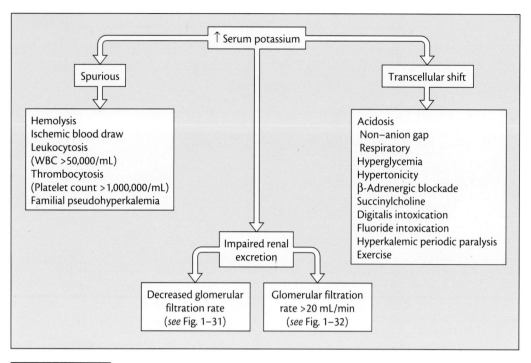

FIGURE 1-30

Approach to hyperkalemia: hyperkalemia without total body potassium excess. Spurious hyperkalemia is suggested by the absence of electrocardiographic (ECG) findings in patients with elevated serum potassium. The most common cause of spurious hyperkalemia is hemolysis, which may be apparent on visual inspection of serum. For patients with extreme leukocytosis or thrombocytosis, potassium levels should be measured in plasma samples that have

been promptly separated from the cellular components since extreme elevations in either leukocytes or platelets results in leakage of potassium from these cells. Familial pseudohyperkalemia is a rare condition of increased potassium efflux from red blood cells in vitro. Ischemia due to tight or prolonged tourniquet application or fist clenching increases serum potassium concentrations by as much as 1.0 to 1.6 mEq/L. Hyperkalemia can also result from decreases in K movement into cells or increases in potassium movement from cells. Hyperchloremic metabolic acidosis (in contrast to organic acid, anion-gap metabolic acidosis) causes potassium ions to flow out of cells. Hypertonic states induced by mannitol, hypertonic saline, or poor blood sugar control promote movement of water and potassium out of cells. Depolarizing muscle relaxants such as succinylcholine increase permeability of muscle cells and should be avoided by hyperkalemic patients. Digitalis impairs function of the Na^+-K^+-ATPase pumps and blocks entry of potassium into cells. Acute fluoride intoxication can be treated with cation-exchange resins or dialysis, as attempts at shifting potassium back into cells may not be successful.

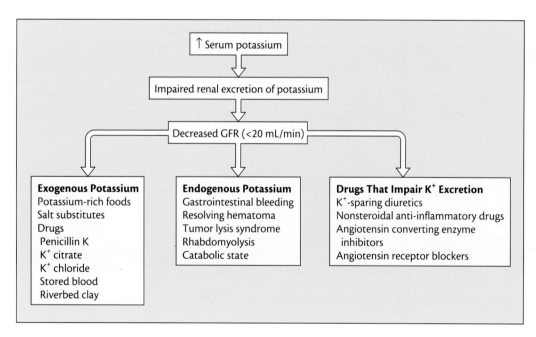

FIGURE 1-31

Approach to hyperkalemia: hyperkalemia with reduced glomerular filtration rate (GFR). Normokalemia can be maintained in patients who consume normal quantities of potassium until GFR decreases to less than 10 mL/min; however, diminished GFR predisposes patients to hyperkalemia from excessive exogenous or endogenous potassium loads. Hidden sources of endogenous and exogenous potassium—and drugs that predispose to hyperkalemia—are listed.

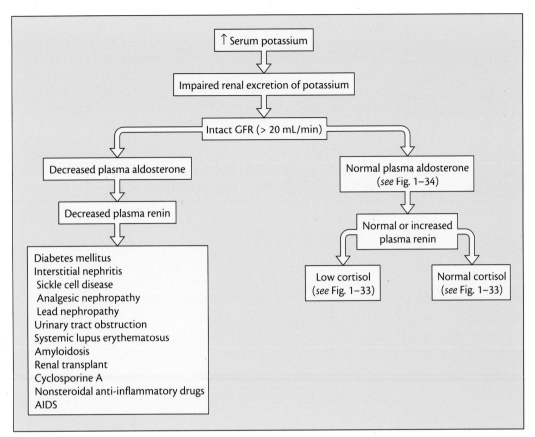

FIGURE 1-32

Approach to hyperkalemia: hyporeninemic hypoaldosteronism. Hyporeninemic hypoaldosteronism accounts for the majority of cases of unexplained hyperkalemia in patients with reduced glomerular filtration rate (GFR) whose level of renal insufficiency is not what would be expected to cause hyperkalemia. Interstitial renal disease is a feature of most of the diseases listed. The transtubular potassium gradient can be used to distinguish between primary tubule defects and hyporeninemic hypoaldosteronism. Although the transtubular potassium gradient should be low in both disorders, exogenous mineralocorticoid would normalize transtubular potassium gradient in hyporeninemic hypoaldosteronism.

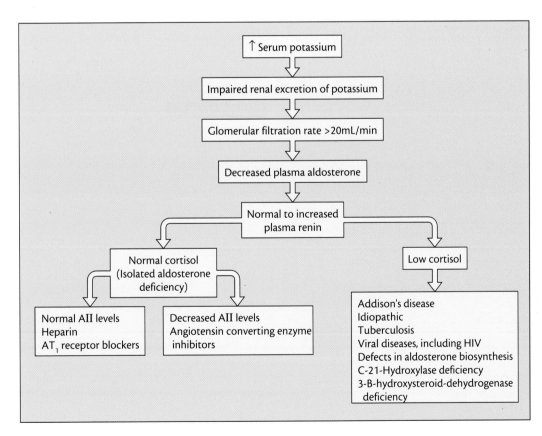

FIGURE 1-33

Approach to hyperkalemia: low aldosterone with normal to increased plasma renin. Heparin impairs aldosterone synthesis by inhibiting the enzyme 18-hydroxylase. Despite its frequent use, heparin is rarely associated with overt hyperkalemia; this suggests that other mechanisms (*eg*, reduced renal potassium secretion) must be present simultaneously for hyperkalemia to manifest itself. Both angiotensin-converting enzyme inhibitors and the angiotensin type 1 receptor blockers (AT_1) receptor blockers interfere with adrenal aldosterone synthesis. Generalized impairment of adrenal cortical function manifested by combined glucocorticoid and mineralocorticoid deficiencies are seen in Addison's disease and in defects of aldosterone biosynthesis.

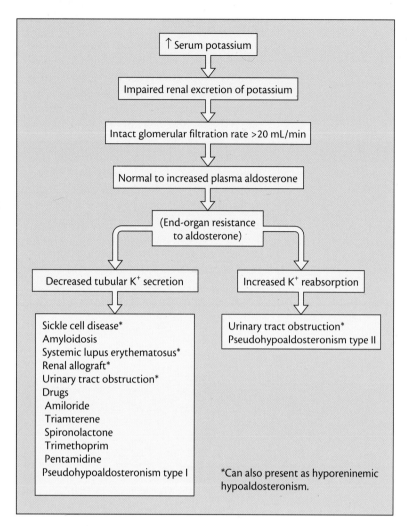

FIGURE 1-34

Approach to hyperkalemia: pseudohypoaldosteronism. The mechanism of decreased potassium excretion is caused either by failure to secrete potassium in the cortical collecting tubule or enhanced reabsorption of potassium in the medullary or papillary collecting tubules. Decreased secretion of potassium in the cortical and medullary collecting duct results from decreases in either apical sodium or potassium channel function or diminished basolateral Na^+-K^+-ATPase activity. Alternatively, potassium may be secreted normally but hyperkalemia can develop because potassium reabsorption is enhanced in the intercalated cells of the medullary collecting duct. The transtubule potassium gradient (TTKG) in both situations is inappropriately low and fails to normalize in response to mineralocorticoid replacement.

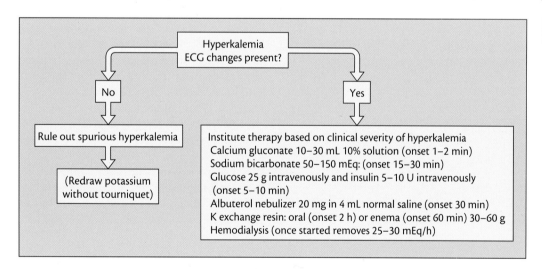

FIGURE 1-35

Treatment of hyperkalemia.

Divalent Cation Metabolism: Magnesium

CAUSES OF MAGNESIUM DEPLETION

Poor Mg intake
- Starvation
- Anorexia
- Protein calorie malnutrition
- No Mg in intravenous fluids

Renal losses

Increased gastrointestinal Mg losses
- Nasogastric suction
- Vomiting
- Intestinal bypass for obesity
- Short-bowel syndrome
- Inflammatory bowel disease
- Pancreatitis
- Diarrhea
- Laxative abuse
- Villous adenoma

Other
- Lactation
- Extensive burns
- Exchange transfusions

FIGURE 1-36

The causes of magnesium (Mg) depletion. Depletion of Mg can develop as a result of low intake or increased losses by way of the gastrointestinal tract, the kidneys, or other routes [12,13,14–19].

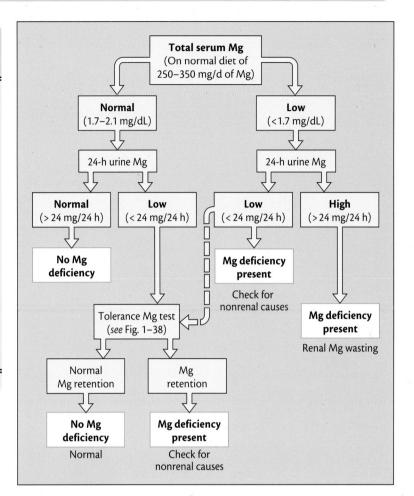

FIGURE 1-37

Evaluation in suspected magnesium (Mg) deficiency. Serum Mg levels may not always indicate total body stores. More refined tools used to assess the status of Mg in erythrocytes, muscle, lymphocytes, bone, isotope studies, and indicators of intracellular Mg, are not routinely available. Screening for Mg deficiency relies on the fact that urinary Mg decreases rapidly in the face of Mg depletion in the presence of normal renal function [13–19,20,21]. (*Adapted from* Al-Ghamdi *et al.* [17].)

MAGNESIUM TOLERANCE TEST FOR PATIENTS WITH NORMAL SERUM MAGNESIUM

Time	Action
0 (baseline)	Urine (spot or timed) for molar Mg:Cr ratio
0–4 h	IV infusion of 2.4 mg (0.1 mmol) of Mg/kg lean body wt in 50 mL of 50% dextrose
0–24 h	Collect urine (starting with Mg infusion) for Mg and Cr
End	Calculate % Mg retained (%M)

$$\% \, M = 1 - \frac{(24\text{-h urine Mg}) - ([\text{Preinfusion urine Mg:Cr}] \times [24\text{-h urine Cr}])}{\text{Total Mg infused}} \times 100$$

Mg retained, %	Mg deficiency
>50	Definite
20–50	Probable
<20	None

Cr—creatinine; IV—intravenous; Mg—magnesium.

FIGURE 1-38

The magnesium (Mg) tolerance test, in various forms [13–18,20,21], has been advocated to diagnose Mg depletion in patients with normal or near-normal serum Mg levels. All such tests are predicated on the fact that patients with normal Mg status rapidly excrete over 50% of an acute Mg load, whereas patients with depleted Mg retain Mg in an effort to replenish Mg stores. (*Adapted from* Ryzen *et al.* [21].)

MAGNESIUM SALTS USED IN MAGNESIUM REPLACEMENT THERAPY

Magnesium salt	Chemical formula	Mg content, *mg/g*	Examples*	Mg content	Diarrhea[†]
Gluconate	$Cl_2H_{22}MgO_{14}$	58	Magonate°	27-mg tablet 54 mg/5 mL	±
Chloride	$MgCl_2 \cdot (H_2O)_6$	120	Mag-L-100	100-mg capsule	+
Lactate	$C_6H_{10}MgO_6$	120	MagTab SR*	84-mg caplet	+
Citrate	$C_{12}H_{10}Mg_3O_{14}$	53	Multiple	47–56 mg/5 mL	++
Hydroxide	$Mg(OH)_2$	410	Maalox°, Mylanta°, Gelusil° Riopan°	83 mg/ 5 mL and 63-mg tablet 96 mg/5 mL	++
Oxide	MgO	600	Mag-Ox 400° Uro-Mag° Beelith°	241-mg tablet 84.5-mg tablet 362-mg tablet	++
Sulfate	$MgSO_4 \cdot (H_2O)_7$	100	IV IV Oral epsom salt	10%—9.9 mg/mL 50%—49.3 mg/mL 97 mg/g	++ ++
Milk of Magnesia			Phillips' Milk of Magnesia°	168 mg/ 5 mL	++

Data from McLean [16], Al-Ghamdi and coworkers [18], Oster and Epstein [23], and Physicians' Desk Reference [24].

*Magonate°, Fleming & Co, Fenton, MD; MagTab Sr°, Niche Pharmaceuticals, Roanoke, TX; Maalox°, Rhone-Poulenc Rorer Pharmaceutical, Collegeville, PA; Mylanta°, J & J-Merck Consumer Pharm, Ft Washinton, PA; Riopan°, Whitehall Robbins Laboratories, Madison, NJ; Mag-Ox 400° and Uro-Mag°, Blaine, Erlanger, KY; Beelith°, Beach Pharmaceuticals, Conestee, SC; Phillips' Milk of Magnesia, Bayer Corp, Parsippany, NJ.

[†]*Plus signs* indicate likelihood of causing diarrhea: *double plus signs* indicate most likely; ± sign indicates least likely.

FIGURE 1-39

Magnesium (Mg) salts that may be used in Mg replacement therapy.

GUIDELINES FOR MAGNESIUM REPLACEMENT

Life-threatening event (eg, seizures and cardiac arrhythmia)

I. 2–4 g MgSO$_4$ IV or IM stat
(2–4 vials [2 mL each] of 50% MgSO$_4$)
Provides 200–400 mg of Mg (8.3–16.7 mmol Mg)
Closely monitor:
  Deep tendon reflexes
  Heart rate
  Blood pressure
  Respiratory rate
  Serum Mg (<2.5 mmol/L [6.0 mg/dL])
  Serum K

II. IV drip over first 24 h
to provide no more
than 1200 mg (50
mmol) Mg/24 h

Subacute and chronic Mg replacement

I. 400–600 mg (16.7–25 mmol Mg daily for 2–5 d)
IV: continuous infusion
IM: painful
Oral: use divided doses to minimize diarrhea

FIGURE 1-40

Acute Mg replacement for life-threatening events such as seizures or potentially lethal cardiac arrhythmias has been described [14–19,22]. Acute increases in the level of serum Mg can cause nausea, vomiting, cutaneous flushing, muscular weakness, and hyporeflexia. As Mg levels increase above 6 mg/dL (2.5 mmol/L), electrocardiographic changes are followed, in sequence, by hyporeflexia, respiratory paralysis, and cardiac arrest. Mg should be administered with caution in patients with renal failure. In the event of an emergency the acute Mg load should be followed by an intravenous (IV) infusion, providing no more than 1200 mg (50 mmol) of Mg on the first day. This treatment can be followed by another 2 to 5 days of Mg repletion in the same dosage, which is used in less urgent situations. Continuous IV infusion of Mg is preferred to both intramuscular (which is painful) and oral (which causes diarrhea) administration. A continuous infusion avoids the higher urinary fractional excretion of Mg seen with intermittent administration of Mg. Patients with mild Mg deficiency may be treated with oral Mg salts rather than parenteral Mg and may be equally efficacious [14]. Administration of Mg sulfate may cause kaliuresis owing to excretion of the nonreabsorbable sulfate anion; Mg oxide administration has been reported to cause significant acidosis and hyperkalemia [22]. Parenteral Mg also is administered (often in a manner different from that shown here) to patients with preeclampsia, asthma, acute myocardial infarction, and congestive heart failure.

Divalent Cation Metabolism: Calcium

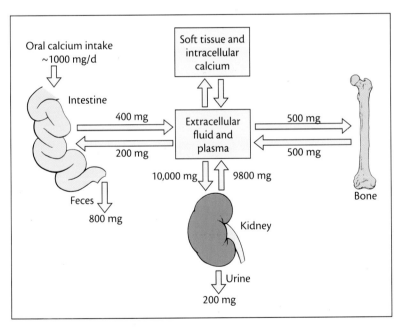

FIGURE 1-41

Calcium (Ca) flux between body compartments. Ca balance is a complex process involving bone, intestinal absorption of dietary Ca, and renal excretion of Ca. The parathyroid glands, by their production of parathyroid hormone, and the liver, through its participation in vitamin D metabolism, also are integral organs in the maintenance of Ca balance. (*Adapted from* Kumar [24].)

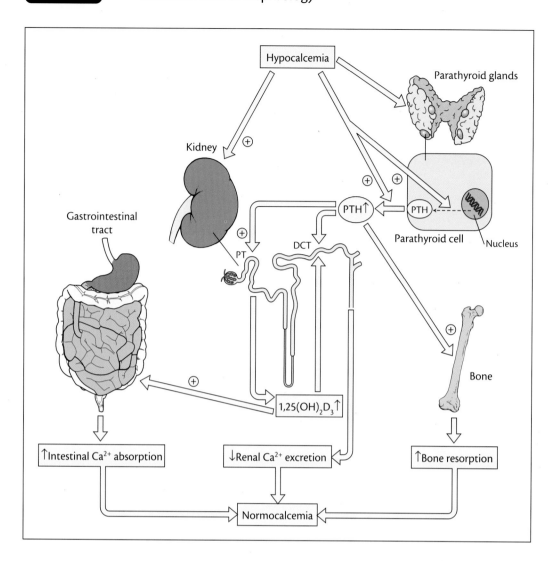

FIGURE 1-42

Physiologic response to hypocalcemia. Hypocalcemia stimulates both parathyroid hormone (PTH) release and PTH synthesis. Both hypocalcemia and PTH increase the activity of the 1-α-hydroxylase enzyme in the proximal tubular (PT) cells of the nephron, which increases the synthesis of 1,25-dihydroxy-vitamin D_3 (1,25[OH]$_2D_3$). PTH increases bone resorption by osteoclasts. PTH and 1,25(OH)$_2D_3$ stimulate Ca reabsorption in the distal convoluted tubule (DCT). 1,25(OH)$_2D_3$ increases the fractional absorption of dietary Ca by the gastrointestinal (GI) tract. All these mechanisms aid in returning the serum Ca to normal levels [24].

FIGURE 1-43

Causes of hypocalcemia (decrease in ionized plasma calcium).

CAUSES OF HYPOCALCEMIA

Lack of parathyroid hormone (PTH)

After thyroidectomy or parathyroidectomy

Hereditary (congenital) hypoparathyroidism

Pseudohypoparathyroidism (lack of effective PTH)

Hypomagnesemia (blocks PTH secretion)

Lack of vitamin D

Dietary deficiency or malabsorption (osteomalacia)

Inadequate sunlight

Defective metabolism

  Anticonvulsant therapy

  Liver disease

  Renal disease

  Vitamin D–resistant rickets

Increased calcium complexation

"Bone hunger" after parathyroidectomy

Rhabdomyolysis

Acute pancreatitis

Tumor lysis syndrome (hyperphosphatemia)

Malignancy (increased osteoblastic activity)

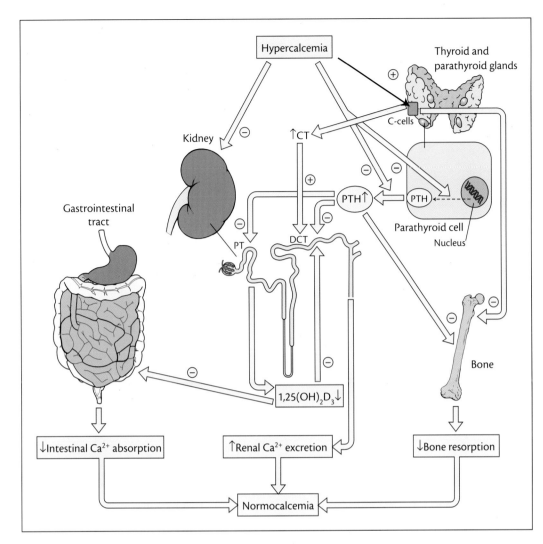

FIGURE 1-44

Physiologic response to hypercalcemia. Hypercalcemia directly inhibits both parathyroid hormone (PTH) release and synthesis. The decrease in PTH and hypercalcemia decrease the activity of the 1-α-hydroxylase enzyme located in the proximal tubular (PT) cells of the nephron, which in turn, decreases the synthesis of 1,25-dihydroxy-vitamin D_3 (1,25[OH]$_2D_3$). Hypercalcemia stimulates the C cells in the thyroid gland to increase synthesis of calcitonin (CT). Bone resorption by osteoclasts is blocked by the increased CT and decreased PTH. Decreased levels of PTH and 1,25(OH)$_2D_3$ inhibit Ca reabsorption in the distal convoluted tubules (DCT) of the nephrons and overwhelm the effects of CT, which augment Ca reabsorption in the medullary thick ascending limb leading to an increase in renal Ca excretion. The decrease in 1,25(OH)$_2D_3$ decreases gastrointestinal (GI) tract absorption of dietary Ca. All of these effects tend to return serum Ca to normal levels [24].

FIGURE 1-45

Causes of hypercalcemia (increase in ionized plasma calcium).

CAUSES OF HYPERCALCEMIA

Excess parathyroid hormone (PTH) production
Primary hyperparathyroidism
"Tertiary" hyperparathyroidism*

Excess 1,25-dihydroxy-vitamin D_3 (1,25[OH]$_2D_3$)
Vitamin D intoxication
Sarcoidosis and granulomatous diseases
Severe hypophosphatemia
Neoplastic production of 1,25(OH)$_2D_3$ (lymphoma)

Increased bone resorption
Metastatic (osteolytic) tumors (*eg*, breast, colon, prostate)
Humoral hypercalcemia
  PTH-related protein (*eg*, squamous cell lung, renal
    cell cancer)
  Osteoclastic activating factor (myeloma)
  1,25 (OH)$_2D_3$ (lymphoma)
  Prostaglandins
Hyperthyroidism
Immobilization
Paget's disease
Vitamin A intoxication

Increased intestinal absorption of calcium
Vitamin D intoxication
Milk-alkali syndrome*

Decreased renal excretion of calcium
Familial hypocalciuric hypercalcemia
Thiazides

Impaired bone formation and incorporation of calcium
Aluminum intoxication*
Adynamic ("low-turnover") bone disease*
Corticosteroids

*Occurs in renal failure.

AVAILABLE THERAPY FOR HYPERCALCEMIA*

Agent	Mechanism of action
Saline and loop diuretics	Increase renal excretion of calcium
Corticosteroids	Block 1,25-dihydroxy-vitamin D_3 synthesis and bone resorption
Ketoconazole	Blocks P450 system, decreases 1, 25-dihydroxy-vitamin D_3
Oral or intravenous phosphate	Complexes calcium
Calcitonin	Inhibits bone resorption
Mithramycin	Inhibits bone resorption
Bisphosphonates	Inhibit bone resorption

*Always identify and treat the primary cause of hypercalcemia.

FIGURE 1-46

Therapy available for the treatment of hypercalcemia.

CALCIUM CONTENT OF ORAL CALCIUM PREPARATIONS

Calcium (Ca) salt	Tablet size, *mg*	Elemental Ca, *mg (%)*
Carbonate	1250	500 (40)
Acetate	667	169 (25)
Citrate	950	200 (21)
Lactate	325	42 (13)
Gluconate	500	4.5 (9)

Fractional intestinal absorption of Ca may differ between Ca salts.
Data from McCarthy and Kumar [25] and *Physicians' Desk Reference* [23].

FIGURE 1-47

Calcium (Ca) content of oral Ca preparations.

VITAMIN D PREPARATIONS AVAILABLE IN THE UNITED STATES

	Ergocalciferol (Vitamin D_2)	Calcifediol (25-hydroxy-vitamin D_3)	Dihydrotachysterol	Calcitriol (1,25-dihydroxy-vitamin D_3)
Commercial name	Calciferol	Calderol® (Organon, Inc, West Orange, NJ)	DHT Intensol® (Roxane Laboratories, Columbus, OH)	Rocaltrol® (Roche Laboratories, Nutley, NJ) Calcijex® (Abbott Laboratories, Abbott Park, NJ)
Oral preparations	50,000 IU tablets	20- and 50-µg capsules	0.125-, 0.2-, 0.4-mg tablets	0.25- and 0.50-µg capsules
Usual daily dose				
Hypoparathyroidism	50,000–500,000 IU	20–200 µg	0.2–1.0 mg	0.25–5.0 µg
Renal failure	Not used	20–40 µg*	0.2-0.4 mg*	0.25–0.50 µg
Time until increase in serum calcium†	4–8 wk	2–4 wk	1–2 wk	4–7 d
Time for reversal of toxic effects	17–60 d	7–30 d	3–14 d	2–10 d

*Not currently advised in patients with chronic renal failure.
†In patients with hypoparathyroidism who have normal renal function.
Data from McCarthy and Kumar [25] and *Physicians' Desk Reference* [23].

FIGURE 1-48

Vitamin D preparations.

Disorders of Acid-Base Balance

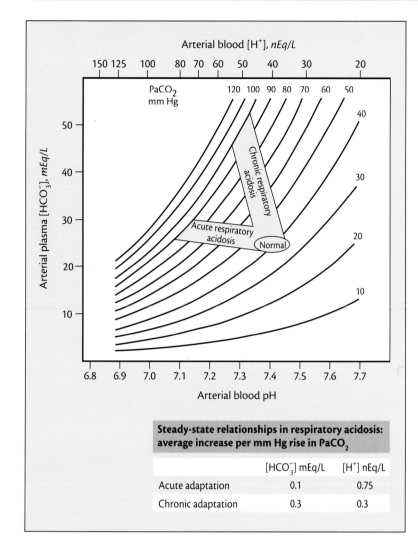

Arterial blood [H⁺], *nEq/L*

Steady-state relationships in respiratory acidosis: average increase per mm Hg rise in PaCO₂

	[HCO₃⁻] mEq/L	[H⁺] nEq/L
Acute adaptation	0.1	0.75
Chronic adaptation	0.3	0.3

FIGURE 1-49

Quantitative aspects of adaptation to respiratory acidosis. Respiratory acidosis, or primary hypercapnia, is the acid-base disturbance initiated by an increase in arterial carbon dioxide tension ($PaCO_2$) and entails acidification of body fluids. Hypercapnia elicits adaptive increments in plasma bicarbonate concentration that should be viewed as an integral part of respiratory acidosis. An immediate increment in plasma bicarbonate occurs in response to hypercapnia. This acute adaptation is complete within 5 to 10 minutes from the onset of hypercapnia and originates exclusively from acidic titration of the nonbicarbonate buffers of the body (hemoglobin, intracellular proteins and phosphates, and to a lesser extent plasma proteins). When hypercapnia is sustained, renal adjustments markedly amplify the secondary increase in plasma bicarbonate, further ameliorating the resulting acidemia. This chronic adaptation requires 3 to 5 days for completion and reflects generation of new bicarbonate by the kidneys as a result of upregulation of renal acidification [26]. Average increases in plasma bicarbonate and hydrogen ion concentrations per mm Hg increase in $PaCO_2$ after completion of the acute or chronic adaptation to respiratory acidosis are shown. Empiric observations on these adaptations have been used for construction of 95% confidence intervals for graded degrees of acute or chronic respiratory acidosis represented by the areas in color in the acid-base template. The ellipse near the center of the figure indicates the normal range for the acid-base parameters [27]. Note that for the same level of $PaCO_2$, the degree of acidemia is considerably lower in chronic respiratory acidosis than it is in acute respiratory acidosis. Assuming a steady state is present, values falling within the areas in color are consistent with but not diagnostic of the corresponding simple disorders. Acid-base values falling outside the areas in color denote the presence of a mixed acid-base disturbance [28].

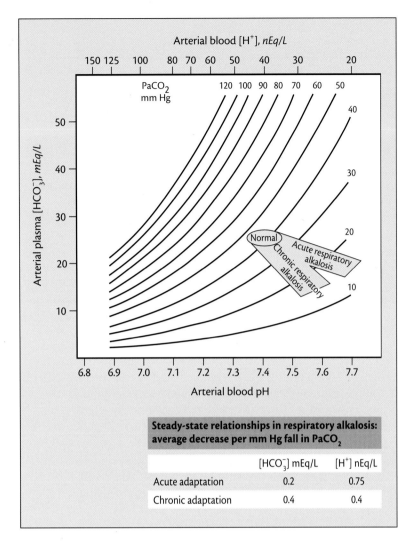

Steps-state relationships in respiratory alkalosis: average decrease per mm Hg fall in PaCO₂

	$[HCO_3^-]$ mEq/L	$[H^+]$ nEq/L
Acute adaptation	0.2	0.75
Chronic adaptation	0.4	0.4

FIGURE 1-50

Adaptation to respiratory alkalosis. Respiratory alkalosis, or primary hypocapnia, is the acid-base disturbance initiated by a decrease in arterial carbon dioxide tension ($PaCO_2$) and entails alkalinization of body fluids. Hypocapnia elicits adaptive decrements in plasma bicarbonate concentration that should be viewed as an integral part of respiratory alkalosis. An immediate decrement in plasma bicarbonate occurs in response to hypocapnia. This acute adaptation is complete within 5 to 10 minutes from the onset of hypocapnia and is accounted for principally by alkaline titration of the nonbicarbonate buffers of the body. To a lesser extent, this acute adaptation reflects increased production of organic acids, notably lactic acid. When hypocapnia is sustained, renal adjustments cause an additional decrease in plasma bicarbonate, further ameliorating the resulting alkalemia. This chronic adaptation requires 2 to 3 days for completion and reflects retention of hydrogen ions by the kidneys as a result of downregulation of renal acidification [26,29]. Shown are the average decreases in plasma bicarbonate and hydrogen ion concentrations per mm Hg decrease in $PaCO_2$ after completion of the acute or chronic adaptation to respiratory alkalosis. Empiric observations on these adaptations have been used for constructing 95% confidence intervals for graded degrees of acute or chronic respiratory alkalosis, which are represented by the areas in color in the acid-base template. The ellipse near the center of the figure indicates the normal range for the acid-base parameters. Note that for the same level of $PaCO_2$, the degree of alkalemia is considerably lower in chronic than it is in acute respiratory alkalosis. Assuming that a steady state is present, values falling within the areas in color are consistent with but not diagnostic of the corresponding simple disorders. Acid-base values falling outside the areas in color denote the presence of a mixed acid-base disturbance [28].

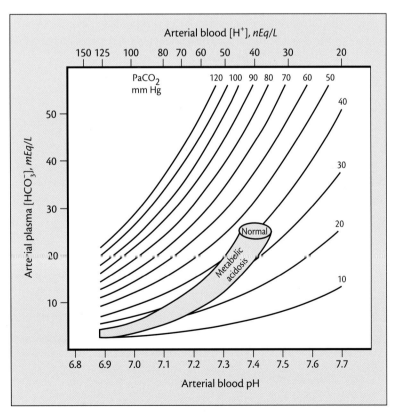

FIGURE 1-51

Ninety-five percent confidence intervals for metabolic acidosis. Metabolic acidosis is the acid-base disturbance initiated by a decrease in plasma bicarbonate concentration ($[HCO_3^-]$). The resultant acidemia stimulates alveolar ventilation and leads to the secondary hypocapnia characteristic of the disorder. Extensive observations in humans encompassing a wide range of stable metabolic acidosis indicate a roughly linear relationship between the steady-state decrease in plasma bicarbonate concentration and the associated decrement in arterial carbon dioxide tension ($PaCO_2$). The slope of the steady state $\Delta PaCO_2$ versus $\Delta[HCO_3^-]$ relationship has been estimated as approximately 1.2 mm Hg per mEq/L decrease in plasma bicarbonate concentration. Such empiric observations have been used for construction of 95% confidence intervals for graded degrees of metabolic acidosis, represented by the area in color in the acid-base template. The ellipse near the center of the figure indicates the normal range for the acid-base parameters [27]. Assuming a steady state is present, values falling within the area in color are consistent with but not diagnostic of simple metabolic acidosis. Acid-base values falling outside the area in color denote the presence of a mixed acid-base disturbance [28]. [H+]—hydrogen ion concentration.

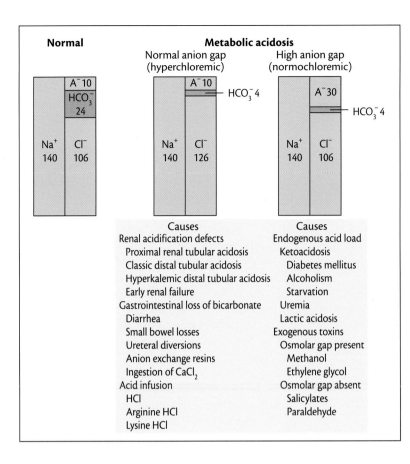

Normal	Metabolic acidosis	
	Normal anion gap (hyperchloremic)	High anion gap (normochloremic)

Causes (Normal anion gap):
Renal acidification defects
  Proximal renal tubular acidosis
  Classic distal tubular acidosis
  Hyperkalemic distal tubular acidosis
  Early renal failure
Gastrointestinal loss of bicarbonate
  Diarrhea
  Small bowel losses
  Ureteral diversions
  Anion exchange resins
  Ingestion of $CaCl_2$
Acid infusion
  HCl
  Arginine HCl
  Lysine HCl

Causes (High anion gap):
Endogenous acid load
  Ketoacidosis
    Diabetes mellitus
    Alcoholism
    Starvation
  Uremia
  Lactic acidosis
Exogenous toxins
  Osmolar gap present
    Methanol
    Ethylene glycol
  Osmolar gap absent
    Salicylates
    Paraldehyde

FIGURE 1-52

Causes of metabolic acidosis tabulated according to the prevailing pattern of plasma electrolyte composition. Assessment of the plasma unmeasured anion concentration (anion gap) is a very useful first step in approaching the differential diagnosis of unexplained metabolic acidosis. The plasma anion gap is calculated as the difference between the sodium concentration and the sum of chloride and bicarbonate concentrations. Under normal circumstances, the plasma anion gap is primarily composed of the net negative charges of plasma proteins, predominantly albumin, with a smaller contribution from many other organic and inorganic anions. The normal value of the plasma anion gap is 12 ± 4 (mean ± 2 SD) mEq/L, where SD is the standard deviation. However, recent introduction of ion-specific electrodes has shifted the normal anion gap to the range of about 6 ± 3 mEq/L. In one pattern of metabolic acidosis, the decrease in bicarbonate concentration is offset by an increase in the concentration of chloride, with the plasma anion gap remaining normal. In the other pattern, the decrease in bicarbonate is balanced by an increase in the concentration of unmeasured anions (*ie*, anions not measured routinely), with the plasma chloride concentration remaining normal.

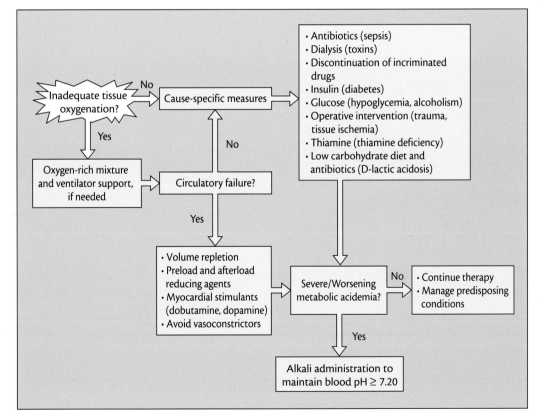

FIGURE 1-53

Lactic acidosis management. Management of lactic acidosis should focus primarily on securing adequate tissue oxygenation and on aggressively identifying and treating the underlying cause or predisposing condition. Monitoring of the patient's hemodynamics, oxygenation, and acid-base status should be used to guide therapy. In the presence of severe or worsening metabolic acidemia, these measures should be supplemented by judicious administration of sodium bicarbonate, given as an infusion rather than a bolus. Alkali administration should be regarded as a temporizing maneuver adjunctive to cause-specific measures. Given the ominous prognosis of lactic acidosis, clinicians should strive to prevent its development by maintaining adequate fluid balance, optimizing cardiorespiratory function, managing infection, and using drugs that predispose to the disorder cautiously. Preventing the development of lactic acidosis is all the more important in patients at special risk for developing it, such as those with diabetes mellitus or advanced cardiac, respiratory, renal, or hepatic disease [30,31–33].

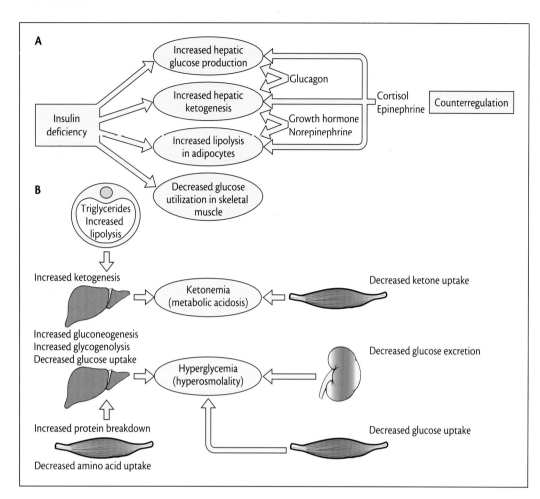

FIGURE 1-54

Role of insulin deficiency and the counter-regulatory hormones, and their respective sites of action, in the pathogenesis of hyperglycemia and ketosis in diabetic ketoacidosis (DKA). **A**, Metabolic processes affected by insulin deficiency, on the one hand, and excess of glucagon, cortisol, epinephrine, norepinephrine, and growth hormone, on the other. **B**, The roles of the adipose tissue, liver, skeletal muscle, and kidney in the pathogenesis of hyperglycemia and ketonemia. Impairment of glucose oxidation in most tissues and excessive hepatic production of glucose are the main determinants of hyperglycemia. Excessive counterregulation and the prevailing hypertonicity, metabolic acidosis, and electrolyte imbalance superimpose a state of insulin resistance. Prerenal azotemia caused by volume depletion can contribute significantly to severe hyperglycemia. Increased hepatic production of ketones and their reduced utilization by peripheral tissues account for the ketonemia typically observed in DKA.

FEATURES OF THE RENAL TUBULAR ACIDOSIS SYNDROMES

Feature	Proximal RTA	Classic Distal RTA	Hyperkalemic Distal RTA
Plasma bicarbonate ion concentration	14–18 mEq/L	Variable, may be < 10 mEq/L	15–20 mEq/L
Plasma chloride ion concentration	Increased	Increased	Increased
Plasma potassium ion concentration	Mildly decreased	Mildly to severely decreased	Mildly to severely increased
Plasma anion gap	Normal	Normal	Normal
Glomerular filtration rate	Normal or slightly decreased	Normal or slightly decreased	Normal to moderately decreased
Urine pH during acidosis	≤5.5	>6.0	≤5.5
Urine pH after acid loading	≤5.5	>6.0	≤5.5
U-B PCO_2 in alkaline urine	Normal	Decreased	Decreased
Fractional excretion of HCO_3^- at normal $[HCO_3^-]_p$	>15%	<5%	<5%
Tm HCO_3^-	Decreased	Normal	Normal
Nephrolithiasis	Absent	Present	Absent
Nephrocalcinosis	Absent	Present	Absent
Osteomalacia	Present	Present	Absent
Fanconi's syndrome*	Usually present	Absent	Absent
Alkali therapy	High dose	Low dose	Low dose

*This syndrome signifies generalized proximal tubule dysfunction and is characterized by impaired reabsorption of glucose, amino acids, phosphate, and urate.

Tm HCO_3^-—maximum reabsorption of bicarbonate; U-B PCO_2—difference between partial pressure of carbon dioxide values in urine and arterial blood.

FIGURE 1-55

Renal tubular acidosis (RTA) defines a group of disorders in which tubular hydrogen ion secretion is impaired out of proportion to any reduction in the glomerular filtration rate. These disorders are characterized by normal anion gap (hyperchloremic) metabolic acidosis. The defects responsible for impaired acidification give rise to three distinct syndromes known as proximal RTA (type 2), classic distal RTA (type 1), and hyperkalemic distal RTA (type 4).

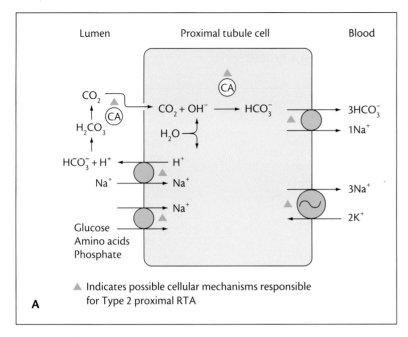

Lumen   Proximal tubule cell   Blood

▲ Indicates possible cellular mechanisms responsible
for Type 2 proximal RTA

A

FIGURE 1-56

Potential defects and causes of proximal renal tubular acidosis
(RTA) (type 2). **A,** Excluding the case of carbonic anhydrase
inhibitors, the nature of the acidification defect responsible for
bicarbonate (HCO_3) wastage remains unknown. It might represent
defects in the luminal sodium ion– hydrogen ion (Na^+-H^+)
exchanger, basolateral Na^+-$3HCO_3^-$ cotransporter, or carbonic
anhydrase activity. Most patients with proximal RTA have additional defects in proximal tubule function (Fanconi's syndrome);
this generalized proximal tubule dysfunction might reflect a defect
in the basolateral Na^+-K^+ adenosine triphosphatase. **B,** Causes of
proximal renal tubular acidosis (RTA) (type 2). An idiopathic form
and cystinosis are the most common causes of proximal RTA in
children. In adults, multiple myeloma and carbonic anhydrase
inhibitors (*eg*, acetazolamide) are the major causes. Ifosfamide is
an increasingly common cause of the disorder in both age groups.
CA—carbonic anhydrase; K^+—potassium ion.

B. CAUSES OF PROXIMAL RENAL TUBULAR ACIDOSIS

Selective defect (isolated bicarbonate wasting)
  Primary (no obvious associated disease)
    Genetically transmitted
    Transient (infants)
  Due to altered carbonic anhydrase activity
    Acetazolamide
    Sulfanilamide
    Mafenide acetate
    Genetically transmitted
    Idiopathic
    Osteopetrosis with carbonic
      anhydrase II deficiency
    York-Yendt syndrome

Generalized defect (associated with multiple
    dysfunctions of the proximal tubule)
  Primary (no obvious associated disease)
    Sporadic
    Genetically transmitted
  Genetically transmitted systemic disease
    Tyrosinemia
    Wilson's disease
    Lowe syndrome
    Hereditary fructose intolerance (during
      administration of fructose)
    Cystinosis
    Pyruvate carboxylate deficiency
    Metachromatic leukodystrophy
    Methylmalonic acidemia

Conditions associated with chronic hypocalcemia
    and secondary hyperparathyroidism
  Vitamin D deficiency or resistance
  Vitamin D dependence

Dysproteinemic states
  Multiple myeloma
  Monoclonal gammopathy

Drug- or toxin-induced
  Outdated tetracycline
  3-Methylchromone
  Streptozotocin
  Lead
  Mercury
  Arginine
  Valproic acid
  Gentamicin
  Ifosfamide

Tubulointerstitial diseases
  Renal transplantation
  Sjögren's syndrome
  Medullary cystic disease

Other renal diseases
  Nephrotic syndrome
  Amyloidosis

Miscellaneous
  Paroxysmal
    nocturnal hemoglobinuria
  Hyperparathyroidism

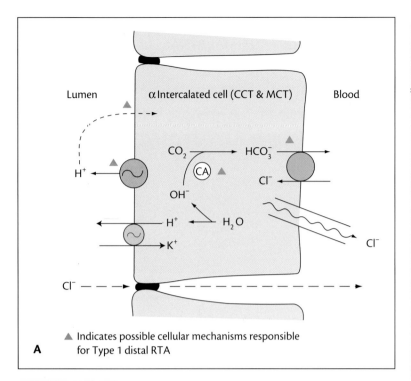

▲ Indicates possible cellular mechanisms responsible
for Type 1 distal RTA

A

FIGURE 1-57

Potential defects and causes of classic distal renal tubular acidosis
(RTA) (type 1). **A,** Potential cellular defects underlying classic distal
RTA include a faulty luminal hydrogen ion–adenosine triphosphatase
(H+ pump failure or secretory defect), an abnormality in the basolateral bicarbonate ion–chloride ion exchanger, inadequacy of carbonic
anhydrase activity, or an increase in the luminal membrane permeability for hydrogen ions (backleak of protons or permeability
defect). **B,** Most of the causes of classic distal RTA likely reflect a
secretory defect, whereas amphotericin B is the only established
cause of a permeability defect. The hereditary form is the most common cause of this disorder in children. Major causes in adults
include autoimmune disorders (*eg,* Sjögren's syndrome) and hypercalciuria [34]. CA—carbonic anhydrase.

B. CAUSES OF CLASSIC DISTAL RENAL TUBULAR ACIDOSIS

Primary (no obvious associated disease)
  Sporadic
  Genetically transmitted

Autoimmune disorders
  Hypergammaglobulinemia
  Hyperglobulinemic purpura
  Cryoglobulinemia
  Familial
  Sjögren's syndrome
  Thyroiditis
  Pulmonary fibrosis
  Chronic active hepatitis
  Primary biliary cirrhosis
  Systemic lupus erythematosus
  Vasculitis

Genetically transmitted systemic disease
  Ehlers-Danlos syndrome
  Hereditary elliptocytosis
  Sickle cell anemia
  Marfan syndrome
  Carbonic anhydrase I deficiency
    or alteration
  Osteopetrosis with carbonic
    anhydrase II deficiency
  Medullary cystic disease
  Neuroaxonal dystrophy

Disorders associated
    with nephrocalcinosis
  Primary or familial hyperparathyroidism
  Vitamin D intoxication
  Milk-alkali syndrome
  Hyperthyroidism
  Idiopathic hypercalciuria
    Genetically transmitted
    Sporadic
  Hereditary fructose intolerance
    (after chronic fructose ingestion)
  Medullary sponge kidney
  Fabry's disease
  Wilson's disease

Drug- or toxin-induced
  Amphotericin B
  Toluene
  Analgesics
  Lithium
  Cyclamate
  Balkan nephropathy

Tubulointerstitial diseases
  Chronic pyelonephritis
  Obstructive uropathy
  Renal transplantation
  Leprosy
  Hyperoxaluria

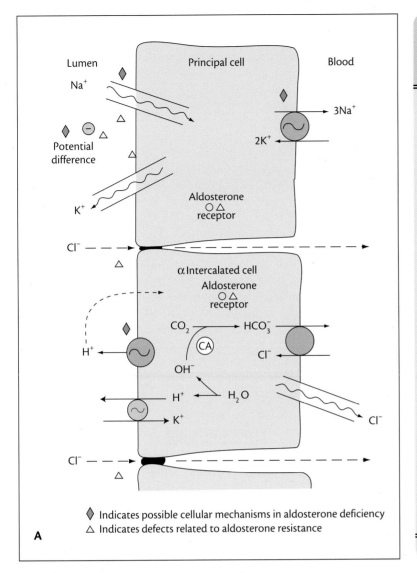

B. CAUSES OF HYPERKALEMIC DISTAL RENAL TUBULAR ACIDOSIS

Deficiency of aldosterone
  Associated with glucocorticoid deficiency
    Addison's disease
    Bilateral adrenalectomy
    Enzymatic defects
      21-Hydroxylase deficiency
      3-β-ol-Dehydrogenase deficiency
      Desmolase deficiency
    Acquired immunodeficiency syndrome
  Isolated aldosterone deficiency
    Genetically transmitted
      Corticosterone methyl
        oxidase deficiency
    Transient (infants)
    Sporadic
    Heparin
    Deficient renin secretion
      Diabetic nephropathy
      Tubulointerstitial renal disease
      Nonsteroidal antiinflammatory drugs
      β-adrenergic blockers
      Acquired immunodeficiency syndrome
      Renal transplantation
  Angiotensin I-converting enzyme inhibition
    Endogenous
    Captopril and related drugs
  Angiotensin AT, receptor blockers

Resistance to aldosterone action
  Pseudohypoaldosteronism type I
    (with salt wasting)
    Childhood forms with
      obstructive uropathy
    Adult forms with
      renal insufficiency
  Spironolactone
  Pseudohypoaldosteronism type II
    (without salt wasting)
  Combined aldosterone deficiency
    and resistance
    Deficient renin secretion
    Cyclosporine nephrotoxicity
    Uncertain renin status
  Voltage-mediated defects
    Obstructive uropathy
    Sickle cell anemia
    Lithium
    Triamterene
    Amiloride
    Trimethoprim, pentamidine
  Renal transplantation

◆ Indicates possible cellular mechanisms in aldosterone deficiency
△ Indicates defects related to aldosterone resistance

A

FIGURE 1-58

Potential defects and causes of hyperkalemic distal renal tubular acidosis (RTA) (type 4). **A,** This syndrome represents the most common type of RTA encountered in adults. The characteristic hyperchloremic metabolic acidosis in the company of hyperkalemia emerges as a consequence of generalized dysfunction of the collecting tubule, including diminished sodium reabsorption and impaired hydrogen ion and potassium secretion. The resultant hyperkalemia causes impaired ammonium excretion that is an important contribution to the generation of the metabolic acidosis. **B,** The causes of this syndrome are broadly classified into disorders resulting in aldosterone deficiency and those that impose resistance to the action of aldosterone. Aldosterone deficiency can arise from hyporeninemia, impaired conversion of angiotensin I to angiotensin II, or abnormal aldosterone synthesis. Aldosterone resistance can reflect the following: blockade of the mineralocorticoid receptor; destruction of the target cells in the collecting tubule (*tubulointerstitial nephropathies*); interference with the sodium channel of the principal cell, thereby decreasing the lumen-negative potential difference and thus the secretion of potassium and hydrogen ions (voltage-mediated defect); inhibition of the basolateral sodium ion, potassium ion–adenosine triphosphatase; and enhanced chloride ion permeability in the collecting tubule, with consequent shunting of the transepithelial potential difference. Some disorders cause combined aldosterone deficiency and resistance [35].

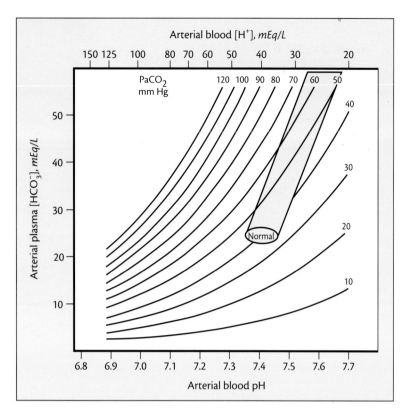

FIGURE 1-59

Ninety-five percent confidence intervals for metabolic alkalosis. Metabolic alkalosis is the acid-base disturbance initiated by an increase in plasma bicarbonate concentration ($[HCO_3^-]$). The resultant alkalemia dampens alveolar ventilation and leads to the secondary hypercapnia characteristic of the disorder. Available observations in humans suggest a roughly linear relationship between the steady-state increase in bicarbonate concentration and the associated increment in the arterial carbon dioxide tension ($PaCO_2$). Although data are limited, the slope of the steady-state $\Delta PaCO_2$ versus $\Delta[HCO_3]$ relationship has been estimated as about a 0.7 mm Hg per mEq/L increase in plasma bicarbonate concentration. The value of this slope is virtually identical to that in dogs that has been derived from rigorously controlled observations [36]. Empiric observations in humans have been used for construction of 95% confidence intervals for graded degrees of metabolic alkalosis represented by the area in color in the acid-base template. The ellipse near the center of the figure indicates the normal range for the acid-base parameters [27]. Assuming a steady state is present, values falling within the area in color are consistent with but not diagnostic of simple metabolic alkalosis. Acid-base values falling outside the area in color denote the presence of a mixed acid-base disturbance [28]. [H^+]—hydrogen ion concentration.

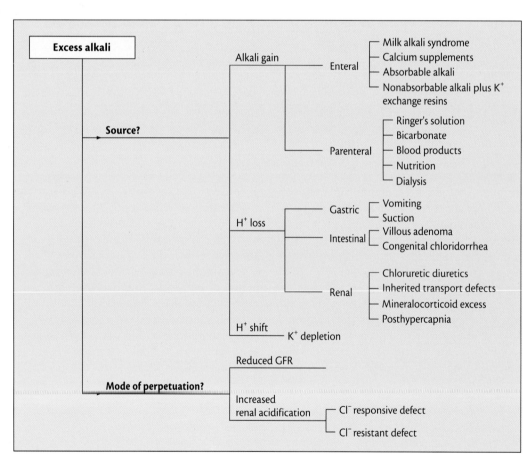

FIGURE 1-60

Pathogenesis of metabolic alkalosis. Two crucial questions must be answered when evaluating the pathogenesis of a case of metabolic alkalosis. 1) What is the source of the excess alkali? Answering this question addresses the primary event responsible for *generating* the hyperbicarbonatemia. 2) What factors perpetuate the hyperbicarbonatemia? Answering this question addresses the pathophysiologic events that *maintain* the metabolic alkalosis.

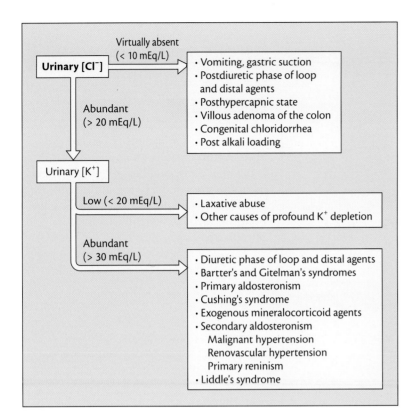

FIGURE 1-61

Urinary composition in the diagnostic evaluation of metabolic alkalosis. Assessing the urinary composition can be an important aid in the diagnostic evaluation of metabolic alkalosis. Measurement of urinary chloride ion concentration ([Cl⁻]) can help distinguish between chloride-responsive and chloride-resistant metabolic alkalosis. The virtual absence of chloride (urine [Cl⁻] < 10 mEq/L) indicates significant chloride depletion. Note, however, that this test loses its diagnostic significance if performed within several hours of administration of chloruretic diuretics, because these agents promote urinary chloride excretion. Measurement of urinary potassium ion concentration ([K⁺]) provides further diagnostic differentiation. With the exception of the diuretic phase of chloruretic agents, abundance of both urinary chloride and potassium signifies a state of mineralocorticoid excess [37].

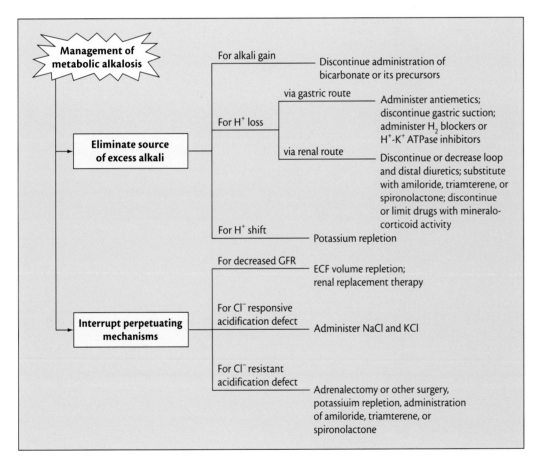

FIGURE 1-62

Metabolic alkalosis management. Effective management of metabolic alkalosis requires sound understanding of the underlying pathophysiology. Therapeutic efforts should focus on eliminating or moderating the processes that generate the alkali excess and on interrupting the mechanisms that perpetuate the hyperbicarbonatemia. Rarely, when the pace of correction of metabolic alkalosis must be accelerated, acetazolamide or an infusion of hydrochloric acid can be used. Treatment of severe metabolic alkalosis can be particularly challenging in patients with advanced cardiac or renal dysfunction. In such patients, hemodialysis or continuous hemofiltration might be required [30].

Disorders of Phosphate Balance _____

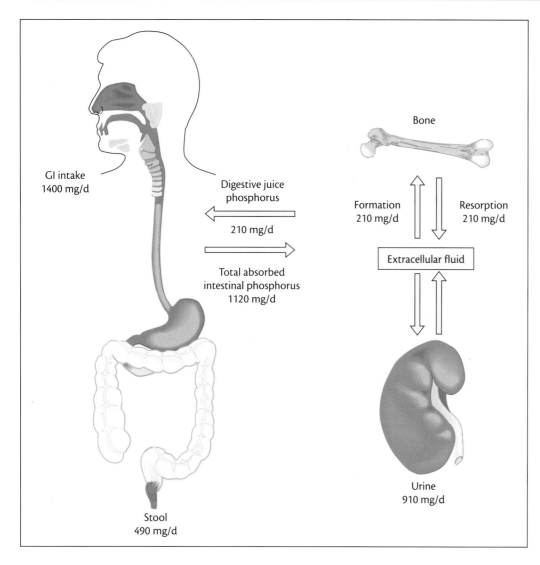

GI intake
1400 mg/d

Digestive juice
phosphorus

210 mg/d

Total absorbed
intestinal phosphorus
1120 mg/d

Stool
490 mg/d

Bone

Formation
210 mg/d

Resorption
210 mg/d

Extracellular fluid

Urine
910 mg/d

FIGURE 1-63

Summary of phosphate metabolism for a normal adult in neutral phosphate balance. Approximately 1400 mg of phosphate is ingested daily, of which 490 mg is excreted in the stool and 910 mg in the urine. The kidney, gastrointestinal (GI) tract, and bone are the major organs involved in phosphorus homeostasis.

CAUSES OF MODERATE HYPOPHOSPHATEMIA

Pseudohypophosphatemia
  Mannitol
  Bilirubin
  Acute leukemia
Decreased dietary intake
Decreased intestinal absorption
  Vitamin D deficiency
  Malabsorption
  Steatorrhea
  Secretory diarrhea
  Vomiting
  PO_4^3-binding antacids
Shift from serum into cells
  Respiratory alkalosis
    Sepsis
    Heat stroke
    Neuroleptic malignant syndrome
    Hepatic coma
    Salicylate poisoning
    Gout
    Panic attacks
    Psychiatric depression

Hormonal effects
  Insulin
  Glucagon
  Epinephrine
  Androgens
  Cortisol
  Anovulatory hormones
Nutrient effects
  Glucose
  Fructose
  Glycerol
  Lactate
  Amino acids
  Xylitol

Cellular uptake syndromes
  Recovery from hypothermia
  Burkitt's lymphoma
  Histiocytic lymphoma
  Acute myelomonocytic leukemia
  Acute myelogenous leukemia
  Chronic myelogenous leukemia
    in blast crisis
  Treatment of pernicious anemia
  Erythropoietin therapy
  Erythrodermic psoriasis
  Hungry bone syndrome
  After parathyroidectomy
  Acute leukemia

Increased excretion into urine
  Hyperparathyroidism
  Renal tubule defects
    Fanconi's syndrome
    X-linked hypophosphatemic rickets
    Hereditary hypophosphatemic rickets
      with hypercalciuria
    Polyostotic fibrous dysphasia
    Panostotic fibrous dysphasia
    Neurofibromatosis
    Kidney transplantation
    Oncogenic osteomalacia
    Recovery from hemolytic-uremic
      syndrome
  Aldosteronism
  Licorice ingestion
  Volume expansion
  Inappropriate secretion of antidiuretic
    hormone
  Mineralocorticoid administration
  Corticosteroid therapy
  Diuretics
  Aminophylline therapy

FIGURE 1-64

Causes of moderate hypophosphatemia. (*Adapted from* Popovtzer *et al.* [38].)

FIGURE 1-65

Causes of severe hypophosphatemia. (*Adapted from* Popovtzer *et al.* [38].)

CAUSES OF SEVERE HYPOPHOSPHATEMIA

Acute renal failure: excessive P binders
Chronic alcoholism and alcohol
  withdrawal
Dietary deficiency and PO_4^3-binding
  antacids
Hyperalimentation
Neuroleptic malignant syndrome
Recovery from diabetic ketoacidosis
Recovery from exhaustive exercise
Kidney transplantation
Respiratory alkalosis
Severe thermal burns
Therapeutic hypothermia

Reye's syndrome
After major surgery
Periodic paralysis
Acute malaria
Drug therapy
  Ifosfamide
  Cisplatin
Acetaminophen intoxication
Cytokine infusions
  Tumor necrosis factor
  Interleukin-2

SIGNS AND SYMPTOMS OF HYPOPHOSPHATEMIA

Central nervous system dysfunction	Cardiac dysfunction	Pulmonary dysfunction	Skeletal and smooth muscle dysfunction	Hematologic dysfunction	Bone disease	Renal effects	Metabolic effects
Metabolic encephalopathy owing to tissue ischemia	Impaired myocardial contractility	Weakness of the diaphragm	Proximal myopathy	Erythrocytes	Increased bone resorption	Decreased glomerular filtration rate	Low parathyroid hormone levels
Irritability	Congestive heart failure	Respiratory failure	Dysphagia and ileus	Increased erythrocyte rigidity	Rickets and osteo-malacia caused by decreased bone mineralization	Decreased tubular transport maximum for bicarbonate	Increased 1,25-dihy-droxy-vitamin D_3 levels
Paresthesias			Rhabdomyolysis	Hemolysis		Decreased renal gluconeogenesis	Increased creatinine phosphokinase levels
Confusion				Leukocytes		Decreased titratable acid excretion	Increased aldolase levels
Delirium				Impaired phagocytosis		Hypercalciuria	
Coma				Decreased granulocyte chemotaxis		Hypermagnesuria	
				Platelets			
				Defective clot retraction			
				Thrombocytopenia			

FIGURE 1-66

Signs and symptoms of hypophosphatemia. (*Adapted from* Hruska and Slatopolsky [39] and Hruska and Gupta [40].)

USUAL DOSAGES FOR PHOSPHORUS REPLETION

Severe symptomatic hypophos-phatemia (plasma phosphate concentration < 1 mg/dL)	Phosphate depletion	Hypophosphatemic rickets
10 mg/kg/d, intravenously, until the plasma phosphate concentration reaches 2 mg/dL	2–4 g/d (64 to 128 mmol/d), orally, in 3 to 4 divided doses	1–4 g/d (32 to 128 mmol/d), orally, in 3 to 4 divided doses

FIGURE 1-67

Usual dosages for phosphorus repletion.

PHOSPHATE PREPARATIONS FOR ORAL USE

Preparation	Phosphate, *mg*	Sodium, *mEq*	Potassium, *mEq*
K-Phos Neutral®, tablet (Beach Pharmaceuticals, Conestee, SC)	250	13	1.1
Neutra-Phos®, capsule or 75-mL solution (Baker Norton Pharmaceuticals, Miami, FL)	250	7.1	7.1
Neutra-Phos K®, capsule or 75-mL solution (Baker Norton Pharmaceuticals, Miami, FL)	250	0	14.2

FIGURE 1-68

Phosphate preparations for oral use.

PHOSPHATE PREPARATIONS FOR INTRAVENOUS USE

Phosphate preparation	Composition, mg/mL	Phosphate, mmol/mL	Sodium, mEq/mL	Potassium, mEq/mL
Potassium	236 mg K_2HPO_4 224 mg KH_2PO_4	3.0	0	4.4
Sodium	142 mg Na_2HPO_4 276 mg $NaH_2PO_4.H_2O$	3.0	4.0	0
Neutral sodium	10.0 mg Na_2HPO 2.7 mg $NaH_2PO_4.H_2O$	0.09	0.2	0
Neutral sodium, potassium	11.5 mg Na_2HPO_4 2.6 mg KH_2PO_4	1.10	0.2	0.02

3 mmol/mL of phosphate corresponds to 93 mg of phosphorus.

FIGURE 1-69

Phosphate preparations for intravenous use. (*Adapted from* Popovtzer *et al.* [38].)

CAUSES OF HYPERPHOSPHATEMIA

Pseudohyperphosphatemia
Multiple myeloma
Extreme hypertriglyceridemia
In vitro hemolysis

Increased exogenous phosphorus load or absorption
Phosphorus-rich cow's milk in premature neonates
Vitamin D intoxication
PO^3_4-containing enemas
Intravenous phosphorus supplements
White phosphorus burns
Acute phosphorus poisoning

Increased endogenous loads
Tumor lysis syndrome
Rhabdomyolysis
Bowel infarction
Malignant hyperthermia
Heat stroke
Acid-base disorders
Organic acidosis
Lactic acidosis
Ketoacidosis
Respiratory acidosis
Chronic respiratory alkalosis

Reduced urinary excretion
Renal failure
Hypoparathyroidism
Hereditary
Acquired
Pseudohypoparathyroidism
Vitamin D intoxication
Growth hormone
Insulin-like growth factor-1
Glucocorticoid withdrawal
Mg^{2+} deficiency
Tumoral calcinosis
Diphosphonate therapy
Hyopophosphatasia

Miscellaneous
Fluoride poisoning
β-Blocker therapy
Verapamil
Hemorrhagic shock
Sleep deprivation

FIGURE 1-70

Causes of hyperphosphatemia. (*Adapted from* Knochel and Agarwal [41].)

TREATMENT OF HYPERPHOSPHATEMIA

Acute hyperphosphatemia in patients with adequate renal function	Chronic hyperphosphatemia in patients with end-stage renal disease
Saline diuresis that causes phosphaturia	Dietary phosphate restriction Phosphate binders to decrease gastrointestinal phosphate reabsorption

FIGURE 1-71

Treatment of hyperphosphatemia.

References

1. Rose BD: Antidiuretic hormone and water balance. In *Clinical Physiology of Acid Base and Electrolyte Disorders*, edn 4. New York: McGraw Hill, 1994.

2. Cogan MG: Normal water homeostasis. In *Fluid & Electrolytes, Physiology and Pathophysiology*. Edited by Cogan MG. Norwalk: Appleton & Lange; 1991:98.

3. Halterman R, Berl T: Therapy of dysnatremic disorders. In *Therapy in Nephrology and Hypertension*. Edited by Brady H, Wilcox C. Philadelphia: WB Saunders, 1999.

4. Ayus JC, Wheeler JM, Arieff AI: Postoperative hyponatremic encephalopathy in menstruant women. *Ann Intern Med* 1992,117:891.

5. Lauriat SM, Berl T: The hyponatremic patient: practical focus on therapy. *J Am Soc Nephrol* 1997, 8(11):1599.

6. Kumar S, Berl T: Disorders of serum sodium concentration. *Lancet* 1999.

7. Gonzalez-Campoy JM, Knox FG: Integrated responses of the kidney to alterations in extracellular fluid volume. In *The Kidney: Physiology and Pathophysiology*, edn 2. Edited by Seldin DW, Giebisch G. New York: Raven Press; 1992:2041–2097.

8. Manning RD, Jr, Coleman TG, Samar RE: Autoregulation, cardiac output, total peripheral resistance and the "quantitative cascade" of the kidney-blood volume system for pressure control. In *Arterial Pressure and Hypertension*. Edited by Guyton AC. Philadelphia: WB Saunders Co; 1980:139–155.

9. Albillos A, Colombato LA, Groszmann RJ: Vasodilation and sodium retention in prehepatic portal hypertension. *Gastroenterology* 1992, 102:931–935.

10. Mitch WE, Wilcox CS: Disorders of body fluids, sodium and potassium in chronic renal failure. *Am J Med* 1982, 72:536–550.

11. Nora NA, Berns AS: Hypokalemic, hypophosphatemic thyrotoxic periodic paralysis. *Am J Kidney Dis* 1989, 13:247–251.

12. de Rouffignac C, Quamme G: Renal magnesium handling and its hormonal control. *Physiol Rev* 1994, 74:305–322.

13. Quamme GA: Magnesium homeostasis and renal magnesium handling. *Miner Electrolyte Metab* 1993, 19:218–225.

14. Whang R, Hampton EM, Whang DD: Magnesium homeostasis and clinical disorders of magnesium deficiency. *Ann Pharmacother* 1994, 28:220–226.

15. McLean RM: Magnesium and its therapeutic uses: a review. *Am J Med* 1994, 96:63–76.

16. Abbott LG, Rude RK: Clinical manifestations of magnesium deficiency. *Miner Electrolyte Metab* 1993, 19:314–322.

17. Al-Ghamdi SMG, Cameron EC, Sutton RAL: Magnesium deficiency: pathophysiologic and clinical overview. *Am J Kid Dis* 1994, 24:737–752.

18. Nadler JL, Rude RK: Disorders of magnesium metabolism. *Endocrinol Metab Clin North Am* 1995, 24:623–641.

19. Kayne LH, Lee DBN: Intestinal magnesium absorption. *Miner Electrolyte Metab* 1993, 19:210–217.

20. Sutton RAL, Domrongkitchaiporn S: Abnormal renal magnesium handling. *Miner Electrolyte Metab* 1993, 19:232–240.

21. Ryzen E, Elbaum N, Singer FR, Rude RK: Parenteral magnesium tolerance testing in the evaluation of magnesium deficiency. *Magnesium* 1985, 4:137–147.

22. Oster JR, Epstein M: Management of magnesium depletion. *Am J Nephrol* 1988, 8:349–354.

23. *Physicians' Desk Reference* (PDR). Montvale, NJ: Medical Economics Company; 1996.

24. Kumar R: Calcium metabolism. In *The Principles and Practice of Nephrology*. Edited by Jacobson HR, Striker GE, Klahr S. St. Louis: Mosby-Year Book; 1995, 964–971.

25. McCarthy JT, Kumar R: Renal osteodystrophy. In *The Principles and Practice of Nephrology*. Edited by Jacobson HR, Striker GE, Klahr S. St. Louis: Mosby-Year Book; 1995, 1032–1045.

26. Madias NE, Adrogué HJ: Acid-base disturbances in pulmonary medicine. In *Fluid, Electrolyte, and Acid-Base Disorders*. Edited by Arieff AI, DeFronzo RA. New York: Churchill Livingstone; 1995:223–253.

27. Madias NE, Adrogué HJ, Horowitz GL, *et al.*: A redefinition of normal acid-base equilibrium in man: carbon dioxide tension as a key determinant of plasma bicarbonate concentration. *Kidney Int* 1979, 16:612–618.

28. Adrogué HJ, Madias NE: Mixed acid-base disorders. In *The Principles and Practice of Nephrology*. Edited by Jacobson HR, Striker GE, Klahr S. St. Louis: Mosby-Year Book; 1995:953–962.

29. Krapf R, Beeler I, Hertner D, Hulter HN: Chronic respiratory alkalosis: the effect of sustained hyperventilation on renal regulation of acid-base equilibrium. *N Engl J Med* 1991, 324:1394–1401.

30. Adrogué HJ, Madias NE: Management of life-threatening acid-base disorders. *N Engl J Med*, 1998, 338:26–34, 107–111.

31. Madias NE: Lactic acidosis. *Kidney Int* 1986, 29:752–774.

32. Kraut JA, Madias NE: Lactic acidosis. In *Textbook of Nephrology*. Edited by Massry SG, Glassock RJ. Baltimore: Williams and Wilkins; 1995:449–457.

33. Hindman BJ: Sodium bicarbonate in the treatment of subtypes of acute lactic acidosis: physiologic considerations. *Anesthesiology* 1990, 72:1064–1076.

34. Bastani B, Gluck SL: New insights into the pathogenesis of distal renal tubular acidosis. *Miner Electrolyte Metab* 1996, 22:396–409.

35. DuBose TD, Jr: Hyperkalemic hyperchloremic metabolic acidosis: pathophysiologic insights. *Kidney Int* 1997, 51:591–602.

36. Madias NE, Bossert WH, Adrogué HJ: Ventilatory response to chronic metabolic acidosis and alkalosis in the dog. *J Appl Physiol* 1984, 56:1640–1646.

37. Gennari FJ: Metabolic alkalosis. In *The Principles and Practice of Nephrology*. Edited by Jacobson HR, Striker GE, Klahr S. St Louis: Mosby-Year Book; 1995:932–942.

38. Popovtzer M, Knochel JP, Kumar R: Disorders of calcium, phosphorus, vitamin D, and parathyroid hormone activity. In *Renal Electrolyte Disorders*, edn 5. Edited by Schrier RW. Philadelphia: Lippincott-Raven; 1997.

39. Hruska KA, Slatopolsky E: Disorders of phosphorus, calcium, and magnesium metabolism. In *Diseases of the Kidney*, edn 6. Edited by Schrier RW, Gottschalk CW. Boston: Little and Brown, 1997.

40. Hruska K, Gupta A: Disorders of phosphate homeostasis. In *Metabolic Bone Disease*, edn 3. Edited by Avioli LV, SM Krane. New York: Academic Press; 1998.

41. Knochel JP, Agarwal R: Hypophosphatemia and hyperphosphatemia. In *The Kidney*, edn 5. Edited by Brenner BM. Philadelphia: WB Saunders; 1996.

Acute Renal Failure

Joseph V. Bonventre

Robert J. Anderson, Robert Bacallao, Marc E. De Broe, Kevin T. Bush,
Wilfred Druml, Brian G. Dwinnell, Michael S. Goligorsky,
Katrina J. Kelly, Fernando Liaño, Wilfred Lieberthal, Ravindra L. Mehta,
Steven B. Miller, Bruce A. Molitoris, Cynthia C. Nast, Sanjay K. Nigam,
Babu J. Padanilam, Julio Pascual, Lorraine C. Racusen, Hiroyuki
Sakurai, Rick G. Schnellmann, Kim Solez, Tatsuo Tsukamoto

Causes and Prognosis

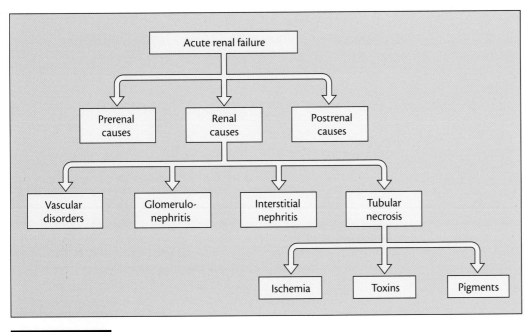

FIGURE 2-1

Classification and diagnosis of acute renal failure (ARF) [1–3]. The most common general
cause of ARF (60% to 70% of cases) is prerenal factors. Prerenal causes include those secondary to renal hypoperfusion, which occurs in the setting of extracellular fluid loss (eg,
with vomiting, nasogastric suctioning, gas-
trointestinal hemorrhage, diarrhea, burns,
heat stroke, diuretics, glucosuria), sequestration of extracellular fluid (eg, with pancreatitis, abdominal surgery, muscle crush
injury, early sepsis), or impaired cardiac
output. Once prerenal forms of ARF have
been ruled out, postrenal forms (ie, obstruction to urine flow) should be considered.
Obstruction to urine flow is a less common
(5% to 15% of cases) cause of ARF but is
nearly always amenable to therapy. The site
of obstruction can be intrarenal (eg, crystals
or proteins obstructing the terminal collecting tubules) or extrarenal (eg, blockade of
the renal pelvis, ureters, bladder, or urethra). After pre- and postrenal forms of
ARF have been considered, attention should
focus on the kidney. When considering
renal forms of ARF, it is helpful to think in
terms of renal anatomic compartments
(vasculature, glomeruli, interstitium, and
tubules). Acute disorders involving any of
these compartments can lead to ARF.

CAUSES OF PRERENAL ACUTE RENAL FAILURE

Decreased effective extracellular volume

Renal losses: hemorrhage, vomiting, diarrhea, burns, diuretics

Redistribution: hepatic disease, nephrotic syndrome, intestinal obstruction, pancreatitis, peritonitis, malnutrition

Decreased cardiac output: cardiogenic shock, valvulopathy, myocarditis, myocardial infarction, arrhythmia, congestive heart failure, pulmonary emboli, cardiac tamponade

Peripheral vasodilation: hypotension, sepsis, hypoxemia, anaphylactic shock, treatment with interleukin 2 or interferons, ovarian hyperstimulation syndrome

Renal vasoconstriction: prostaglandin synthesis inhibition, α-adrenergics, sepsis, hepatorenal syndrome, hypercalcemia

Efferent arteriole vasodilation: angiotensin converting-enzyme inhibitors

FIGURE 2-2

Causes of prerenal acute renal failure (ARF). *Prerenal* ARF supervenes when glomerular filtration rate falls as a consequence of decreased effective renal blood supply. The condition is reversible if the underlying disease is resolved.

CAUSES OF PARENCHYMAL ACUTE RENAL FAILURE

Acute tubular necrosis

Hemodynamic: cardiovascular surgery,* sepsis,* prerenal causes*

Toxic: antimicrobials,* iodide contrast agents,* anesthesics, immunosuppressive or antineoplastic agents,* Chinese herbs, Opiaceous, Extasis, mercurials, organic solvents, venoms, heavy metals, mannitol, radiation

Intratubular deposits: acute uric acid nephropathy, myeloma, severe hypercalcemia, primary oxalosis, sulfadiazine, fluoride anesthesics

Organic pigments (endogenous nephrotoxins):

Myoglobin rhabdomyolysis: muscle trauma; infections; dermatopolymyositis; metabolic alterations; hyperosmolar coma; diabetic ketoacidosis; severe hypokalemia; hyper- or hyponatremia; hypophosphatemia; severe hypothyroidism; malignant hyperthermia; toxins such as ethylene glycol, carbon monoxide, mercurial chloride, stings; drugs such as fibrates, statins, opioids and amphetamines; hereditary diseases such as muscular dystrophy, metabolopathies, McArdle disease and carnitine deficit

Hemoglobinuria: malaria; mechanical destruction of erythrocytes with extracorporeal circulation or metallic prosthesis, transfusion reactions, or other hemolysis; heat stroke; burns; glucose-6-phosphate dehydrogenase; nocturnal paroxystic hemoglobinuria; chemicals such as aniline, quinine, glycerol, benzene, phenol, hydralazine; insect venoms

Acute tubulointerstitial nephritis (see Fig. 2-4)

Vascular occlusion

Principal vessels: bilateral (unilateral in solitary functioning kidney) renal artery thrombosis or embolism, bilateral renal vein thrombosis

Small vessels: atheroembolic disease, thrombotic microangiopathy, hemolytic-uremic syndrome or thrombotic thrombocytopenic purpura, postpartum acute renal failure, antiphospholipid syndrome, disseminated intravascular coagulation, scleroderma, malignant arterial hypertension, radiation nephritis, vasculitis

Acute glomerulonephritis

Postinfectious: streptococcal or other pathogen associated with visceral abscess, endocarditis, or shunt

Henoch-Schönlein purpura

Essential mixed cryoglobulinemia

Systemic lupus erythematosus

Immunoglobulin A nephropathy

Mesangiocapillary

With antiglomerular basement membrane antibodies with lung disease (Goodpasture's syndrome) or without it

Idiopathic, rapidly progressive, without immune deposits

Cortical necrosis, abruptio placentae, septic abortion, disseminated intravascular coagulation

FIGURE 2-3

Causes of parenchymal acute renal failure (ARF). When the sudden decrease in glomerular filtration rate that characterizes ARF is secondary to intrinsic renal damage mainly affecting tubules, interstitium, glomeruli and/or vessels, we are facing a *parenchymal* ARF. The most frequent causes are marked with an asterisk.

MOST FREQUENT CAUSES OF ACUTE TUBULOINTERSTITIAL NEPHRITIS

Antimicrobials
  Penicillin
  Ampicillin
  Rifampicin
  Sulfonamides
Analgesics, anti-inflammatories
  Fenoprofen
  Ibuprofen
  Naproxen
  Amidopyrine
  Glafenine
Other drugs
  Cimetidine
  Allopurinol

Immunological
  Systemic lupus erythematosus
  Rejection
Infections (at present quite rare)
Neoplasia
  Myeloma
  Lymphoma
  Acute leukemia
Idiopathic
  Isolated
  Associated with uveitis

FIGURE 2-4

Most common causes of tubulointerstitial nephritis. Acute tubulo-interstitial nephritis is increasing in importance as a cause of acute renal failure. For decades, infections were the most important cause. At present, antimicrobials and other drugs are the most common causes.

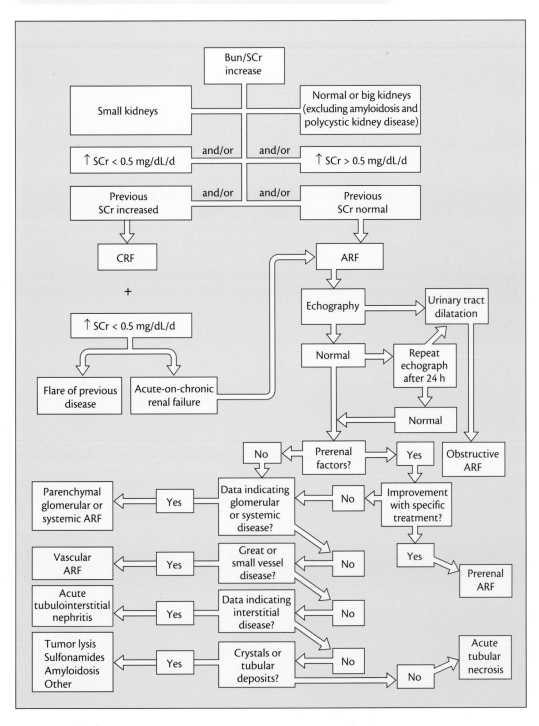

FIGURE 2-5

Discovering the cause of acute renal failure (ARF). This is a great challenge for clinicians. This algorithm could help to determine the cause of the increase in blood urea nitrogen (BUN) or serum creatinine (SCr) in a given patient.

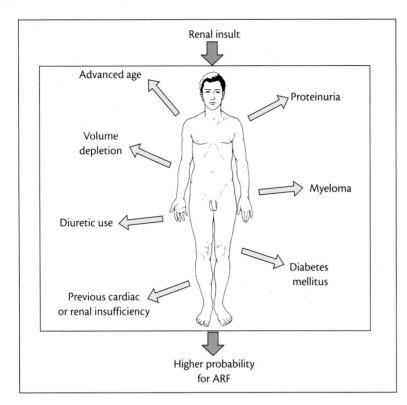

FIGURE 2-6

Factors that predispose to acute renal failure (ARF). Some of them act synergistically when they occur in the same patient. Advanced age and volume depletion are particularly important.

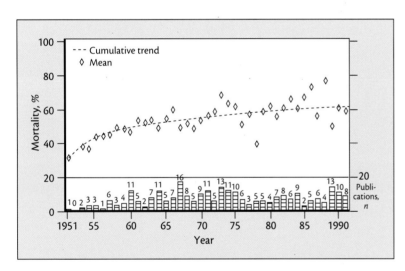

FIGURE 2-7

Mortality trends in acute renal failure (ARF). This figure shows the evolution of mortality during a 40-year period, starting in 1951. The graphic was elaborated after reviewing the outcome of 32,996 ARF patients reported in 258 published papers. As can be appreciated, mortality rate increases slowly but constantly during this follow-up, despite theoretically better availability of therapeutic armamentarium (mainly antibiotics and vasoactive drugs), deeper knowledge of dialysis techniques, and wider access to intensive care facilities. This improvement in supporting measures allows the physician to keep patients alive for longer periods of time. A complementary explanation could be that the patients treated now are usually older, sicker, and more likely to be treated more aggressively. (*Adapted from* Kierdorf and Sieberth [4].)

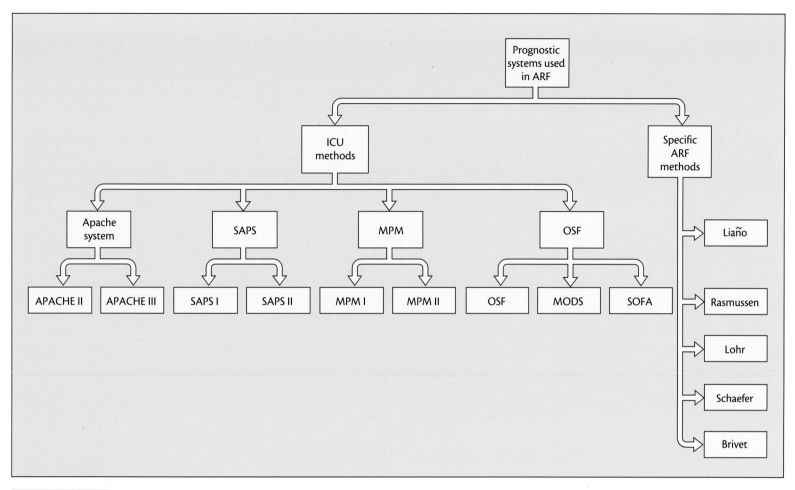

FIGURE 2-8

Ways of estimating prognosis in acute renal failure (ARF). This can be done using either general intensive care unit (ICU) score systems or methods developed specifically for ARF patients. ICU systems include Acute Physiological and Chronic Health Evaluation (APACHE) [5,6], Simplified Physiologic Score (SAPS)[7,8], Mortality Prediction Model (MPM) [9,10], and Organ System Failure scores (OSF) [11]. Multiple Organ Dysfunction Score (MODS) [12] and Sepsis-Related Organ Failure Assessment Score (SOFA) [13] are those that seem most suitable for this purpose. APACHE II used to be most used. Other systems have been used in ARF. On the other hand, at least 17 specific ARF prognostic methods have been developed [4,14]. The figure shows only those that have been used after their publication [15], plus one recently published system which is not yet in general use [16].

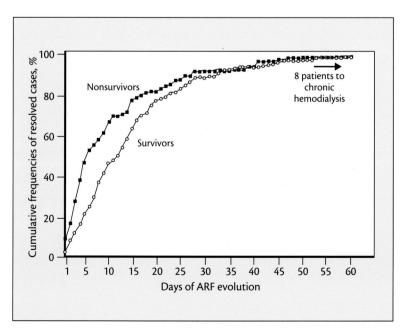

FIGURE 2-9

Duration and resolution of acute renal failure (ARF). Most of the episodes of ARF resolved in the first month of evolution. Mean duration of ARF was 14 days. Seventy-eight percent of the patients with ARF who died did so within 2 weeks after the renal insult. Similarly, 60% of survivors had recovered renal function at that time. After 30 days, 90% of the patients had had a final resolution of the ARF episode, one way or the other. Patients who finally lost renal function and needed to be included in a chronic periodic dialysis program usually had severe forms of glomerulonephritis, vasculitis, or systemic disease. (*Adapted from* Liaño *et al.* [1].)

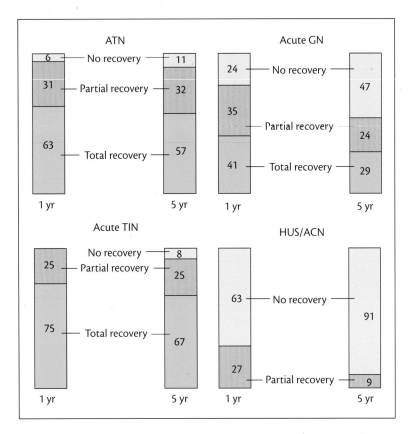

FIGURE 2-10

Outcome of acute renal failure (ARF). Long-term outcome of ARF has been studied only in some series of intrinsic or parenchymal ARF. The figure shows the different long-term prognoses for intrinsic ARF of various causes. *Left*, The percentages of recovery rate of renal function 1 year after the acute episode of renal failure. *Right*, The situation of renal function 5 years after the ARF episode. Acute tubulointerstitial nephritis (TIN) carries the better prognosis: the vast majority of patients had recovered renal function after 1 and 5 years. Two thirds of the patients with acute tubule necrosis (ATN) recovered normal renal function, 31% showed partial recovery, and 6% experienced no functional recovery. Some patients with ATN lost renal function over the years. Patients with ARF due to glomerular lesions have a poorer prognosis; 24% at 1 year and 47% at 5 years show terminal renal failure. The poorest evolution is observed with severe forms of acute cortical necrosis or hemolytic-uremic syndrome. GN—glomerulonephritis; HUS—hemolytic-uremic syndrome; ACN—acute cortical necrosis. (*Data from* Bonomini *et al.* [17].)

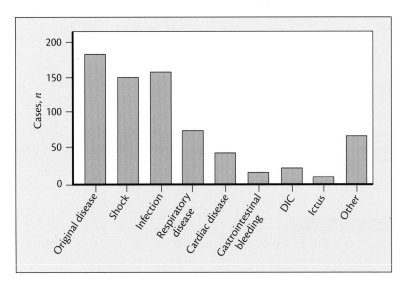

FIGURE 2-11

Causes of death. The causes of death from acute renal failure (ARF) were analyzed in 337 patients in the Madrid ARF Study [1]. In this work all the potential causes of death were recorded; thus, more than one cause could be present in a given patient. In fact, each dead patient averaged two causes, suggesting multifactorial origin. This could be the expression of a high presence of multiple organ dysfunction syndrome (MODS) among the nonsurviving patients. The main cause of death was the original disease, which was present in 55% of nonsurviving patients. Infection and shock were the next most common causes of death, usually concurrent in septic patients. It is worth noting that, if we exclude from the mortality analysis patients who died as a result of the original disease, the corrected mortality due to the ARF episode itself and its complications drops to 27%. DIC—disseminated intravascular coagulation.

Renal Histopathology, Urine Cytology, and Cytopathology of Acute Renal Failure

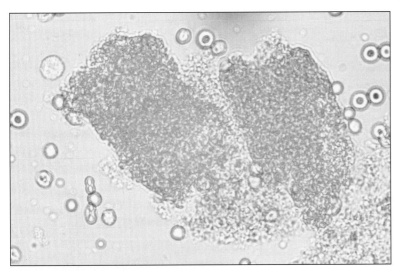

FIGURE 2-12 (*see* Color Plates)

Urine sediment of a patient with acute renal failure revealing red blood cells and some red blood cell casts (original magnification × 600). Biopsy in this case revealed crescentic glomerulonephritis. However, hematuria may be seen in any proliferative glomerulonephritis or with parenchymal infarcts. The "casts" assume the cylindrical shape of the renal tubules, and confirm an intrarenal source of the blood in the urine. Fragmented or dysmorphic red blood cells may be seen when the red cells have traversed through damaged glomerular capillaries.

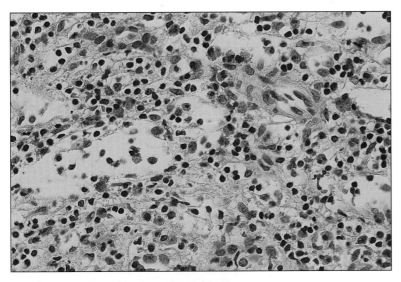

FIGURE 2-14 (*see* Color Plates)

Numerous eosinophils in an interstitial inflammatory infiltrate. Eosinophils may be diffuse within the infiltrate, but may also be clustered, forming "eosinophilic abscesses," as in this area (hematoxylin and eosin, original magnification × 400). Eosinophils may also be demonstrated in the urine sediment. Drugs most commonly producing acute interstitial nephritis as part of a hypersensitivity reaction include penicillins, sulfonamides, and nonsteroidal anti-inflammatory drugs [18]. The patient had recently undergone a course of therapy with methicillin. The interstitial nephritis may be part of a systemic reaction that includes fever, rash, and eosinophilia.

FIGURE 2-13 (*see* Color Plates)

Numerous polymorphonuclear leukocytes (PML) in the urine sediment of a patient with acute pyelonephritis (hematoxylin and eosin, original magnification × 400). Some red blood cells and tubular cells are seen in the background of this cytospin preparation. PML may be found in the urine with acute infection of the lower urinary tract as well, or as a contaminant from vaginal secretions in females. PML casts, on the other hand, are evidence that the cells are from the kidney.

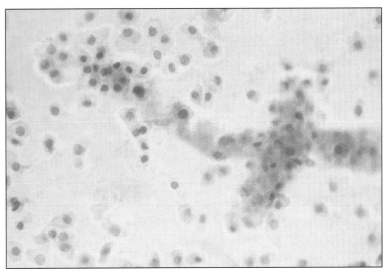

FIGURE 2-15 (*see* Color Plates)

Urine sediment from a patient with acute tubular injury showing tubular cells and cell casts (Papanicolaou stain, original magnification × 250). Many of these cells are morphologically intact, even by electron microscopy. Studies have shown that a significant percentage of the cells shed into the urine may exclude vital dyes, and may even grow when placed in culture, indicating that they remain viable. Such cells clearly detached from tubular basement membrane as a manifestation of sublethal injury [19].

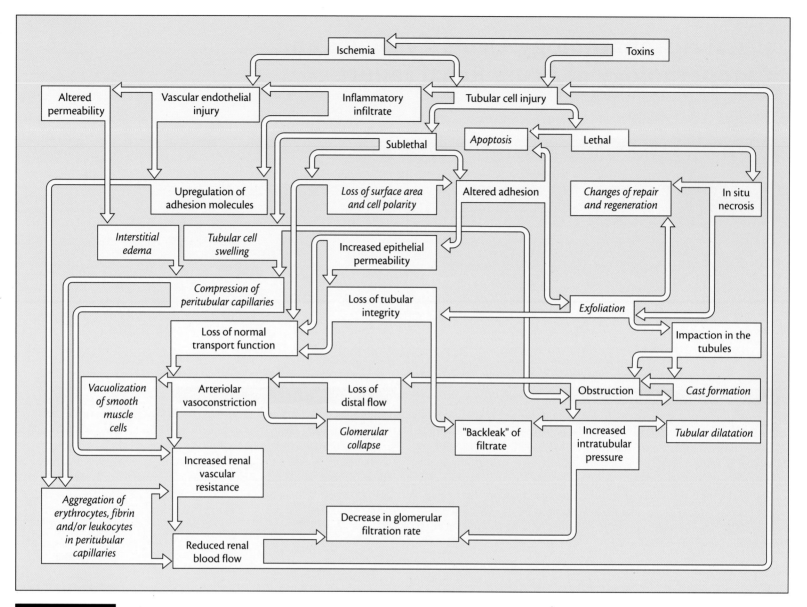

FIGURE 2-16

A schematic showing the relationship between morphologic and functional changes with injury to the renal tubule due to ischemia or nephrotoxins. Morphologic changes are shown in italics. Histology reflects the altered hemodynamics, epithelial derangements, and obstruction that contribute to loss of renal function. (*Adapted from* Racusen [20].)

Acute Renal Failure in the Transplanted Kidney

DIAGNOSTIC POSSIBILITIES IN TRANSPLANT-RELATED ACUTE RENAL FAILURE

Acute (cell-mediated) rejection

Delayed-appearing antibody-mediated rejection

Acute tubular necrosis

Cyclosporine or FK506 toxicity

Urine leak

Obstruction

Viral infection

Posttransplant lymphoproliferative disorder

Vascular thrombosis

Prerenal azotemia

FIGURE 2-17

Diagnostic possibilities in transplant-related acute renal failure.

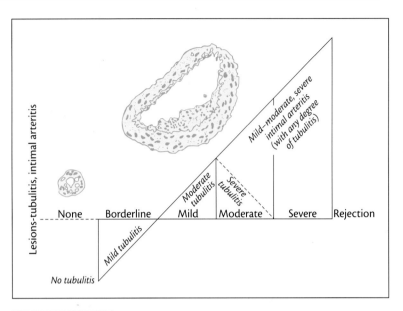

FIGURE 2-18

Diagnosis of rejection in the Banff classification makes use of two basic lesions: tubulitis and intimal arteritis. The 1993–1995 Banff classification depicted in this figure is the standard in use in virtually all current clinical trials and in many individual transplant units. In this construct, rejection is regarded as a continuum of mild, moderate, and severe forms. The 1997 Banff classification is similar, having the same threshold for rejection diagnosis, but it recognizes three different histologic types of acute rejection: tubulointersititial, vascular, and transmural. The quotation marks emphasize the possible overlap of features of the various types (*eg*, the finding of tubulitis should not dissuade the pathologist from conducting a thorough search for intimal arteritis).

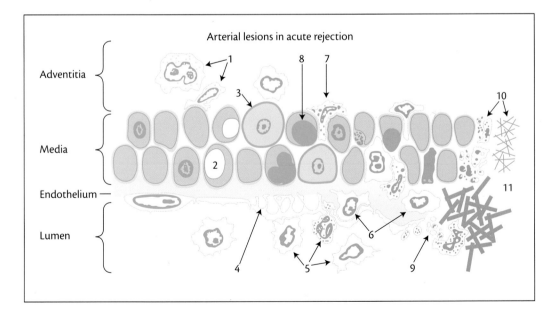

Arterial lesions in acute rejection

FIGURE 2-19

Diagram of arterial lesions of acute rejection. The initial changes (1–5) before intimal arteritis (6) occurs are completely nonspecific. These early changes are probably mechanistically related to the diagnostic lesions but can occur as a completely self-limiting phenomenon unrelated to clinical rejection. Lesions 7 to 10 are those characteristic of "transmural" rejection. Lesion 1 is perivascular inflammation; lesion 2, myocyte vacuolization; lesion 3, apoptosis; lesion 4, endothelial activation and prominence; lesion 5, leukocyte adherence to the endothelium; lesion 6 (specific), penetration of inflammatory cells under the endothelium (intimal arteritis); lesion 7, inflammatory cell penetration of the media; lesion 8, necrosis of medial smooth muscle cells; lesion 9, platelet aggregation; lesion 10, fibrinoid change; lesion 11 is thrombosis.

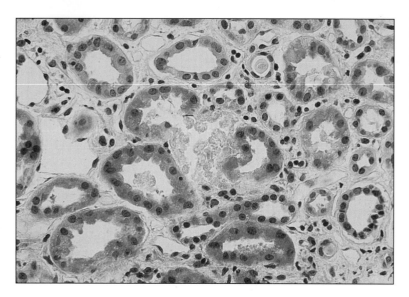

FIGURE 2-20 (*see* Color Plates)

Acute tubular necrosis in the allograft. Unlike "acute tubule necrosis" in native kidney, in this condition actual necrosis appears in the transplanted kidney but in a very small proportion of tubules, often less than one in 300 tubule cross-sections. Where the necrosis does occur it tends to affect the entire tubule cross-section, as in the center of this field [21].

FEATURES OF TRANSPLANT ATN THAT DIFFERENTIATE IT FROM NATIVE KIDNEY ATN

Apparently intact proximal tubular brush border

Occasional foci of necrosis of entire tubular cross-sections

More extensive calcium oxalate deposition

Significantly fewer tubular casts

Significantly more interstitial inflammation

Less cell-to-cell variation in size and shape ("tubular cell unrest")

FIGURE 2-21

Features of transplant acute tubular necrosis that differentiate it from the same condition in native kidney [21].

Renal Injury Due to Environmental Toxins, Drugs, and Contrast Agents

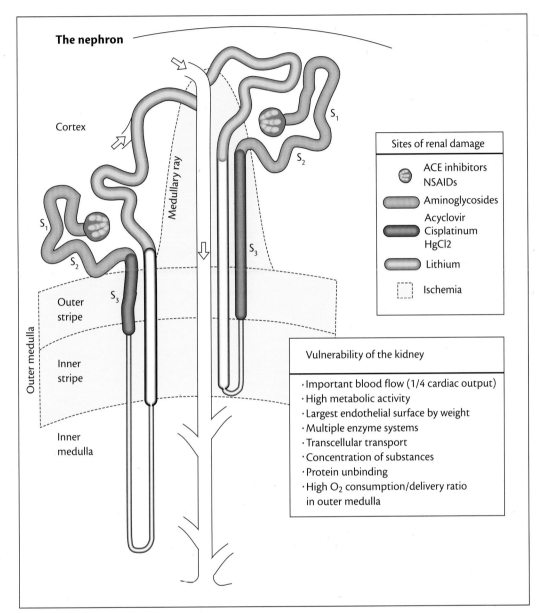

The nephron

Cortex

S_1

S_2

S_1

S_2

S_3

S_3

Medullary ray

Outer stripe

Inner stripe

Outer medulla

Inner medulla

Sites of renal damage

ACE inhibitors
NSAIDs

Aminoglycosides

Acyclovir
Cisplatinum
HgCl2

Lithium

Ischemia

Vulnerability of the kidney

· Important blood flow (1/4 cardiac output)
· High metabolic activity
· Largest endothelial surface by weight
· Multiple enzyme systems
· Transcellular transport
· Concentration of substances
· Protein unbinding
· High O_2 consumption/delivery ratio
 in outer medulla

FIGURE 2-22

Sites of renal damage, including factors that contribute to the kidney's susceptibility to damage. ACE—angiotensin-converting enzyme; $HgCl_2$—mercuric chloride; NSAID—nonsteroidal anti-inflammatory drugs.

DRUGS AND CHEMICALS ASSOCIATED WITH ACUTE RENAL FAILURE

Mechanisms

M1 Reduction in renal perfusion through alteration of intrarenal hemodynamics

M2 Direct tubular toxicity

M3 Heme pigment–induced toxicity (rhabdomyolysis)

M4 Intratubular obstruction by precipitation of the agents or its metabolites or byproducts

M5 Allergic interstitial nephritis

M6 Hemolytic-uremic syndrome

M1	M2	M3	M4	M5*	M6	Drugs
✓	✓				✓	Cyclosporine, tacrolimus
✓	✓					Amphotericin B, radiocontrast agents
✓				✓		Nonsteroidal anti-inflammatory drugs
✓						Angiotensin-converting enzyme inhibitors, interleukin-2†
✓	✓		✓			Methotrexate§
	✓					Aminoglycosides, cisplatin, foscarnet, heavy metals, intravenous immunoglobulin¶, organic solvents, pentamidine
		✓			✓	Cocaine
		✓				Ethanol, lovastatin**
			✓	✓		Sulfonamides
			✓			Acyclovir, Indinavir, chemotherapeutic agents, ethylene glycol***
				✓		Allopurinol, cephalosporins, cimetidine, ciprofloxacin, furosemide, penicillins, phenytoin, rifampin, thiazide diuretics
					✓	Conjugated estrogens, mitomycin, quinine

* Many other drugs in addition to the ones listed can cause renal failure by this mechanism.

† Interleukin-2 produces a capillary leak syndrome with volume contraction.

§ Uric acid crystals form as a result of tumor lysis.

¶ The mechanism of this agent is unclear but may be due to additives.

** Acute renal failure is most likely to occur when lovastatin is given in combination with cyclosporine.

*** Ethylene glycol–induced toxicity can cause calcium oxalate crystals.

FIGURE 2-23

Drugs and chemicals associated with acute renal failure. (*Adapted from* Thadhani *et al.* [22].)

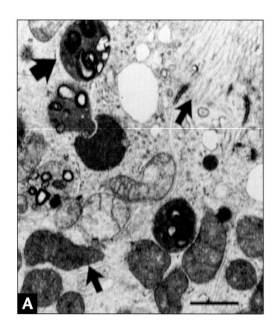

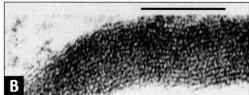

FIGURE 2-24

Ultrastructural appearance of proximal tubule cells in aminoglycoside-treated patients (4 days of therapeutic doses). Lysosomes (*large arrow*) contain dense lamellar and concentric structures. Brush border, mitochondria (*small arrows*), and peroxisomes are unaltered. At higher magnification the structures in lysosomes show a periodic pattern. The bar in **part A** represents 1 µm; in **part B**, 0.1 µm [23].

RISK FACTORS FOR AMINOGLYCOSIDE NEPHROTOXICITY

Patient-Related Factors	Aminoglycoside-Related Factors	Other Drugs
Older age*	Recent aminoglycoside therapy	Amphotericin B
Preexisting renal disease		Cephalosporins
Female gender	Larger doses*	Cisplatin
Magnesium, potassium, or calcium deficiency*	Treatment for 3 days or more*	Clindamycin
Intravascular volume depletion*		Cyclosporine
Hypotension*	Dose regimen*	Foscarnet
Hepatorenal syndrome		Furosemide
Sepsis syndrome		Piperacillin
		Radiocontrast agents
		Thyroid hormone

* Similar to experimental data.

FIGURE 2-25

Risk factors for aminoglycoside nephrotoxicity. Several risk factors have been identified and classified as patient related, aminoglycoside related, or related to concurrent administration of certain drugs.

The usual recommended aminoglycoside dose may be excessive for older patients because of decreased renal function and decreased regenerative capacity of a damaged kidney. Preexisting renal disease clearly can expose patients to inadvertent overdosing if careful dose adjustment is not performed. Hypomagnesemia, hypokalemia, and calcium deficiency may be predisposing risk factors for consequences of aminoglycoside-induced damage [24]. Liver disease is an important clinical risk factor for aminoglycoside nephrotoxicity, particularly in patients with cholestasis [24]. Acute or chronic endotoxemia amplifies the nephrotoxic potential of the aminoglycosides [25].

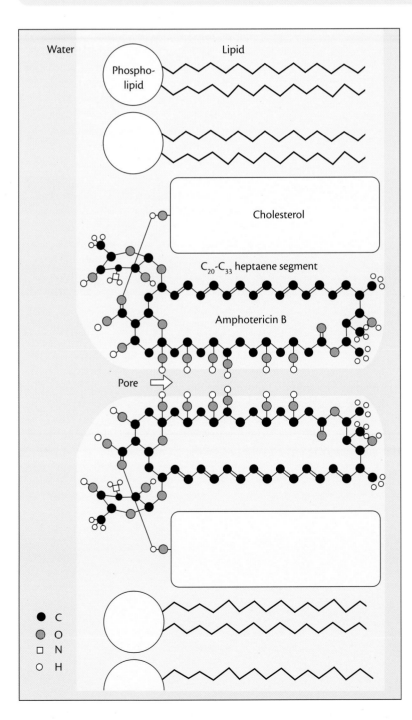

FIGURE 2-26

Proposed partial model for the amphotericin B (AmB)–induced pore in the cell membrane. AmB is an amphipathic molecule: its structure enhances the drug's binding to sterols in the cell membranes and induces formation of aqueous pores that result in weakening of barrier function and loss of protons and cations from the cell. The drug acts as a counterfeit phospholipid, with the C_{15} hydroxyl, C_{16} carboxyl, and C_{19} mycosamine groups situated at the membrane-water interface, and the C_1 to C_{14} and C_{20} to C_{33} chains aligned in parallel within the membrane. The heptaene chain seeks a hydrophobic environment, and the hydroxyl groups seek a hydrophilic environment. Thus, a cylindrical pore is formed, the inner wall of which consists of the hydroxyl-substituted carbon chains of the AmB molecules and the outer wall of which is formed by the heptaene chains of the molecules and by sterol nuclei [26].

RISK FACTORS IN THE DEVELOPMENT OF AMPHOTERICIN NEPHROTOXICITY

Age

Concurrent use of diuretics

Abnormal baseline renal function

Larger daily doses

Hypokalemia

Hypomagnesemia

Other nephrotoxic drugs (aminoglycosides, cyclosporine)

FIGURE 2-27

Risk factors for development of amphotericin B (AmB) nephrotoxicity. Nephrotoxicity of AmB is a major problem associated with clinical use of this important drug. Disturbances in both glomerular and tubule function are well described. The nephrotoxic effect of AmB is initially a distal tubule phenomenon, characterized by a loss of urine concentration, distal renal tubule acidosis, and wasting of potassium and magnesium, but it also causes renal vasoconstriction leading to renal ischemia. Initially, the drug binds to membrane sterols in the renal vasculature and epithelial cells, altering its membrane permeability. AmB-induced vasoconstriction and ischemia to very vulnerable sections of the nephron, such as medullary thick ascending limb, enhance the cell death produced by direct toxic action of AmB on those cells. This potentially explains the salutary effect on AmB nephrotoxicity of salt loading, furosemide, theophylline, or calcium channel blockers, all of which improve renal blood flow or inhibit transport in the medullary thick ascending limb.

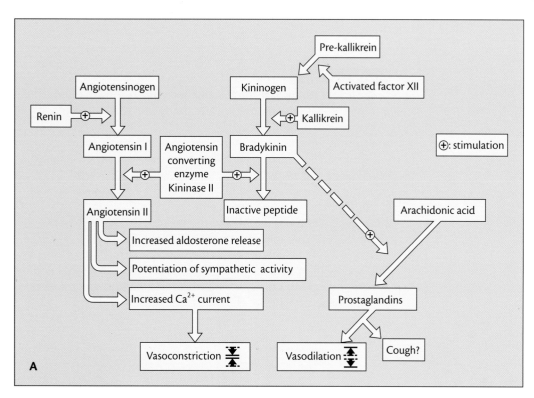

A

FIGURE 2-28

Soon after the release of this useful class of antihypertensive drugs, the syndrome of functional acute renal insufficiency was described as a class effect. This phenomenon was first observed in patients with renal artery stenosis, particularly when the entire renal mass was affected, as in bilateral renal artery stenosis or in renal transplants with stenosis to a solitary kidney [27]. Acute renal dysfunction appears to be related to loss of postglomerular efferent arteriolar vas-

cular tone and in general is reversible after withdrawing the angiotensin-converting enzyme (ACE) inhibitor [28].

Inhibition of the ACE kininase II results in at least two important effects: depletion of angiotensin II and accumulation of bradykinin [29]. The role of the latter effect on renal perfusion pressure is not clear (**part A**).

To understand the angiotensin I converting enzyme inhibitor–induced drop in glomerular filtration rate, it is important to understand the physiologic role of the renin-angiotensin system in the regulation of renal hemodynamics (**part B**). When renal perfusion drops, renin is released into the plasma and lymph by the juxtaglomerular cells of the kidneys. Renin cleaves angiotensinogen to form angiotensin I, which is cleaved further by converting enzyme to form angiotensin II, the principal effector molecule in this system. Angiotensin II participates in glomerular filtration rate regulation in a least two ways. First, angiotensin II increases arterial pressure directly and acutely by causing vasoconstriction and more "chronically" by increasing body fluid volumes through stimulation of renal sodium retention; *directly* through an effect on the tubules, as well as by stimulating thirst, and *indirectly* via aldosterone.

(*Continued on next page*)

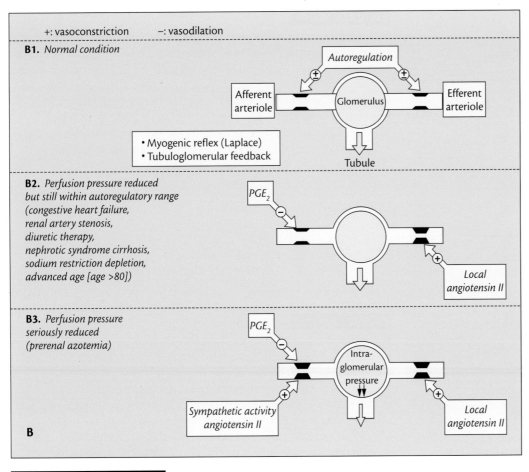

+: vasoconstriction   –: vasodilation

B1. *Normal condition*

Autoregulation

Afferent arteriole   Glomerulus   Efferent arteriole

• Myogenic reflex (Laplace)
• Tubuloglomerular feedback

Tubule

B2. *Perfusion pressure reduced but still within autoregulatory range (congestive heart failure, renal artery stenosis, diuretic therapy, nephrotic syndrome cirrhosis, sodium restriction depletion, advanced age [age >80])*

PGE_2

Local angiotensin II

B3. *Perfusion pressure seriously reduced (prerenal azotemia)*

PGE_2

Intra-glomerular pressure

Sympathetic activity angiotensin II

Local angiotensin II

B

FIGURE 2-28 (*continued*)

Second, angiotensin II preferentially constricts the efferent arteriole, thus helping to preserve glomerular capillary hydrostatic pressure and, consequently, glomerular filtration rate.

When arterial pressure or body fluid volumes are sensed as subnormal, the renin-angiotensin system is activated and plasma renin activity and angiotensin II levels increase. This may occur in the context of clinical settings such as renal artery stenosis, dietary sodium restriction or sodium depletion as during diuretic therapy, congestive heart failure, cirrhosis, and nephrotic syndrome. When activated, this renin-angiotensin system plays an important role in the maintenance of glomerular pressure and filtration through preferential angiotensin II–mediated constriction of the efferent arteriole. Thus, under such conditions the kidney becomes sensitive to the effects of blockade of the renin-angiotensin system by angiotensin I–converting enzyme inhibitor or angiotensin II receptor antagonist.

The highest incidence of renal failure in patients treated with ACE inhibitors was associated with bilateral renovascular disease [28]. In patients with already compromised renal function and congestive heart failure, the incidence of serious changes in serum creatinine during ACE inhibition depends on the severity of the pretreatment heart failure and renal failure.

Volume management, dose reduction, use of relatively short-acting ACE inhibitors, diuretic holiday for some days before initiating treatment, and avoidance of concurrent use of nonsteroidal anti-inflammatory drug (hyperkalemia) are among the appropriate measures for patients at risk.

Acute interstitial nephritis associated with angiotensin I–converting enzyme inhibition has been described [30]. (*Adapted from* Opie [31].)

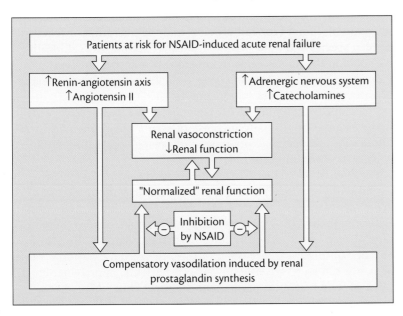

Patients at risk for NSAID-induced acute renal failure

↑Renin-angiotensin axis
↑Angiotensin II

↑Adrenergic nervous system
↑Catecholamines

Renal vasoconstriction
↓Renal function

"Normalized" renal function

Inhibition by NSAID

Compensatory vasodilation induced by renal prostaglandin synthesis

FIGURE 2-29

Mechanism by which nonsteroidal anti-inflammatory drugs (NSAIDs) disrupt the compensatory vasodilatation response of renal prostaglandins to vasoconstrictor hormones in patients with prerenal conditions. Most of the renal abnormalities encountered clinically as a result of NSAIDs can be attributed to the action of these compounds on prostaglandin production in the kidney [32].

Sodium chloride and water retention are the most common side effects of NSAIDs. This should not be considered drug toxicity because it represents a modification of a physiologic control mechanism without the production of a true functional disorder in the kidney.

RISK FACTORS THAT PREDISPOSE TO CONTRAST-ASSOCIATED NEPHROPATHY

Confirmed	Suspected	Disproved
Chronic renal failure	Hypertension	Myeloma
Diabetic nephropathy	Generalized atherosclerosis	Diabetes without
Severe congestive heart failure	Abnormal liver function tests	nephropathy
Amount and frequency of contrast media	Hyperuricemia	
Volume depletion or hypotension	Proteinuria	

FIGURE 2-30

Risk factors that predispose to contrast-associated nephropathy. In random populations undergoing radiocontrast imaging, the incidence of contrast-associated nephropathy (defined by a change in serum creatinine of more than 0.5 mg/dL or a greater than 50% increase over baseline) is between 2% and 7%. For confirmed high-risk patients (baseline serum creatinine values greater than 1.5 mg/dL) it rises to 10% to 35%. In addition, suspected risk factors that should be considered when assessing the value of contrast-enhanced imaging.

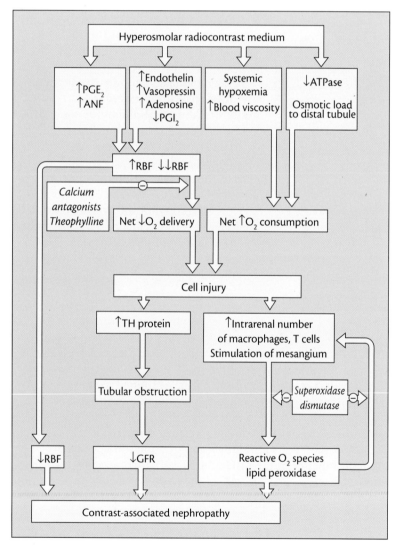

FIGURE 2-31

A proposed model of the mechanisms involved in radiocontrast medium–induced renal dysfunction. Based on experimental models, a consensus is developing to the effect that contrast-associated nephropathy involves combined toxic and hypoxic insults to the kidney [33]. The initial glomerular vasoconstriction that follows the injection of radiocontrast medium induces the liberation of both vasoconstrictor (endothelin, vasopressin) and vasodilator (prostaglandin E_2 [PGE_2], adenosine, atrionatiuretic factor [ANP]) substances. The net effect is reduced oxygen delivery to tubule cells, especially those in the thick ascending limb of Henle. Because of the systemic hypoxemia, raised blood viscosity, inhibition of sodium-potassium–activated ATPase and the increased osmotic load to the distal tubule at a time of reduced oxygen delivery, the demand for oxygen increases, resulting in cellular hypoxia and, eventually, cell death. Additional factors that contribute to the acute renal dysfunction of contrast-associated nephropathy are the tubule obstruction that results from increased secretion of Tamm-Horsfall proteins and the liberation of reactive oxygen species and lipid peroxidation that accompany cell death. As noted in the figure, calcium antagonists and theophylline (adenosine receptor antagonist) are thought to diminish the degree of vasoconstriction induced by contrast medium.

The clinical presentation of contrast-associated nephropathy involves an asymptomatic increase in serum creatinine within 24 hours of a radiographic imaging study using contrast medium, with or without oliguria [34].

The clinical outcome of 281 patients with contrast-associated nephropathy was compared in patient with or without oliguric acute renal failure at the time of diagnosis. Of oliguric acute renal failure patients, 32% have persistent elevations of serum creatinine at recovery and half require permanent dialysis. In the absence of oliguric acute renal failure, the serum creatinine value does not return to baseline in 24% of patients, approximately a third of whom require permanent dialysis. Thus, this is not a benign condition but rather one whose defined risks are not only permanent dialysis but also death. GFR—glomerular filtration rate; RBF—renal blood flow; TH—Tamm Horsfall protein.

Diagnostic Evaluation of the Patient with Acute Renal Failure

BLOOD UREA NITROGEN (BUN)-CREATININE RATIO

> 10	< 10
Increased protein intake	Starvation
Catabolic state	Advanced liver disease
Fever	Postdialysis state
Sepsis	Drugs that impair tubular secretion
Trauma	Cimetidine
Corticosteroids	Trimethoprim
Tissue necrosis	Rhabdomyolysis
Tetracyclines	
Diminished urine flow	
Prerenal state	
Postrenal state	

FIGURE 2-32

The blood urea nitrogen (BUN)-creatinine ratio. The BUN-creatinine ratio often deviates from the usual value of about 10:1. These deviations may have modest diagnostic implications. As an example, for reasons as yet unclear, tubular reabsorption of urea nitrogen is enhanced in low urine flow states. Thus, a high BUN-creatinine ratio often occurs in prerenal and postrenal (*see* Fig. 2-33) forms of renal failure. Similarly, enhanced delivery of amino acids to the liver (as with catabolism, corticosteroids, etc.) can enhance urea nitrogen formation and increase the BUN-creatinine ratio. A BUN-creatinine ratio lower than 10:1 can occur because of decreased urea nitrogen formation (*eg*, in protein malnutrition, advanced liver disease), enhanced creatinine formation (*eg*, with rhabdomyolysis), impaired tubular secretion of creatinine (*eg*, secondary to trimethoprim, cimetidine), or relatively enhanced removal of the small substance urea nitrogen by dialysis.

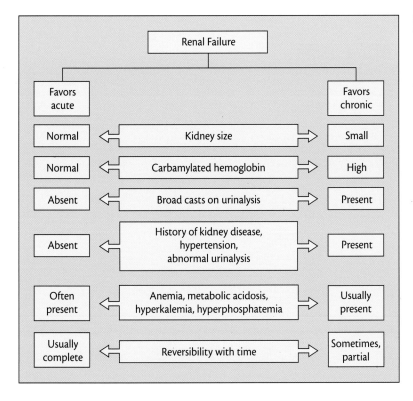

FIGURE 2-33

Categories of renal failure. Once the presence of renal failure is ascertained by elevated blood urea nitrogen (BUN) or serum creatinine value, the clinician must decide whether it is acute or chronic. When previous values are available for review, this judgment is made relatively easily. In the absence of such values, the factors depicted here may be helpful. Hemoglobin potentially undergoes nonenzymatic carbamylation of its terminal valine [35]. Thus, similar to the hemoglobin A1C value as an index of blood sugar control, the level of carbamylated hemoglobin is an indicator of the degree and duration of elevated BUN, but this test is not yet widely available. The presence of small kidneys strongly suggests that renal failure is at least in part chronic. From a practical standpoint, because even chronic renal failure often is partially reversible, the clinician should assume and evaluate for the presence of acute reversible factors in all cases of acute renal failure.

FIRST STEP IN EVALUATION OF ACUTE RENAL FAILURE

History

Disorders that suggest or predispose to renal failure: hypertension, diabetes mellitus, HIV, vascular disease, abnormal urinalyses, family history of renal disease, medication use, toxin or environmental exposure, infection, heart failure, vasculitis, cancer

Disorders that suggest or predispose to volume depletion: vomiting, diarrhea, pancreatitis, gastrointestinal bleeding, burns, heat stroke, fever, uncontrolled diabetes mellitus, diuretic use, orthostatic hypotension, nothing-by-mouth status, nasogastric suctioning

Disorders that suggest or predispose to obstruction: stream abnormalities, nocturia, anticholingeric medications, stones, urinary tract infections, bladder or prostate disease, intra-abnominal malignancy, suprapubic or flank pain, anuria, fluctuating urine volumes

Symptoms of renal failure: anorexia, vomiting, reversed sleep pattern, pruritus

Record review

Recent events (procedures, surgery)

Medications

Vital signs

Intake and output

Body weights

Blood chemistries and hemogram

Physical examination

Skin: rash suggestive of allergy, palpable purpura of vasculitis, livedo reticularis and digital infarctions suggesting atheroemboli

Eyes: hypertension, diabetes mellitus, Hollenhorst plaques, vasculitis, candidemia

Lungs: rales, rubs

Heart: evidence of heart failure, pericardial disease, jugular venous pressure

Vascular system: bruits, pulses, abdominal aortic aneurysm

Abdomen: flank or suprapubic masses, ascites, costovertebral angle pain

Extremities: edema, pulses, compartment syndromes

Nervous system: focal findings, asterixis, mini-mental status examination

Consider bladder catheterization

Urinalysis

FIGURE 2-34

First step in evaluation of acute renal failure.

SECOND STEP IN EVALUATION OF ACUTE RENAL FAILURE

Urine diagnostic indices (*see* Fig. 2-37)

Consider need for further evaluation for obstruction

Ultrasonography, computed tomography, or magnetic resonance imaging

Consider need for additional blood tests

Vasculitis/glomerulopathy: HIV infections, antineutrophilic cytoplasmic antibodies, antinuclear antibodies, serologic tests for hepatitis, systemic bacterial endocarditis and streptococcal infections, rheumatoid factor, complement, cryoglobins

Plasma cell disorders: urine for light chains, serum analysis for abnormal proteins

Drug screen/level, additional chemical tests

Consider need for evaluation of renal vascular supply

Isotope scans, Doppler sonography, angiography

Consider need for more data to assess volume and cardiac status

Swan-Ganz catheterization

FIGURE 2-35

Second step in evaluation of acute renal failure.

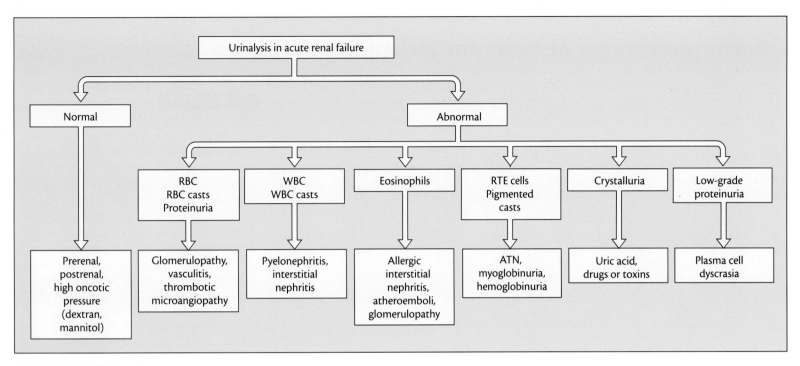

FIGURE 2-36

Urinalysis in acute renal failure (ARF). A normal urinalysis suggests a prerenal or postrenal form of ARF; however, many patients with ARF of postrenal causes have some cellular elements on urinalysis. Relatively uncommon causes of ARF that usually present with oligoanuria and a normal urinalysis are mannitol toxicity and large doses of dextran infusion. In these disorders, a "hyperoncotic state" occurs in which glomerular capillary oncotic pressure, combined with the intratubular hydrostatic pressure, exceeds the glomerular capillary hydrostatic pressure and stop glomerular filtration. Red blood cells (RBCs) can be seen with all renal forms of ARF. When RBC casts are present, glomerulonephritis or vasculitis is most likely.

White blood cells (WBCs) can also be present in small numbers in the urine of patients with ARF. Large numbers of WBCs and WBC casts strongly suggest the presence of either pyelonephritis or acute interstitial nephritis. Eosinolphiluria (Hansel's stain) is often present in either allergic interstitial nephritis or atheroembolic disease [36, 37]. Renal tubular epithelial (RTE) cells and casts and pigmented granular casts typically are present in pigmenturia-associated ARF and in established acute tubular necrosis (ATN). The presence of large numbers of crystals on urinalysis, in conjunction with the clinical history, may suggest uric acid, sulfonamides, or protease inhibitors as a cause of the renal failure.

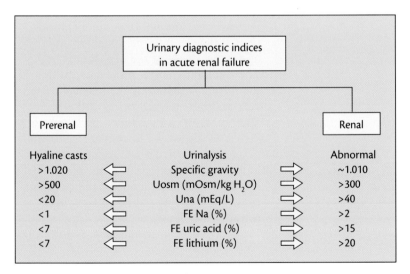

FIGURE 2-37

Urinary diagnostic indices in acute renal failure (ARF). These indices have traditionally been used in the setting of oliguria to help differentiate between prerenal (intact tubular function) and acute tubular necrosis (ATN, impaired tubular function). Several caveats to interpretation of these indices are in order [38]. First, none of these is completely sensitive or specific in differentiating the prerenal from the ATN form of ARF. Second, often a continuum exists between early prerenal conditions and late prerenal conditions that lead to ischemic ATN. Most of the data depicted here are derived from patients relatively late in the progress of ARF when the serum creatinine concentrations were 3 to 5 mg/dL. Third, there is often a relatively large "gray area," in which the various indices do not give definitive results. Finally, some of the indices (*eg*, fractional excretion of endogenous lithium [FE lithium]) are not readily available in the clinical setting. The fractional excretion (FE) of a substance is determined by this formula: FE = U/P substance ÷ U/P creatinine × 100. U/P—urine-plasma ratio.

Pathophysiology of Ischemic Acute Renal Failure

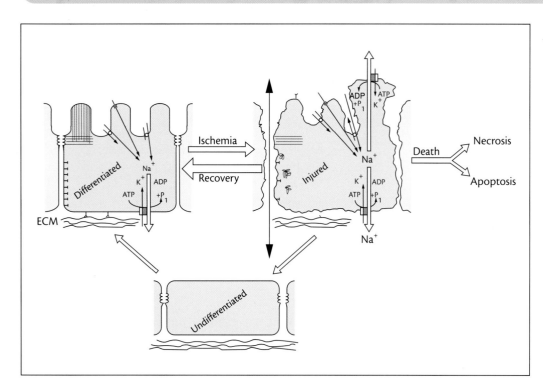

FIGURE 2-38

Fate of an injured proximal tubule cell. The fate of a proximal tubule cell after an ischemic episode depends on the extent and duration of the ischemia. Cell death can occur immediately via necrosis or in a more programmed fashion (apoptosis) hours to days after the injury. Fortunately, most cells recover either in a direct fashion or via an intermediate undifferentiated cellular pathway. Again, the severity of the injury determines the route taken by a particular cell. Adjacent cells are often injured to varying degrees, especially during mild to moderate ischemia. It is believed that the rate of organ functional recovery relates directly to the severity of cell injury during the initiation phase. ECM—extracellular membrane; K^+—potassium ion; Na^+—sodium ion; P_1—phosphate.

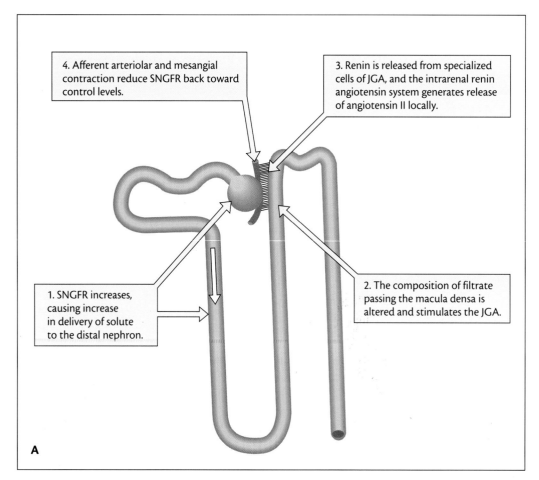

A

FIGURE 2-39

The tubuloglomerular (TG) feedback mechanism. **A,** Normal TG feedback. In the normal kidney, the TG feedback mechanism is a sensitive device for the regulation of the single nephron glomerular filtration rate (SNGFR). *Step 1:* An increase in SNGFR increases the amount of sodium chloride (NaCl) delivered to the juxtaglomerular apparatus (JGA) of the nephron. *Step 2:* The resultant change in the composition of the filtrate is sensed by the macula densa cells and initiates activation of the JGA. *Step 3:* The JGA releases renin, which results in the local and systemic generation of angiotensin II. *Step 4:* Angiotensin II induces vasoconstriction of the glomerular arterioles and contraction of the mesangial cells. These events return SNGFR back toward basal levels.

(Continued on next page)

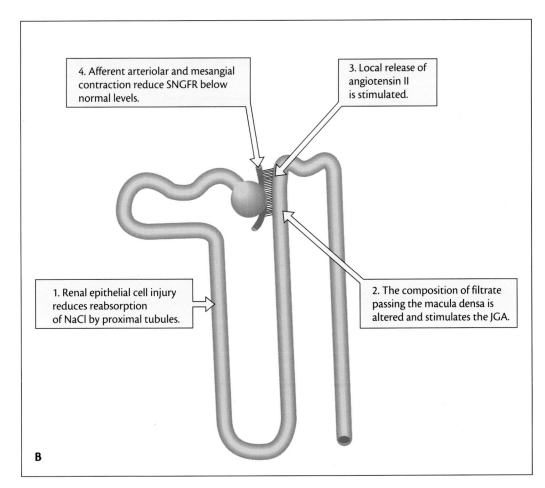

B

FIGURE 2-39 *(continued)*

B, TG feedback in ARF. *Step 1*: Ischemic or toxic injury to renal tubules leads to impaired reabsorption of NaCl by injured tubular segments proximal to the JGA. *Step 2*: The composition of the filtrate passing the macula densa is altered and activates the JGA. *Step 3*: Angiotensin II is released locally. *Step 4*: SNGFR is reduced below normal levels. It is likely that vasoconstrictors other than angiotensin II, as well as vasodilator hormones (such as PGI_2 and nitric oxide) are also involved in modulating TG feedback. Abnormalities in these vasoactive hormones in ARF may contribute to alterations in TG feedback in ARF.

In the figure:

4. Afferent arteriolar and mesangial contraction reduce SNGFR below normal levels.

3. Local release of angiotensin II is stimulated.

1. Renal epithelial cell injury reduces reabsorption of NaCl by proximal tubules.

2. The composition of filtrate passing the macula densa is altered and stimulates the JGA.

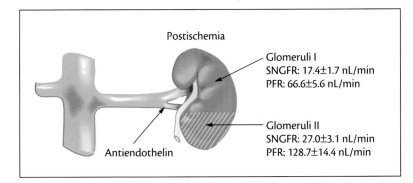

Postischemia

Glomeruli I
SNGFR: 17.4 ± 1.7 nL/min
PFR: 66.6 ± 5.6 nL/min

Glomeruli II
SNGFR: 27.0 ± 3.1 nL/min
PFR: 128.7 ± 14.4 nL/min

Antiendothelin

FIGURE 2-40

Endothelin (ET) has been implicated as an important vasoconstrictor in ARF. Function in separate populations of glomeruli within the same kidney. Endothelin (ET) is a potent renal vasoconstrictor. ET is a 21-amino-acid peptide of which three isoforms—ET-1, ET-2 and ET-3—have been described, all of which have been shown to be present in renal tissue. However, only the effects of ET-1 on the kidney have been clearly elucidated. ET-1 is the most potent vasoconstrictor known. Infusion of ET-1 into the kidney induces profound and long-lasting vasoconstriction of the renal circulation.

The entire kidney underwent 25 minutes of ischemia 48 hours before micropuncture. Glomeruli I are nephrons not exposed to endothelin antibody; Glomeruli II are nephrons that received infusion with antibody through the inferior branch of the main renal artery. SNGFR—single nephron glomerular filtration rate; PFR—glomerular renal plasma flow rate. (*Adapted from* Kon *et al.* [39].)

A. VASODILATORS USED IN EXPERIMENTAL ACUTE RENAL FAILURE

Vasodilator	ARF Disorder	Time Given in Relation to Induction	Observed Effect
Propranolol	Ischemic	Before, during, after	↓Scr, BUN if given before, during; no effect if given after
Phenoxybenzamine	Toxic	Before, during, after	Prevented fall in RBF
Clonidine	Ischemic	After	↓Scr, BUN
Bradykinin	Ischemic	Before, during	↑RBF, GFR
Acetylcholine	Ischemic	Before, after	↑RBF; no change in GFR
Prostaglandin E_1	Ischemic	After	↑RBF; no change in GFR
Prostaglandin E_2	Ischemic, toxic	Before, during	↑GFR
Prostaglandin I_2	Ischemic	Before, during, after	↑GFR
Saralasin	Toxic, ischemic	Before	↑RBF; no change in Scr, BUN
Captopril	Toxic, ischemic	Before	↑RBF; no change in Scr, BUN
Verapamil	Ischemic, toxic	Before, during, after	↑RBF, GFR in most studies
Nifedipine	Ischemic	Before	↑GFR
Nitrendipine	Toxic	Before, during	↑GFR
Diliazem	Toxic	Before, during, after	↑GFR; ↓recovery time
Chlorpromazine	Toxic	Before	↑GFR; ↓recovery time
Atrial natriuretic peptide	Ischemic, toxic	After	↑RBF, GFR

BUN—blood urea nitrogen; GFR—glomerular filtration rate; RBF—renal blood flow; Scr–serum creatinine.

B. VASODILATORS USED TO ALTER COURSE OF CLINICAL ACUTE RENAL FAILURE

Vasodilator	ARF Disorder	Observed Effect	Remarks
Dopamine	Ischemic, toxic	Improved V, Scr if used early	Combined with furosemide
Phenoxybenzamine	Ischemic, toxic	No change in V, RBF	
Phentolamine	Ischemic, toxic	No change in V, RBF	
Prostaglandin A_1	Ischemic	No change in V, Scr	Used with dopamine
Prostaglandin E_1	Ischemic	↑RBF, no change v, C_{cr}	Used with NE
Dihydralazine	Ischemic, toxic	↑RBF, no change V, Scr	
Verapamil	Ischemic	↑C_{cr} or no effect	
Diltiazem	Transplant, toxic	↑C_{cr} or no effect	Prophylactic use
Nifedipine	Radiocontrast	No effect	
Atrial natriuretic peptide	Ischemic	↑C_{cr}	

C_{cr}—creatinine clearance; NE—norepinephrine; RBF—renal blood flow; Scr—serum creatinine; V—urine flow rate.

FIGURE 2-41

Vasodilators used in acute renal failure (ARF). **A,** Vasodilators used in experimental acute ARF. **B,** Vasodilators used to alter the course of clinical ARF. (*Adapted from* Conger [40].)

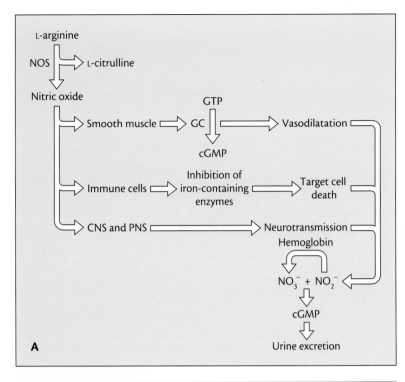

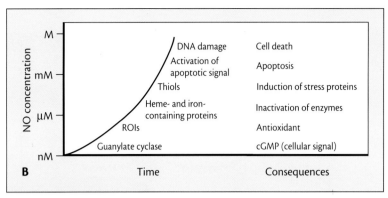

FIGURE 2-42

Major organ, and cellular, targets of nitric oxide (NO). NO has been implicated in the pathophysiology of ARF. It may have beneficial, as well as detrimental, effects. **A,** Synthesis and function of NO. **B,** Intracellular targets for NO and pathophysiologic consequences of its action. **C,** Endothelium-dependent vasodilators, such as acetylcholine and the calcium ionophore A23187, act by stimulating eNOS activity, thereby increasing endothelium-derived nitric oxide (EDNO) production. In contrast, other vasodilators act independently of the endothelium. Some endothelium-independent vasodilators such as nitroprusside and nitroglycerin induce vasodilation by directly releasing nitric oxide in vascular smooth muscle cells. NO released by these agents, like EDNO, induces vasodilation by stimulating the production of cyclic guanosine monophosphate (cGMP) in vascular smooth muscle (VSM) cells. Atrial natriuretic peptide (ANP) is also an endothelium-independent vasodilator but acts differently from NO. ANP directly stimulates an isoform of guanylyl cyclase (GC) distinct from soluble GC (called particulate GC) in VSM. CNS—central nervous system; GTP—guanosine triphosphate; NOS—nitric oxide synthase; PGC—particulate guanylyl cyclase; PNS—peripheral nervous system; ROI—reduced oxygen intermediates; SGC—soluble guanylyl cyclase. (*Adapted from* Reyes *et al.* [41] and Kim *et al.* [42].)

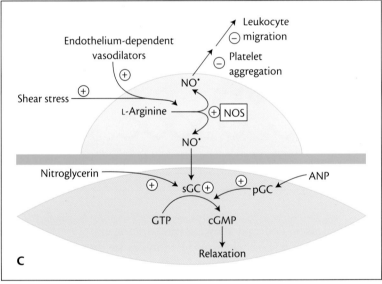

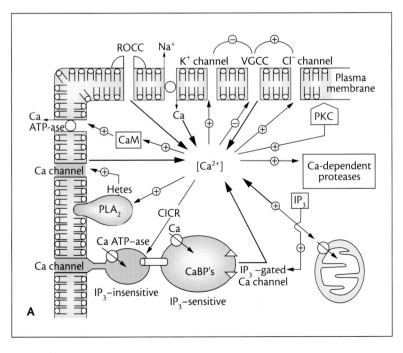

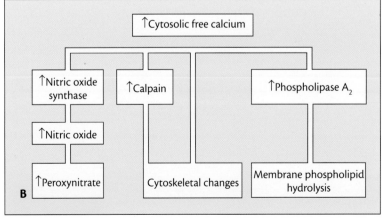

FIGURE 2-43

Cellular calcium metabolism and potential targets of the elevated cytosolic calcium. **A,** Pathways of calcium mobilization. **B,** Pathophysiologic mechanisms ignited by the elevation of cytosolic calcium concentration. (*Adapted from* Goligorsky [43] and Edelstein and Schrier [44].)

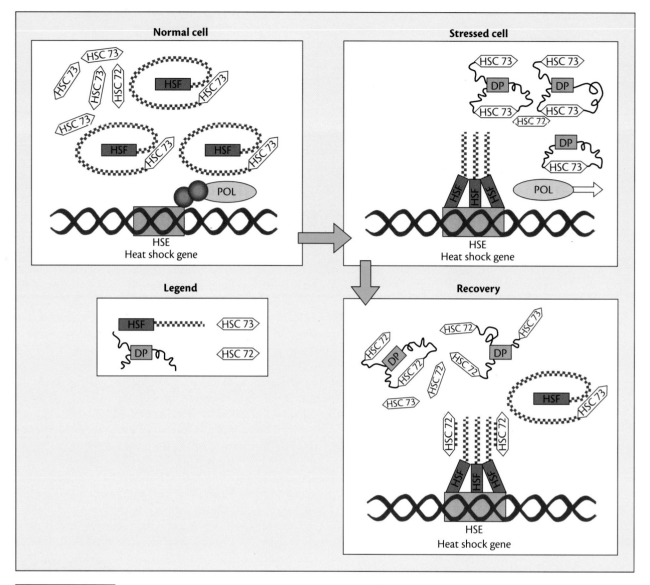

FIGURE 2-44

Dynamics of heat shock proteins (HSP) in stressed cells. Mechanisms of activation and feedback control of the inducible heat shock gene. In the normal unstressed cell, heat shock factor (HSF) is rendered inactive by association with the constitutively expressed HSP70. After hypoxia or ATP depletion, partially denatured proteins (DP) become preferentially associated with HSC73, releasing HSF and allowing trimerization and binding to the heat shock element (HSE) to initiate the transcription of the heat shock gene. After translation, excess inducible HSP (HSP72) interacts with the trimerized HSF to convert it back to its monomeric state and release it from the HSE, thus turning off the response. (*Adapted from* Kashgarian [45].)

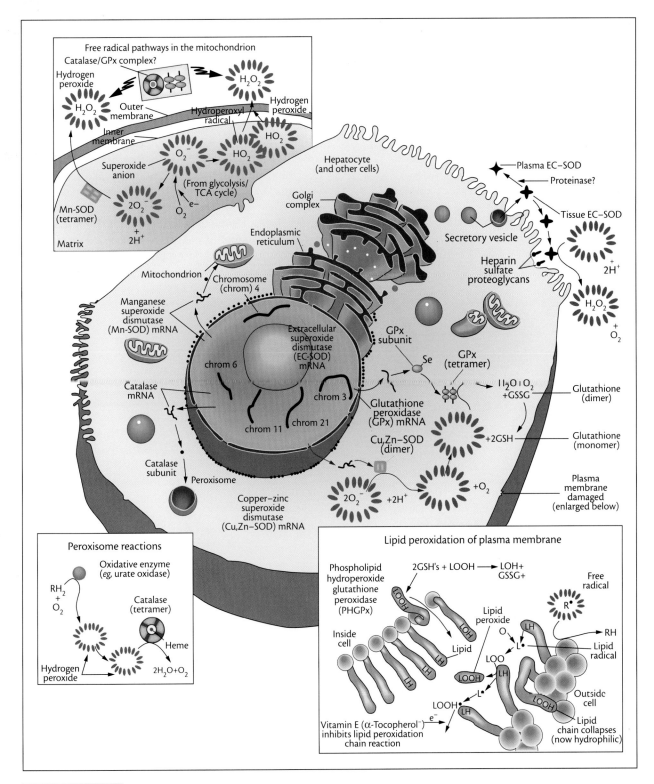

FIGURE 2-45

Cellular sources of reactive oxygen species (ROS) defense systems from free radicals. Superoxide and hydrogen peroxide are produced during normal cellular metabolism. ROS are constantly being produced by the normal cell during a number of physiologic reactions. Mitochondrial respiration is an important source of superoxide production under normal conditions and can be increased during ischemia-reflow or gentamycin-induced renal injury. A number of enzymes generate superoxide and hydrogen peroxide during their catalytic cycling. These include cycloxygenases and lipoxygenes that catalyze prostanoid and leukotriene synthesis. Some cells (such as leukocytes, endothelial cells, and vascular smooth muscle cells) have NADH or NADPH oxidase enzymes in the plasma membrane that are capable of generating superoxide. Xanthine oxidase, which converts hypoxathine to xanthine, has been implicated as an important source of ROS after ischemia-reperfusion injury. Cytochrome p450, which is bound to the membrane of the endoplasmic reticulum, can be increased by the presence of high concentrations of metabolites that are oxidized by this cytochrome or by injurious events that uncouple the activity of the p450. Finally, the oxidation of small molecules including free heme, thiols, hydroquinines, catecholamines, flavins, and tetrahydropterins also contribute to intracellular superoxide production.

EVIDENCE SUGGESTING A ROLE FOR REACTIVE OXYGEN METABOLITES IN ISCHEMIC ACUTE RENAL FAILURE

Enhanced generation of reactive oxygen metabolites and xanthine oxidase and increased conversion of xanthine dehydrogenase to oxidase occur in in vitro and in vivo models of injury.

Lipid peroxidation occurs in in vitro and in vivo models of injury, and this can be prevented by scavengers of reactive oxygen metabolites, xanthine oxidase inhibitors, or iron chelators.

Glutathione redox ratio, a parameter of "oxidant stress," decreases during ischemia and markedly increases on reperfusion.

Scavengers of reative oxygen metabolites, antioxidants, xanthine oxidase inhibitors, and iron chelators protect against injury.

A diet deficient in selenium and vitamin E increases susceptibility to injury.

Inhibition of catalase exacerbates injury, and transgenic mice with increased superoxide dismutase activity are less susceptible to injury.

FIGURE 2-46

Evidence suggesting a role for reactive oxygen metabolites in acute renal failure. The increased ROS production results from two major sources: the conversion of hypoxanthine to xanthine by xanthine dehydrogenase and the oxidation of NADH by NADH oxidase(s). During the period of ischemia, oxygen deprivation results in the massive dephosphorylation of adenine nucleotides to hypoxanthine. Normally, hypoxanthine is metabolized by xanthine dehydrogenase, which uses NAD^+ rather than oxygen as the acceptor of electrons and does not generate free radicals. However, during ischemia, xanthine dehydrogenase is converted to xanthine oxidase. When oxygen becomes available during reperfusion, the metabolism of hypoxanthine by xanthine oxidase generates superoxide. Conversion of NAD^+ to its reduced form, NADH, and the accumulation of NADH occurs during ischemia. During the reperfusion period, the conversion of NADH back to NAD^+ by NADH oxidase also results in a burst of superoxide production. (*Adapted from* Ueda *et al.* [46].)

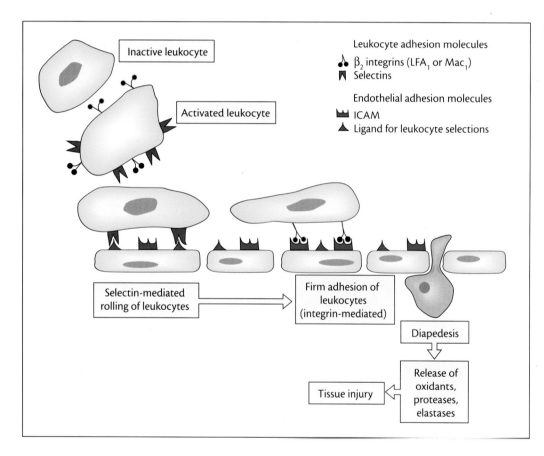

FIGURE 2-47

Role of adhesion molecules in mediating leukocyte attachment to endothelium. **A,** The normal inflammatory response is mediated by the release of cytokines that induce leukocyte chemotaxis and activation. The initial interaction of leukocytes with endothelium is mediated by the selectins and their ligands, both of which are present on leukocytes and endothelial cells.

FIGURE 2-48

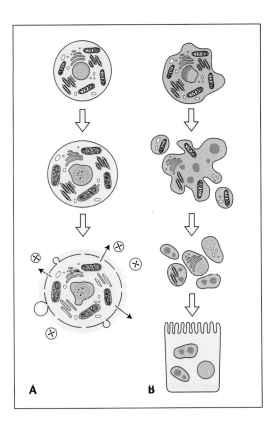

Apoptosis and necrosis: two distinct morphologic forms of cell death. **A,** Necrosis. Cells undergoing necrosis become swollen and enlarged. The mitochondria become markedly abnormal. The main morphoplogic features of mitochondrial injury include swelling and flattening of the folds of the inner mitochondrial membrane (the christae). The cell plasma membrane loses its integrity and allows the escape of cytosolic contents including lyzosomal proteases that cause injury and inflammation of the surrounding tissues. **B,** Apoptosis. In contrast to necrosis, apoptosis is associated with a progressive decrease in cell size and maintenance of a functionally and structurally intact plasma membrane. The decrease in cell size is due to both a loss of cytosolic volume and a decrease in the size of the nucleus. The most characteristic and specific morphologic feature of apoptosis is condensation of nuclear chromatin. Initially the chromatin condenses against the nuclear membrane. Then the nuclear membrane disappears, and the condensed chromatin fragments into many pieces. The plasma membrane undergoes a process of "budding," which progresses to fragmentation of the cell itself. Multiple plasma membrane–bound fragments of condensed DNA called apoptotic bodies are formed as a result of cell fragmentation. The apoptotic cells and apoptotic bodies are rapidly phagocytosed by neighboring epithelial cells as well as professional phagocytes such as macrophages. The rapid phagocytosis of apoptotic bodies with intact plasma membranes ensures that apoptosis does not cause any surrounding inflammatory reaction.

FIGURE 2-49

Hypothetical schema of cellular events triggering apoptotic cell death. (*Adapted from* Kroemer *et al.* [47].)

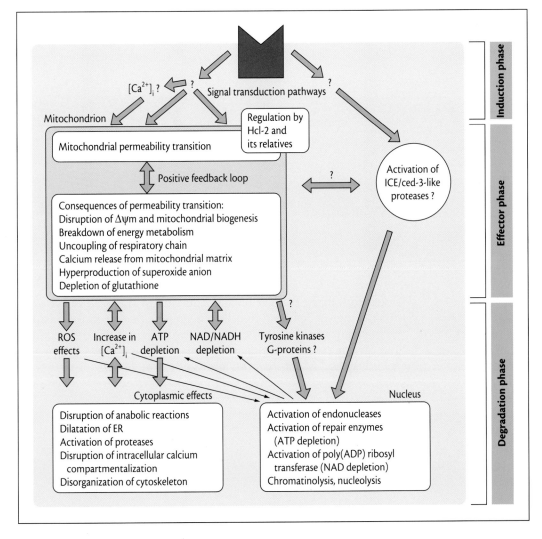

Pathophysiology of Nephrotoxic Acute Renal Failure _____

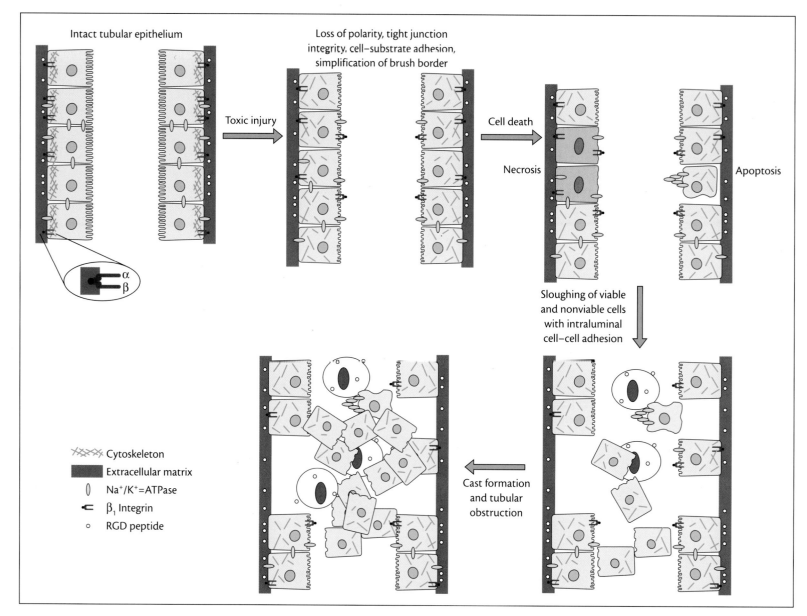

Intact tubular epithelium

Toxic injury

Loss of polarity, tight junction integrity, cell–substrate adhesion, simplification of brush border

Cell death

Necrosis

Apoptosis

Sloughing of viable and nonviable cells with intraluminal cell–cell adhesion

Cast formation and tubular obstruction

α
β

XXXX Cytoskeleton

Extracellular matrix

Na⁺/K⁺=ATPase

β₁ Integrin

RGD peptide

FIGURE 2-50

After injury, alterations can occur in the cytoskeleton and in the normal distribution of membrane proteins such as Na+, K+-ATPase and β_1 integrins in sublethally injured renal tubular cells. These changes result in loss of cell polarity, tight junction integrity, and cell–substrate adhesion. Lethally injured cells undergo oncosis or apoptosis, and both dead and viable cells may be sloughed into the tubular lumen. Adhesion of sloughed cells to other sloughed cells and to cells remaining adherent to the basement membrane may result in cast formation, tubular obstruction, and further compromise the glomerular filtration rate. (*Adapted from* Fish and Molitoris [48], and Gailit *et al.* [49].)

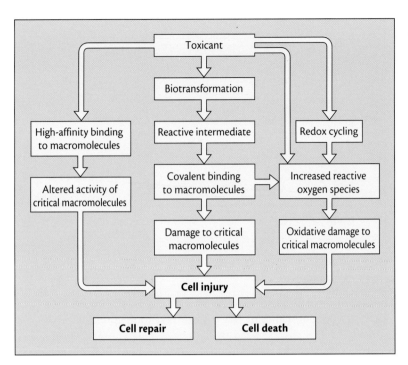

FIGURE 2-51

Covalent and noncovalent binding versus oxidative stress mechanisms of cell injury. Nephrotoxicants are generally thought to produce cell injury and death through one of two mechanisms, either alone or in combination. In some cases the toxicant may have a high affinity for a specific macromolecule or class of macromolecules that results in altered activity (increase or decrease) of these molecules, resulting in cell injury. Alternatively, the parent nephrotoxicant may not be toxic until it is biotransformed into a reactive intermediate that binds covalently to macromolecules and in turn alters their activity, resulting in cell injury. Finally, the toxicant may increase reactive oxygen species in the cells directly, after being biotransformed into a reactive intermediate or through redox cycling. The resulting increase in reactive oxygen species results in oxidative damage and cell injury.

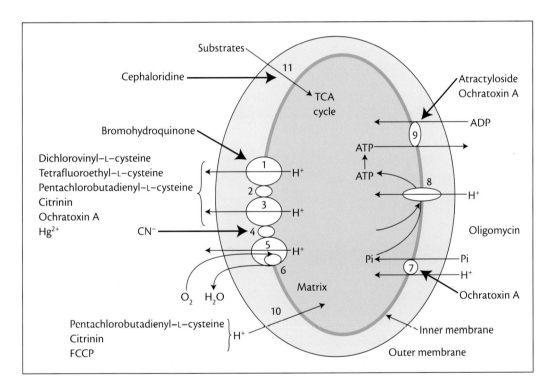

FIGURE 2-52

Some of the mitochondrial targets of nephrotoxicants: 1) nicotinamide adenine dinucleotide (NADH) dehydrogenase; 2) succinate dehydrogenase; 3) coenzyme Q–cytochrome C reductase; 4) cytochrome C; 5) cytochrome C oxidase; 6) cytochrome Aa_3; 7) H^+-Pi contransporter; 8) F_0F_1-ATPase; 9) adenine triphosphate/diphosphate (ATP/ADP) translocase; 10) protonophore (uncoupler); 11) substrate transporters.

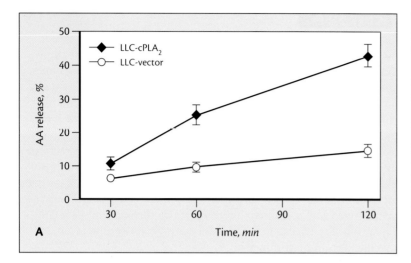

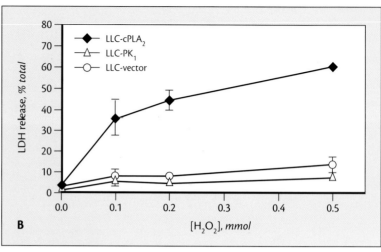

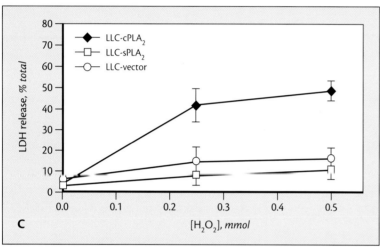

FIGURE 2-53

The importance of the cytosolic phospholipase A_2 in oxidant injury. **A,** Time-dependent release of arachidonic acid (AA) from LLC-PK_1 cells exposed to hydrogen peroxide (0.5 mM). **B** and **C,** The concentration-dependent effects of hydrogen peroxide on LLC-PK_1 cell death (using lactate dehydrogenase [LDH] release as marker) after 3 hours' exposure. Cells were transfected with 1) the cytosolic PLA_2 (LLC-$cPLA_2$), 2) the secretory PLA_2 (LLC-$sPLA_2$), 3) vector (LLC-vector), or 4) were not transfected (LLC-PK_1). Cells transfected with cytosolic PLA_2 exhibited greater AA release and cell death in response to oxidant exposure than cells transfected with the vector or secretory PLA_2 or not transfected. These results suggest that activation of cytosolic PLA_2 during oxidant injury contributes to cell injury and death. (*Adapted from* Sapirstein *et al.* [50].)

Cellular Features of Injury and Repair

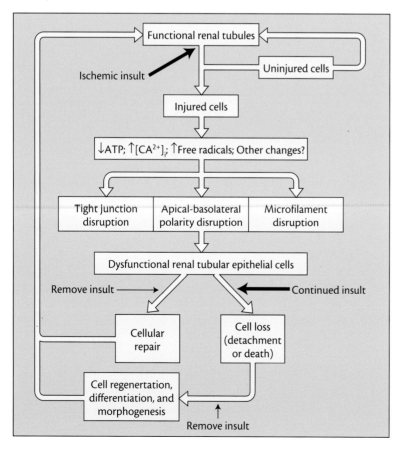

FIGURE 2-54

Ischemic acute renal failure (ARF). This flow chart illustrates the cellular basis of ischemic ARF. Renal tubule epithelial cells undergo a variety of biochemical and structural changes in response to ischemic insult. If the duration of the insult is sufficiently short, these alterations are readily reversible, but if the insult continues it ultimately leads to cell detachment and/or cell death. Interestingly, unlike other organs in which ischemic injury often leads to permanent cell loss, a kidney severely damaged by ischemia can regenerate and replace lost epithelial cells to restore renal tubular function virtually completely, although it remains unclear how this happens.

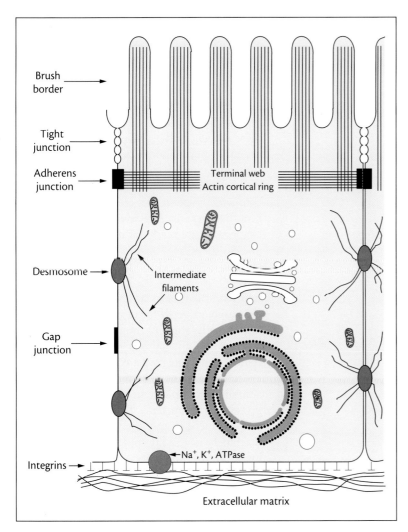

Brush border

Tight junction

Adherens junction

Terminal web
Actin cortical ring

Desmosome

Intermediate filaments

Gap junction

Na⁺, K⁺, ATPase

Integrins

Extracellular matrix

FIGURE 2-55

Typical renal epithelial cell. Diagram of a typical renal epithelial cell. Sublethal injury to polarized epithelial cells leads to multiple lesions, including loss of the permeability barrier and apical-basolateral polarity [51–56]. To recover, cells must reestablish intercellular junctions and repolarize to form distinct apical and basolateral domains characteristic of functional renal epithelial cells. These junctions include those necessary for maintaining the permeability barrier (*ie*, tight junctions), maintaining cell-cell contact (*ie*, adherens junctions and desmosomes), and those involved in cell-cell communication (*ie*, gap junctions). In addition, the cell must establish and maintain contact with the basement membrane through its integrin receptors. Thus, to understand how kidney cells recover from sublethal ischemic injury, it is necessary to understand how renal epithelial cells form these junctions. Furthermore, after lethal injury to tubule cells, new cells may have to replace those lost during the ischemic insult, and these new cells must differentiate into epithelial cells to restore proper function to the tubules.

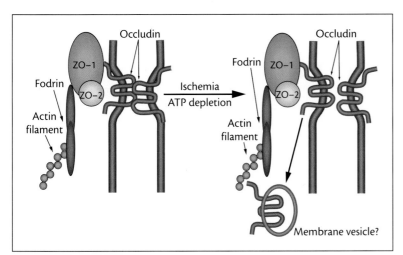

Occludin

ZO-1

Fodrin

ZO-2

Actin filament

Ischemia
ATP depletion

Occludin

Fodrin   ZO-1

ZO-2

Actin filament

Membrane vesicle?

FIGURE 2-56

Depletion of ATP causes disruption of tight junctions. This diagram shows the changes induced in tight junction structure by ATP depletion. ATP depletion causes the cytoplasmic tight junction proteins zonula occludens 1 (ZO-1) and ZO-2 to form large insoluble complexes, probably in association with the cytoskeletal protein fodrin [56], though aggregation may also be significant. Furthermore, occludin, the transmembrane protein of the tight junction, becomes localized to the cell interior, probably in membrane vesicles. These kinds of studies have begun to provide insight into the biochemical basis of tight junction disruption after ATP depletion, although how the tight junction reassembles during recovery of epithelial cells from ischemic injury remains unclear.

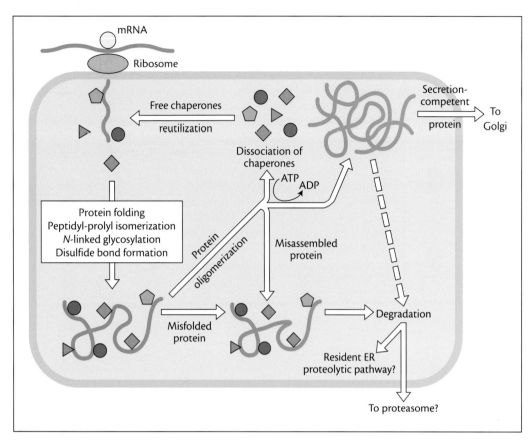

factors) proteins. The ER is the initial site of synthesis of all membrane and secreted proteins. As a protein is translocated into the lumen of the ER it begins to interact with a group of resident ER proteins called molecular chaperones [57,58–61]. Molecular chaperones bind transiently to and interact with these nascent polypeptides as they fold, assemble, and oligomerize [57,58,62]. Upon successful completion of folding or assembly, the molecular chaperones and the secretion-competent protein part company via a reaction that requires ATP hydrolysis, and the chaperones are ready for another round of protein folding [57,63–65]. If a protein is recognized as being misfolded or misassembled it is retained within the ER via stable association with the molecular chaperones and is ultimately targeted for degradation [66]. Interestingly, some of the more characteristic features of epithelial ischemia include loss of cellular functions mediated by proteins that are folded and assembled in the ER (*ie*, cell adhesion molecules, integrins, tight junctional proteins, transporters). This suggests that proper functioning of the protein-folding machinery of the ER could be critically important to the ability of epithelial cells to withstand and recover from ischemic insult. ADP—adenosine diphosphate.

FIGURE 2-57

Protein processing in the endoplasmic reticulum (ER). To recover from serious injury, cells must synthesize and assemble new membrane (tight junction proteins) and secreted (growth

Molecular Responses and Growth Factors ⎯⎯⎯⎯⎯⎯⎯⎯

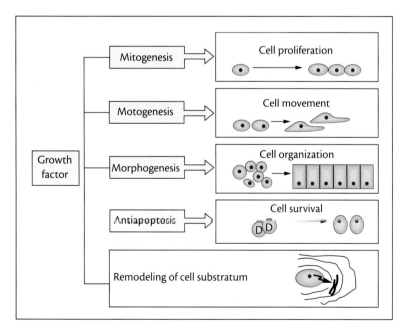

FIGURE 2-58

Cellular response to growth factors. Schematic representation of the pleiotrophic effects of growth factors, which share several properties and are believed to be important in the development and morphogenesis of organs and tissues, such as those of the kidney. Among these properties are the ability to regulate or activate numerous cellular signaling responses, including proliferation (mitogenesis), motility (motogenesis), and differentiation (morphogenesis). These characteristics allow growth factors to play critical roles in a number of complex biological functions, including embryogenesis, angiogenesis, tissue regeneration, and malignant transformation [67].

GROWTH FACTORS IN DEVELOPMENTAL AND RENAL RECOVERY

Growth Factor	Expression Following Renal Ischemia	Effect of Exogenous Administration	Branching/Tubulogenic Activity
HGF	Increased [68]	Enhanced recovery [74]	Facilatory [80,81]
EGF	Unclear [69,70]	Enhanced recovery [75,76]	Facilatory [82]
HB-EGF	Increased [71]	Undetermined	Facilatory [82]
TGF-α	Unclear	Enhanced recovery [77]	Facilatory [82]
IGF	Increased [72]	Enhanced recovery [78,79]	Facilatory [83,84]
KGF	Increased [73]	Undetermined	Undetermined
bFGF	Undetermined	Undetermined	Facilatory [83]
GDNF	Undetermined	Undetermined	Facilatory [85]
TGF-β	Increased† [69]	Undetermined	Inhibitory for branching [86]
PDGF	Increased† [69]	Undetermined	No effect [83]

*Increase in endogenous biologically active EGF probably from preformed sources; increase in EGF-receptor mRNA

†Chemoattractants for macrophages and monocytes (important source of growth promoting factors)

FIGURE 2-59

Growth factors in development and renal recovery. This table describes the roles of different growth factors in renal injury or in branching tubulogenesis. A large variety of growth factors have been tested for their ability either to mediate ureteric branching tubulogenesis or to affect recovery of kidney tubules after ischemic or other injury. Interestingly, growth factors that facilitate branching tubulogenesis in vitro also enhance the recovery of injured renal tubules.

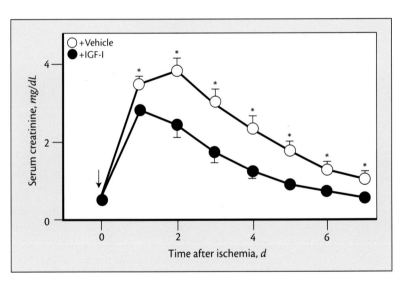

FIGURE 2-60

Serial serum creatinine values in rats with ischemic acute renal failure (ARF) treated with insulin-like growth factor (IGF-I) or vehicle. This is the original animal experiment that demonstrated a benefit from IGF-I in the setting of ARF. In this study, IGF-I was administered beginning 30 minutes after the ischemic insult (*arrow*). Data are expressed as mean ± standard error. Significant differences between groups are indicated by asterisks.

This experiment has been reproduced, with variations, by several groups, with similar findings. IGF-I has now been demonstrated to be beneficial when administered prophylactically before an ischemic injury and when started as late as 24 hours after reperfusion when injury is established. It has also been reported to improve outcomes for a variety of toxic injuries and is beneficial in a model of renal transplantation with delayed graft function and in cyclosporine-induced acute renal insufficiency. (*Adapted from* Miller *et al.* [87].)

MOLECULAR RESPONSE TO RENAL ISCHEMIC/REPERFUSION INJURY

Genes		Response Interval			References
	1 Hour	1 Day	2 Days	5 Days	
Transcription factors					
c-jun	↑	↔			Bardella *et al.* [88]
c-fos	↑	↔			Ouellette *et al.* [89]
Egr-1	↑	↔			Bonventre *et al.* [90]
Kid 1	↔	↓	↓	↓	Witzgall *et al.* [91]
Cytokines					
JE	↑	↑	↑	↑	Safirstein *et al.* [92]
KC	↑	↔			"
IL-2				↑	Goes *et al.* [93]
IL-10			↑	↑	"
IFN-γ				↑	"
GM-CSF			↑	↑	"
MIP-2	↑	↑			Singh *et al.* [94]
IL-6	↑	↑			"
IL-11	↑	↑			"
LIF	↑	↑			"
PTHrP	↑	↑	↔	↔	Soifer *et al.* [95]
Endothelin 1	↑ (6 h)	↑	↑		Firth and Ratcliffe [96]
Endothelin 3	↓ (6 h)	↓	↓		"

(Table continued on next page)

FIGURE 2-61

A list of genes whose expression is induced at various time points by ischemic renal injury. The molecular response of the kidney to an ischemic insult is complex and is the subject of investigations by several laboratories.

(*Continued on next page*)

MOLECULAR RESPONSE TO RENAL ISCHEMIC/REPERFUSION INJURY (continued)

Genes	1 Hour	1 Day	2 Days	5 Days	References
			Response Interval		
Cell cycle markers					
PCNA			↑	↑	Witzgall et al. [97]
Vimentin			↑	↑	"
Apoptosis					
Clusterin	↑	↑	↑		Witzgall et al. [97]
Bcl2	↔	↑	↑	↔	Basile et al. [98]
Bax	↔	↑	↑	↑	"
Growth factors and receptors					
IGF-I			↑	↑	Matejka et al. [99]
HGF	↑ (6 h)	↔	↔		Ishibashi et al. [100]
HGF-R (c-met)	↑ (6 h)	↔	↔		"
EGF	↓	↓	↓	↓	Safirstein et al. [101]
TGF-β1		↑	↑	↑	Basile et al. [102]
Signal transduction					
RACK1		↑	↑	↑	Padanilam et al. [103]
PKC-α		↑			La Porta and Comolli [104]
SAPK	↑	↔	↔	↔	Pombo et al. [105]
c-ros		↑			Safirstein et al. [106]
Heat shock proteins					
HSP-32 (heme oxygenase-1)		↑	↔		Raju et al. [107]
HSP-70	↑	↔			Van Why et al. [108]
HSP-72	↑	↑	↑		"
ECM Components					
Osteopontin		↑	↑	↑	Padanilam et al. [109]
Laminin		↓	↓	↑	Walker [110]
Fibronectin	↑	↑	↑	↑	"
Collagen type IV		↔	↔	↔	"
Others					
Na+-K+-ATPase	↓	↓			Van Why et al. [111]
H-K-ATPase	↑	↔			Wang et al. [112]
Na/H exchanger (NHE3)	↓	↓			"
Tamm Horsfall protein	↔	↓	↓		Safirstein et al. [101]
Annexin I (p35)			↑		McKanna et al. [112]
PLA2	↑				Nakamura et al. [114]
Calcyclin		↑	↑	↑	Lewington et al. [115]

FIGURE 2-61 (continued)

Several genes have already been identified to be induced or downregulated after ischemia and reperfusion. This table lists genes whose expression is altered as a result of ischemic injury. It is not clear at present if the varied expression of these genes plays a role in cell injury, survival, or proliferation.

Nutrition and Metabolism in Acute Renal Failure

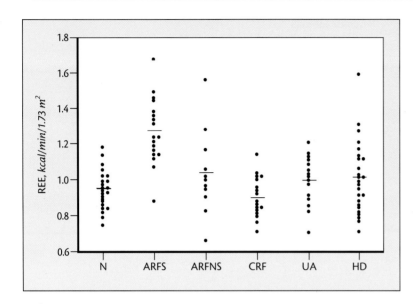

FIGURE 2-62

Energy metabolism in acute renal failure (ARF). In experimental animals ARF decreases oxygen consumption even when hypothermia and acidosis are corrected (uremic hypometabolism) [116]. In contrast, in the clinical setting oxygen consumption of patients with various form of renal failure is remarkably little changed [117]. In subjects with chronic renal failure (CRF), advanced uremia (UA), patients on regular hemodialysis therapy (HD) but also in patients with uncomplicated ARF (ARFNS) resting energy expenditure (REE) was comparable to that seen in controls (N). However, in patients with ARF and sepsis (ARFS) REE is increased by approximately 20%.

Thus, energy expenditure of patients with ARF is more determined by the underlying disease than acute uremic state. Taken together, these data indicate that when uremia is well-controlled by hemodialysis or hemofiltration, there is little if any change in energy metabolism in ARF. In contrast to many other acute disease processes, ARF might rather decrease than increase REE because in multiple organ dysfunction syndrome oxygen consumption was significantly higher in patients without impairment of renal function than in those with ARF [118]. (*Adapted from* Schneeweiss *et al.* [117].)

ESTIMATION OF ENERGY REQUIREMENTS

Calculation of resting energy expenditure (REE) (Harris Benedict equation):

Males: $66.47 \div (13.75 \times BW) \div (5 \times height) - (6.76 \times age)$

Females: $655.1 \div (9.56 \times BW) \div (1.85 \times height) - (4.67 \times age)$

The average REE is approximately 25 kcal/kg BW/day

Stress factors to correct calculated energy requirement for hypermetabolism:

Postoperative (no complications) 1.0

Long bone fracture 1.15–1.30

Cancer 1.10–1.30

Peritonitis/sepsis 1.20–1.30

Severe infection/polytrauma 1.20–1.40

Burns (= approxim. REE + % burned body surface area) 1.20–2.00

Corrected energy requirements (kcal/d) = REE × stress factor]

FIGURE 2-63

Estimation of energy requirements. Energy requirements of patients with acute renal failure (ARF) have been grossly overestimated in the past and energy intakes of more than 50 kcal/kg of body weight (BW) per day (*ie*, about 100% above resting energy expenditure (REE) have been advocated [119]. Adverse effects of overfeeding have been extensively documented during the last decades, and it should be noted that energy intake must not exceed the actual energy consumption. Energy requirements can be calculated with sufficient accuracy by standard formulas such as the Harris Benedict equation. Calculated REE should be multiplied with a stress factor to correct for hypermetabolic disease; however, even in hypercatabolic conditions such as sepsis or multiple organ dysfunction syndrome, energy requirements rarely exceed 1.3 times calculated REE [120].

CONTRIBUTING FACTORS TO PROTEIN CATABOLISM IN ACUTE RENAL FAILURE

Impairment of metabolic functions by uremia toxins
Endocrine factors
    Insulin resistance
    Increased secretion of catabolic hormones (catecholamines,
        glucagon, glucocorticoids)
    Hyperparathyroidism
    Suppression of release or resistance to growth factors
Acidosis
Systemic inflammatory response syndrome (activation of cytokine network)
Release of proteases
Inadequate supply of nutritional substrates
Loss of nutritional substrates (renal replacement therapy)

FIGURE 2-64

Protein catabolism in acute renal failure (ARF): contributing factors. The causes of hypercatabolism in ARF are complex and multifold and present a combination of nonspecific mechanisms induced by the acute disease process and underlying illness and associated complications, specific effects induced by the acute loss of renal function, and, finally, the type and intensity of renal replacement therapy.

CAUSES OF ELECTROLYTE DERANGEMENTS IN ACUTE RENAL FAILURE

Hyperkalemia	Hyperphosphatemia
Decreased renal elimination	Decreased renal elimination
Increased release during catabolism	Increased release from bone
2.38 mEq/g nitrogen	Increased release during catabolism:
0.36 mEq/g glycogen	2 mmol/g nitrogen
Decreased cellular uptake/ increased release	Decreased cellular uptake/utilization and/or increased release from cells
Metabolic acidosis: 0.6 mmol/L rise/0.1 decrease in pH	

FIGURE 2-65

Electrolytes in acute renal failure (ARF): causes of hyperkalemia and hyperphosphatemia. ARF frequently is associated with hyperkalemia and hyperphosphatemia. Causes are not only impaired renal excretion of electrolytes but release during catabolism, altered distribution in intracellular and extracellular spaces, impaired cellular uptake, and acidosis. Thus, the type of underlying disease and degree of hypercatabolism also determine the occurrence and severity of electrolyte abnormalities. Either hypophosphatemia or hyperphosphatemia can predispose to the development and maintenance of ARF [127].

A major stimulus of muscle protein catabolism in ARF is insulin resistance. In muscle, the maximal rate of insulin-stimulated protein synthesis is depressed by ARF and protein degradation is increased even in the presence of insulin [121].

Acidosis was identified as an important factor in muscle protein breakdown. Metabolic acidosis activates the catabolism of protein and oxidation of amino acids independently of azotemia, and nitrogen balance can be improved by correcting the metabolic acidosis [122]. These findings were not uniformly confirmed for ARF in animal experiments [123].

Several additional catabolic factors are operative in ARF. The secretion of catabolic hormones (catecholamines, glucagon, glucocorticoids), hyperparathyroidism which is also present in ARF (see Fig. 2-66), suppression of or decreased sensitivity to growth factors, the release of proteases from activated leukocytes—all can stimulate protein breakdown. Moreover, the release of inflammatory mediators such as tumor necrosis factor and interleukins have been shown to mediate hypercatabolism in acute disease [121,124].

The type and frequency of renal replacement therapy can also affect protein balance. Aggravation of protein catabolism, certainly, is mediated in part by the loss of nutritional substrates, but some findings suggest that, in addition, both activation of protein breakdown and inhibition of muscular protein synthesis are induced by hemodialysis [125].

Last (but not least), of major relevance for the clinical situation is the fact that inadequate nutrition contributes to the loss of lean body mass in ARF. In experimental animals, starvation potentiates the catabolic response of ARF [126].

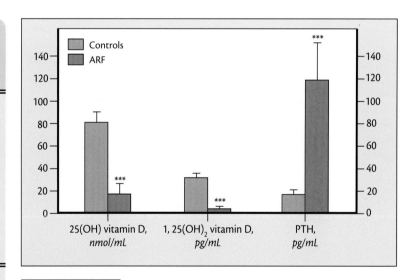

FIGURE 2-66

Hypocalcemia and the vitamin D–parathyroid hormone (PTH) axis in acute renal failure (ARF). ARF is also frequently associated with hypocalcemia secondary to hypoalbuminemia, elevated serum phosphate, plus skeletal resistance to calcemic effect of PTH and impairment of vitamin D activation. Plasma concentration of PTH is increased. Plasma concentrations of vitamin D metabolites, 25-OH vitamin D_3 and 1,25-$(OH)_2$ vitamin D_3, are decreased [128]. In ARF caused by rhabdomyolysis rebound hypercalcemia may develop during the diuretic phase. (*Adapted from* Druml *et al.* [128].)

PATIENT CLASSIFICATION AND SUBSTRATE REQUIREMENTS IN PATIENTS WITH ACUTE RENAL FAILURE

	Extent of Catabolism		
	Mild	Moderate	Severe
Excess urea appearance (above nitrogen intake)	>6 g	6–12 g	>12 g
Clinical setting (examples)	Drug toxicity	Elective surgery ± infection	Severe injury or sepsis
Mortality	20 %	60%	>80%
Dialysis or hemofiltration frequency	Rare	As needed	Frequent
Route of nutrient administration	Oral	Enteral or parenteral	Enteral or parenteral
Energy recommendations (kcal/kg BW/d)	25	25–30	25–35
Energy substrates	Glucose	Glucose + fat	Glucose + fat
Glucose (g/kg BW/d)	3.0–5.0	3.0–5.0	3.0–5.0 (max. 7.0)
Fat (g/kg BW/d)		0.5–1.0	0.8–1.5
Amino acids/protein (g/kg/d)	0.6–1.0	0.8–1.2	1.0–1.5
	EAA (+NEAA)	EAA + NEAA	EAA + NEAA
Nutrients used	Foods	Enteral formulas	Enteral formulas
		Glucose 50%–70% + fat emulsions 10% or 20%	Glucose 50%–70% + fat emulsions 10% or 20%
	EAA + specific NEAA solutions (general or "nephro")		
	Multivitamin and multitrace element preparations		

FIGURE 2-67

Patient classification: substrate requirements. Ideally, a nutritional program should be designed for each individual acute renal failure (ARF) patient. In clinical practice, it has proved useful to distinguish three groups of patients based on the extent of protein catabolism associated with the underlying disease and resulting levels of dietary requirements.

Group I includes patients without excess catabolism and a UNA of less than 6 g of nitrogen above nitrogen intake per day. ARF is usually caused by nephrotoxins (aminoglycosides, contrast media, mismatched blood transfusion). In most cases, these patients are fed orally and the prognosis for recovery of renal function and survival is excellent.

Group II consists of patients with moderate hypercatabolism and a UNA exceeding nitrogen intake 6 to 12 g of nitrogen per day. Affected patients frequently suffer from complicating infections, peritonitis, or moderate injury in association with ARF. Tube feeding or intravenous nutritional support is generally required, and dialysis or hemofiltration often becomes necessary to limit waste product accumulation.

Group III are patients who develop ARF in association with severe trauma, burns, or overwhelming infection. UNA is markedly elevated (more than 12 g of nitrogen above nitrogen intake). Treatment strategies are usually complex and include parenteral nutrition, hemodialysis or continuous hemofiltration plus blood pressure and ventilatory support. To reduce catabolism and avoid protein depletion nutrient requirements are high and dialysis is used to maintain fluid balance and blood urea nitrogen below 100 mg/dL. Mortality in this group of patients exceeds 60% to 80%, but it is not the loss of renal function that accounts for the poor prognosis; rather, the cause is superimposed hypercatabolism and the severity of the underlying illness. BW—body weight; EAA—essential amino acids; NEAA—nonessential amino acids. (*Adapted from* Druml [120].)

SPECIFIC ENTERAL FORMULAS FOR NUTRITIONAL SUPPORT OF PATIENTS WITH RENAL FAILURE

	Amin-Aid	Travasorb renal*	Salvipeptide nephro†	Survimed renal‡	Suplena§	Nepro§
Volume (mL)	750	1050	500	1000	500	500
Calories (kcal)	1467	1400	1000	1320	1000	1000
(cal/mL)	1.96	1.35	2.00	1.32	2.00	2.00
Energy distribution						
Protein:fat:carbohydrates (%)	4:21:75	7:12:81	8:22:70	6:10:84	6:43:51	14:43:43
kcal/g N	832:1	389:1	313:1	398:1	418:1	179:1
Proteins (g)	14.6	24.0	20.0	20.8	15.0	35
EAA (%)	100	60	23			
NEAA (%)	—	30	20			
Hydrolysate (%)	—	—	23	100		
Full protein (%)	—	—	34	—	100	100
Nitrogen (g)	1.76	3.6	3.2	3.32	2.4	5.6
Carbohydrates (g)	274	284	175	276	128	108
Monodisaccharides (%)	100	100	3		10	12
Oligosaccharides (%)	—	—	28			
Polysaccharides (%)	—	—	69	88		90
Fat (g)	34.6	18.6	24	15.2	48	47.8
LCT (%)		30	50		100	100
Essential GA (%)		18	31	52	22	
MCT (%)		70	50	30	0	0
Nonprotein (cal/g N)	502	363	288	374	393	154
Osmol (mOsm/kg)	1095	590	507	600	635	615
Sodium (mmol/L)	11	—	7.2	15.2	32	34.0
Potassium (mmol/L)	—	—	1.5	8	27.0	28.5
Phosphate (mmol)	—	16.1	6.13	6.4	11.0	11.0
Vitamins¶	b	a	a	a	a	a
Minerals¶	b	b	a	a	a	a

* 3 bags + 810 mL = 1050 mL

† component I + component II + 350 mL = 500 mL

‡ 4 bags + 800 mL = 1000 mL

§ Liquid formula, 8-oz cans (237.5 mL), supplemented with carnitine, taurine with a low-protein (Suplena) or moderate-protein content (Nepro)

¶ *Letter a* indicates that 2000 kcal/d meets RDA for most vitamins and trace elements; *letter b* indicates that vitamins or minerals must be added.

FIGURE 2-68

Enteral feeding formulas. There are standardized tube feeding formulas designed for subjects with normal renal function that can also be given to patients with acute renal failure (ARF). Unfortunately, the fixed composition of nutrients, including proteins and high content of electrolytes (especially potassium and phosphate) often limits their use for ARF.

Alternatively, enteral feeding formulas designed for nutritional therapy of patients with chronic renal failure (CRF) can be used. The preparations listed here may have advantages also for patients with ARF. The protein content is lower and is confined to high-quality proteins (in part as oligopeptides and free amino acids), the electrolyte concentrations are restricted. Most formulations contain recommended allowances of vitamins and minerals.

In part, these enteral formulas are made up of components that increase the flexibility in nutritional prescription and enable adaptation to individual needs. The diets can be supplemented with additional electrolytes, protein, and lipids as required. Recently, ready-to-use liquid diets have also become available for renal failure patients. EAA—essential amino acids; FA—fatty acids; LCT—long-chain triglycerides; MCT—medium-chain triglycerides; N—nitrogen; NEAA—nonessential amino acids.

Supportive Therapies

DIALYSIS MODALITIES FOR ACUTE RENAL FAILURE

Intermittent therapies	Continuous therapies
Hemodialysis (HD)	Peritoneal (CAPD, CCPD)
Single-pass	Ultrafiltration (SCUF)
Sorbent-based	Hemofiltration (CAVH, CVVH)
Peritoneal (IPD)	Hemodialysis (CAVHD, CVVHD)
Hemofiltration (IHF)	Hemodiafiltration (CAVHDF, CVVHDF)
Ultrafiltration (UF)	CVVHDF

FIGURE 2-69

Several methods of dialysis are available for renal replacement therapy. While most of these have been adapted from dialysis procedures developed for end-stage renal disease, several variations are available specifically for ARF patients [129] .

Of the intermittent procedures, intermittent hemodialysis (IHD) is currently the standard form of therapy worldwide for treatment of ARF in both intensive care unit (ICU) and non-ICU settings. The vast majority of IHD is performed using single-pass systems with moderate blood flow rates (200 to 250 mL/min) and countercurrent dialysate flow rates of 500 mL/min. Although this method is very efficient, it is also associated with hemodynamic instability resulting from the large shifts of solutes and fluid over a short time. Sorbent system IHD that regenerates small volumes of dialysate with an in-line Sorbent cartridge have not been very popular; however, they are a useful adjunct if large amounts of water are not available or in disasters [2]. These systems depend on a sorbent cartridge with multiple layers of different chemicals to regenerate the dialysate. In addition to the advantage of needing a small amount of water (6 L for a typical

run) that does not need to be pretreated, the unique characteristics of the regeneration process allow greater flexibility in custom tailoring the dialysate. In contrast to IHD, intermittent hemodiafiltration (IHF), which uses convective clearance for solute removal, has not been used extensively in the United States, mainly because of the high cost of the sterile replacement fluid [130]. Several modifications have been made in this therapy, including the provision of on-line preparation of sterile replacement solutions. Proponents of this modality claim a greater degree of hemodynamic stability and improved middle molecule clearance, which may have an impact on outcomes.

As a more continuous technique, peritoneal dialysis (PD) is an alternative for some patients. In ARF patients two forms of PD have been used. Most commonly, dialysate is infused and drained from the peritoneal cavity by gravity. More commonly a variation of the procedure for continuous ambulatory PD termed continuous equilibrated PD is utilized [131]. Dialysate is instilled and drained manually and continuously every 3 to 6 hours, and fluid removal is achieved by varying the concentration of dextrose in the solutions. Alternatively, the process can be automated with a cycling device programmed to deliver a predetermined volume of dialysate and drain the peritoneal cavity at fixed intervals. The cycler makes the process less labor intensive, but the utility of PD in treating ARF in the ICU is limited because of 1) its impact on respiratory status owing to interference with diaphragmatic excursion; 2) technical difficulty of using it in patients with abdominal sepsis or after abdominal surgery; 3) relative inefficiency in removing waste products in "catabolic" patients; and 4) a high incidence of associated peritonitis. Several continuous renal replacement therapies (CRRT) have evolved that differ only in the access utilized (arteriovenous [nonpumped: SCUF, CAVH, CAVHD, CAVHDF] versus venovenous [pumped: CVVH, CVVHD, CVVHDF]), and, in the principal method of solute clearance (convection alone [UF and H], diffusion alone [hemodialyis (HD)], and combined convection and diffusion [hemodiafiltration (HDF)]).

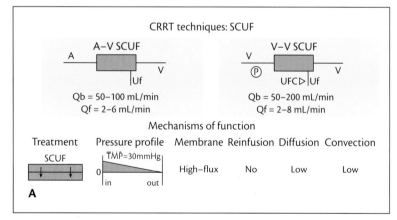

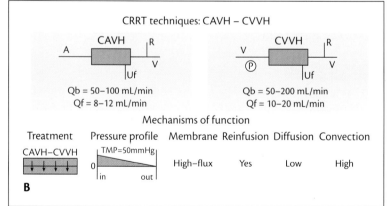

FIGURE 2-70

Schematics of different CRRT techniques. **A,** Schematic representation of SCUF therapy. **B,** Schematic representation of continuous arteriovenous or venovenous hemofiltration (CAVH/CVVH) therapy.

(*Continued on next page*)

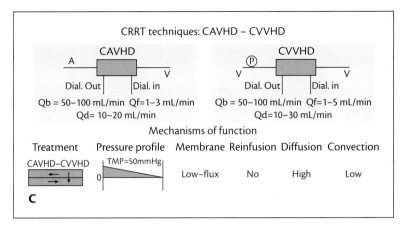

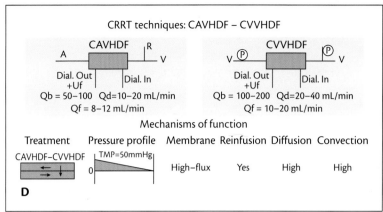

FIGURE 2-70 *(continued)*

C, Schematic representation of continuous arteriovenous/venovenous hemodialysis (CAVHD-CVVHD) therapy.
D, Schematic representation of continuous arteriovenous/venovenous hemodiafiltration (CAVHDF/CVVHDF) therapy.
A—artery; Dial—dialysate; in—dilyzer inlet; out—dialyzer outlet;
P—peristaltic pump; Qb—blood flow; Qd—dialysate flow rate; Qf—ultrafiltration rate; R—replacement fluid; TMP—transmembrane pressure; Uf—ultrafiltrate; UFC—ultrafiltration control system; V—vein. (*Adapted from* Bellomo *et al.* [132].)

CONTINUOUS RENAL REPLACEMENT THERAPY: COMPARISON OF TECHNIQUES

	SCUF	CAVH	CVVH	CAVHD	CAVHDF	CVVHD	CVVHDF	PD
Access	AV	AV	VV	AV	AV	VV	VV	Perit. Cath.
Pump	No	No	Yes	No	No	Yes	Yes	No†
Filtrate (mL/h)	100	600	1000	300	600	300	800	100
Filtrate (L/d)	2.4	14.4	24	7.2	14.4	7.2	19.2	2.4
Dialysate flow (L/h)	0	0	0	1.0	1.0	1.0	1.0	0.4
Replacement fluid (L/d)	0	12	21.6	4.8	12	4.8	16.8	0
Urea clearance (mL/min)	1.7	10	16.7	21.7	26.7	21.7	30	8.5
Simplicity*	1	2	3	2	2	3	3	2
Cost*	1	2	4	3	3	4	4	3

* 1 = most simple and least expensive; 4 = most difficult and expensive.

† Cycler can be used to automate exchanges, but they add to the cost and complexity.

FIGURE 2-71

In contrast to intermittent techniques, until recently, the terminology for continuous renal replacement therapy (CRRT) techniques has been subject to individual interpretation. Recognizing this lack of standardization an international group of experts have proposed standardized terms for these therapies [132]. The basic premise in the development of these terms is to link the nomenclature to the operational characteristics of the different techniques. In general all these techniques use highly permeable synthetic membranes and differ in the driving force for solute removal. When arteriovenous (AV) circuits are used, the mean arterial pressure provides the pumping mechanism. Alternatively, external pumps generally utilize a venovenous (VV) circuit and permit better control of blood flow rates. The letters AV or VV in the terminology serve to identify the driving force in the technique. Solute removal in these techniques is achieved by convection, diffusion, or a combination of these two. Convective techniques include ultrafiltration (UF) and hemofiltration (H) and depend on solute removal by solvent drag [133].

Diffusion-based techniques similar to intermittent hemodialysis (HD) are based on the principle of a solute gradient between the blood and the dialysate. If both diffusion and convection are used in the same technique, the process is termed hemodiafiltration (HDF). In this instance, both dialysate and a replacement solution are used, and small and middle molecules can both be removed easily. The letters UF, H, HD, and HDF identify the operational characteristics in the terminology. Based on these principles, the terminology for these techniques is easier to understand. As shown in Figure 2-69, the letter C in all the terms describes the continuous nature of the methods; the next two letters (AV or VV) depict the driving force, and the remaining letters (UF, H, HD, HDF) represent the operational characteristics. The only exception to this is the acronym SCUF (slow continuous ultrafiltration), which remains as a reminder of the initiation of these therapies as simple techniques harnessing the power of AV circuits. (*Adapted from* Mehta [134].)

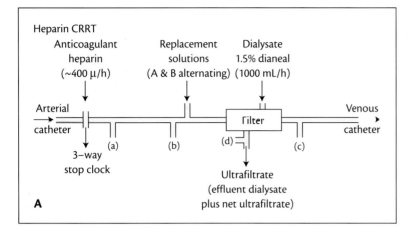

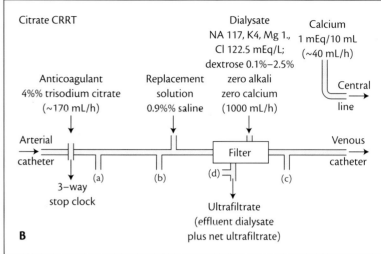

FIGURE 2-72

Modalities for anticoagulation for continuous renal replacement therapy. While systemic heparin is the anticoagulant most commonly used for dialysis, other modalities are available. The utilization of these modalities is largely influenced by prevailing local experience. Schematic diagrams for heparin (A) and citrate (B) anticoagulation techniques for continuous renal replacement therapy (CRRT). Regional citrate anticoagulation minimizes the major complication of bleeding associated with heparin, but it requires monitoring of ionized calcium. It is now well-recognized that the longevity of pumped or nonpumped CRRT circuits is influenced by

maintaining the filtration fraction at less than 20%. Nonpumped circuits (CAVH/HD/HDF) have a decrease in efficacy over time related to a decrease in blood flow (BFR), whereas in pumped circuits (CVVH/HD/HDF) blood flow is maintained; however, the constant pressure across the membrane results in a layer of protein forming over the membrane reducing its efficacy. This process is termed concentration repolarization [135]. CAVH/CVVH—continuous arteriovenous/venovenous hemofiltration. (*Adapted from* Mehta *et al.* [136].)

DETERMINANTS OF SOLUTE REMOVAL IN DIALYSIS TECHNIQUES FOR ACUTE RENAL FAILURE

	IHD	CRRT	PD
Small solutes (MW <300)	Diffusion:	Diffusion:	Diffusion:
	Q_b	Q_d	Q_d
	Membrane width	Convection:	Convection:
	Qd	Q_f	Q_f
Middle molecules (MW 500–5000)	Diffusion		
	Convection:	Convection:	Convection:
	Q_f	Q_f	Q_f
	SC	SC	SC
LMW proteins (MW 5000–50,000)	Convection	Convection	Convection
	Diffusion	Adsorption	
	Adsorption		
Large proteins (MW >50,000)	Convection	Convection	Convection

FIGURE 2-73

Determinants of solute removal in dialysis techniques for acute renal failure. Solute removal in these techniques is achieved by convection, diffusion, or a combination of these two. Convective techniques include ultrafiltration (UF) and hemofiltration (H) and they depend on solute removal by solvent drag [133]. As solute removal is solely dependent on convective clearance it can be enhanced only by increasing the volume of ultrafiltrate produced. While ultrafiltration requires fluid removal only, to prevent significant volume loss and resulting hemodynamic compromise, hemofiltration necessitates partial or total replacement of the fluid removed. Larger molecules are removed more efficiently by this process and, thus, middle molecular clearances are superior. In intermittent hemodialysis (IHD) ultrafiltration is achieved by modifying the transmembrane pressure and generally does not contribute significantly to solute removal. In peritoneal dialysis (PD) the UF depends on the osmotic gradient achieved by the concentration of dextrose solution (1.55% to 4.25%) uti-

lized the number of exchanges and the dwell time of each exchange. In continuous arteriovenous and venovenous hemodialysis in most situations ulrafiltration rates of 1 to 3 L/hour are utilized; however, recently high-volume hemofiltration with 6 L of ultrafiltrate produced every hour has been utilized to remove middle– and large–molecular weight cytokines in sepsis [137]. Fluid balance is achieved by replacing the ultrafiltrate removed by a replacement solution. The composition of the replacement fluid can be varied and the solution can be infused before or after the filter.

Diffusion-based techniques (hemodialysis) are based on the principle of a solute gradient between the blood and the dialysate. In IHD, typically dialysate flow rates far exceed blood flow rates (200 to 400 mL/min, dialysate flow rates 500 to 800 mL/min) and dialysate flow is single pass. However, unlike IHD, the dialysate flow rates are significantly slower than the blood flow rates (typically, rates are 100 to 200 mL/min, dialysate flow rates are 1 to 2 L/h [17 to 34mL/min]), resulting in complete saturation of the dialysate. As a consequence, dialysate flow rates become the limiting factor for solute removal and provide an opportunity for clearance enhancement. Small molecules are preferentially removed by these methods. If both diffusion and convection are used in the same technique (hemodiafiltration, HDF) both dialysate and a replacement solution are used and small and middle molecules can both be easily removed.

RELATIVE ADVANTAGES AND DISADVANTAGES OF CRRT, IHD, AND PD

Variable	CRRT	IHD	PD
Continuous renal replacement	+	−	+
Hemodynamic stability	+	−	+
Fluid balance achievement	+	−	−
Unlimited nutrition	+	−	−
Superior metabolic control	+	−	−
Continuous removal of toxins	+	−	+
Simple to perform	±	−	+
Stable intracranial pressure	+	−	+
Rapid removal of poisons	−	+	−
Limited anticoagulation	−	+	+
Need for intensive care nursing support	+	−	+
Need for hemodialysis nursing support	±	+	+
Patient mobility	−	+	−

FIGURE 2-74

Advantages (*plus sign*) and disadvantages (*minus sign*) of dialysis techniques. CRRT—continuous renal replacement therapy; IHD—intermittent hemodialysis; PD—peritoneal dialysis.

MORTALITY IN ACUTE RENAL FAILURE: COMPARISON OF CRRT VERSUS IHD

Investigator	Type of Study	IHD No	IHD Mortality, %	CRRT No	CRRT Mortality, %	Change, %	P Value
Mauritz et al. [144]	Retrospective	31	90	27	70	−20	NS
Alarabi et al. [145]	Retrospective	40	55	40	45	−10	NS
McDonald and Mehta [146]	Retrospective	24	85	18	72	−13	NS
Kierdorf [147]	Retrospective	73	93	73	77	−16	< 0.05
Bellomo et al. [148]	Retrospective	167	70	84	59	−11	NS
Bellomo and Boyce [149]	Retrospective	84	70	76	45	−25	< 0.01
Kruczynski et al. [150]	Retrospective	23	82	12	33	−49	< 0.01
Simpson and Allison [151]	Prospective	58	82	65	70	−12	NS
Kierdorf [152]	Prospective	47	65	48	60	−4.5	NS
Mehta et al. [153]	Prospective	82	41.5	84	59.5	+18	NS

FIGURE 2-75

Continuous renal replacement therapy (CRRT) versus intermittent hemodialysis (IHD): effect on mortality. Despite significant advances in the management of acute renal failure (ARF) over the last four decades, the perception is that the associated mortality has not changed significantly [138]. Recent publications suggest that there may have been some improvement during the last decade [139]. Both IHD and peritoneal dialysis (PD) were the major therapies until a decade ago, and they improved the outcome from the 100% mortality of ARF to its current level. The effect of continuous renal replacement therapy on overall patient outcome is still unclear [140]. The major studies done in this area do not show a survival advantage for CRRT [141,142]. Although several investigators have not been able to demonstrate an advantage of these therapies in influencing mortality, we believe this may represent the difficulty in changing a global outcome that is impacted by several other factors [143]. It is probably more relevant to focus on other outcomes such as renal functional recovery rather than mortality. We believe that continued research is required in this area; however, there appears to be enough evidence to support the use of CRRT techniques as an alternative that may be preferable to IHD in treating ARF in an intensive care setting. NS–not significant.

References

1. Liaño F, Pascual J the Madrid ARF Study Group: Epidemiology of acute renal failure: A prospective, multicenter, community-based study. *Kidney Int* 1996, 50:811–818.

2. McGregor E, Brown I, Campbell H, *et al*.: Acute renal failure. A prospective study on incidence and outcome (Abstract). XXIX Congress of EDTA-ERA, Paris, 1992, p 54.

3. Lunding M, Steiness I, Thaysen JH: Acute renal failure due to tubular necrosis. Immediate prognosis and complications. *Acta Med Scand* 1964, 176:103–119.

4. Kierdorf H, Sieberth HG: Continuous treatment modalities in acute renal failure. *Nephrol Dial Transplant* 1995; 10:2001–2008.

5. Knaus WA, Draper EA, Wagner DP, Zimmerman JE: APACHE II: A severity of disease classification system. *Crit Care Med* 1985, 13:818–829.

6. Knaus WA, Wagner DP, Draper EA, *et al*.: The APACHE III prognostic system: Risk prediction of hospital mortality for critically ill hospitalized adults. *Chest* 1991, 100:1619–1636.

7. Le Gall JR, Loirat P, Alperovitch A, *et al*.: A simplified acute physiology score for ICU patients. *Crit Care Med* 1984, 12:975–977.

8. Le Gall, Lemeshow S, Saulnier F: A new Simplified Acute Phisiology Score (SAPS II) based on a European/North American multicenter study. *JAMA* 1993, 270:2957–2963.

9. Lemeshow S, Teres D, Pastides H, *et al*.: A method for predicting survival and mortality of ICU patients using objectively derived weights. *Crit Care Med* 1985, 13:519–525.

10. Lemeshow S, Teres D, Klar J, *et al*.: Mortality probability models (MPM II) based on an international cohort of intensive care unit patients. *JAMA* 1993, 270:2478–2486.

11. Knaus WA, Draper EA, Wagner DP, Zimmerman JE: Prognosis in acute organ-system failure. *Ann Surg* 1985, 202:685–693.

12. Marshall JC, Cook DJ, Christou NV, *et al*.: Multiple organ dysfunction score: A reliable descriptor of a complex clinical outcome. *Crit Care Med* 1995, 23:1638–1652.

13. Vincent JL, Moreno R, Takala J, *et al*.: The SOFA (sepsis-related organ failure assessment) score to describe organ dysfunction/failure. *Intensive Care Med* 1996, 22:707–710.

14. Liaño F, Pascual J: Acute renal failure, critical illness and the artificial kidney: Can we predict outcome? *Blood Purif* 1997, 15:346–353.

15. Douma CE, Redekop WK, Van der Meulen JHP, *et al*.: Predicting mortality in intensive care patients with acute renal failure treated with dialysis. *J Am Soc Nephrol* 1997, 8:111–117.

16. Brivet FG, Kleinknecht DJ, Loirat P, *et al*.: Acute renal failure in intensive care units—causes, outcome and prognostic factors of hospital mortality: A prospective, multicenter study. *Crit Care Med* 1995, 24:192–197.

17. Bonomini V, Stefoni S, Vangelista A: Long-term patient and renal prognosis in acute renal failure. *Nephron* 1984, 36:169–172.

18. Nadasdy T, Racusen LC: Renal injury caused by therapeutic and diagnostic agents, and abuse of analgesics and narcotics. In *Heptinstalls Pathology of the Kidney*, edn. 5. Edited by Jennette JC, JL Olson, MM Schwartz, FG Silva. New York:Lippincott-Raven, 1998.

19. Racusen LC, Fivush BA, Li Y-L, *et al*.: Dissociation of tubular detachment and tubular cell death in clinical and experimental "acute tubular necrosis." *Lab Invest* 1991, 64:546–556.

20. Racusen LC: Pathology of acute renal failure: Structure/function correlations. *Advances in Renal Replacement Therapy*, 1997 4(Suppl. 2): 3–16.

21. Solez K, Racusen LC, Marcussen N, *et al*.: Morphology of ischemic acute renal failure, normal function, and cyclosporine toxicity in cyclosporine-treated renal allograft recipients. *Kidney Int* 1993, 43(5):1058–1067.

22. Thadhani R, Pascual M, Bonventre JV: Acute renal failure. *N Engl J Med* 1996, 334:1448–1460.

23. De Broe ME, Paulus GJ, Verpooten GA, *et al*.: Early effects of gentamicin, tobramycin, and amikacin on the human kidney. *Kidney Int* 1984, 25:643–652.

24. Moore RD, Smith CR, Lipsky JJ, *et al*.: Risk factors for nephrotoxicity in patients treated with aminoglycosides. *Ann Intern Med* 1984, 100:352–357.

25. Zager RA: A focus of tissue necrosis increases renal susceptibility to gentamicin administration. *Kidney Int* 1988; 33:84–90.

26. Andreoli TE: On the anatomy of amphotericin B-cholesterol pores in lipid bilayer membranes. *Kidney Int* 1973, 4:337–45.

27. Hricik DE, Browning PJ, Kopelman R, *et al*.: Captopril-induced functional renal insufficiency in patients with bilateral renal artery stenosis or renal artery stenosis in a solitary kidney. *N Engl J Med* 1983, 308:373–376.

28. Textor SC: ACE inhibitors in renovascular hypertension. *Cardiovasc Drugs Ther* 1990; 4:229–235.

29. de Jong PE, Woods LL: Renal injury from angiotensin I converting enzyme inhibitors. In *Clinical nephrotoxins—renal injury from drugs and chemicals*. Edited by De Broe ME, Porter GA, Bennett WM, Verpooten GA. Dordrecht: Kluwer Academic, 1998:239–250.

30. Smith WR, Neil J, Cusham WC, Butkus DE: Captopril associated acute interstitial nephritis. *Am J Nephrol* 1989, 9:230–235.

31. Opie LH: *Angiotensin-converting enzyme inhibitors*. New York: Willy-Liss, 1992; 3.

32. Whelton A, Watson J: Nonsteroidal anti-inflammatory drugs: effects on kidney function. In *Clinical Nephrotoxins—Renal Injury From drugs and Chemicals*. Edited by De Broe ME, Porter GA, Bennett WM, Verpooten GA. Dordrecht: Kluwer Academic, 1998:203–216.

33. Heyman SN, Rosen S, Brezis M: Radiocontrast nephropathy: a paradigm for the synergism between toxic and hypoxic insults in the kidney. *Exp Nephrol* 1994, 2:153.

34. Porter GA, Kremer D: Contrast associated nephropathy: presentation, pathophysiology and management. In *Clinical nephrotoxins—Renal Injury From Drugs and Chemicals*. Edited by De Broe ME, Porter GA, Bennett WM, Verpooten GA. Dordrecht: Kluwer Academic, 1998:317–331.

35. Davenport A: Differentiation of acute from chronic renal impairment by detection of carbamylated hemoglobin. *Lancet* 1993, 341:1614–1616.

36. Nolan CR, Anger MS, Kelleher SP: Eosinophiluria —a new method of detection and definition of the clinical spectrum. *N Engl J Med* 1986, 315:1516–1519.

37. Wilson DM, Salager TL, Farkouh ME: Eosinophiluria in atheroembolic renal disease. *Am J Med* 1991, 91:186–191.

38. Anderson RJ, Schrier RW: Acute renal failure. In *Diseases of the Kidney*. Edited by Schrier RW, Gottschalk CW. Boston: Little, Brown; 1997:1069–1113.

39. Kon V, *et al*.: Glomerular actions of endothelin in vivo. *J Clin Invest* 1989, 83:1762–1767.

40. Conger J: NO in acute renal failure. In: *Nitric Oxide and the Kidney*. Edited by Goligorsky M, Gross S. New York: Chapman and Hall, 1997.

41. Reyes A, Karl I, Klahr S: Role of arginine in health and in renal disease. *Am J Physiol* 1994, 267:F331–F346.

42. Kim Y-M, Tseng E, Billiar TR: Role of NO and nitrogen intermediates in regulation of cell functions. In: *Nitric Oxide and the Kidney*. Edited by Goligorsky M, Gross S. New York: Chapman and Hall, 1997.

43. Goligorsky MS: Cell biology of signal transduction. In: *Hormones, autacoids, and the kidney*. Edited by Goldfarb S, Ziyadeh F. New York: Churchill Livingstone, 1991.

44. Edelstein C, Schrier RW: The role of calcium in cell injury. In: *Acute Renal Failure: New Concepts and Therapeutic Strategies*. Edited by Goligorsky MS, Stein JH. New York: Churchill Livingstone, 1995.

45. Kashgarian M: Stress proteins induced by injury to epithelial cells. In: *Acute Renal Failure: New Concepts and therapeutic strategies*. Edited by Goligorsky MS, Stein JH. New York: Churchill Livingstone, 1995.

46. Ueda N, Walker P, Shah SV: Oxidant stress in acute renal failure. In: *Acute Renal Failure: New Concepts and Therapeutic Strategies*. Edited by Goligorsky MS, Stein JH. New York: Churchill Livingstone, 1995.

47. Kroemer G, Petit P, Zamzami N, *et al.*: The biochemistry of programmed cell death. *FASEB J* 1995, 9:1277–1287.

48. Fish EM, Molitoris BA: Alterations in epithelial polarity and the pathogenesis of disease states. *N Engl J Med* 1994, 330:1580.

49. Gailit J, Colfesh D, Rabiner I, *et al.*: Redistribution and dysfunction of integrins in cultured renal epithelial cells exposed to oxidative stress. *Am J Physiol* 1993, 264:F149.

50. Sapirstein A, Spech RA, Witzgall R, Bonventre JV: Cytosolic phospholipase A$_2$ (PLA$_2$), but not secretory PLA$_2$, potentiates hydrogen peroxide cytotoxicity in kidney epithelial cells. *J Biol Chem* 1996, 271:21505.

51. Edelstein CL, Ling H, Schrier RW: The nature of renal cell injury. *Kidney Int* 1997, 51:1341–1351.

52. Fish EM, Molitoris BA: Alterations in epithelial polarity and the pathogenesis of disease states. *N Engl J Med* 1994, 330:1580–1587.

53. Mandel LJ, Bacallao R, Zampighi G: Uncoupling of the molecular 'fence' and paracellular 'gate' functions in epithelial tight junctions. *Nature* 1993, 361:552–555.

54. Goligorsky MS, Lieberthal W, Racusen L, Simon EE: Integrin receptors in renal tubular epithelium: New insights into pathophysiology of acute renal failure. *Am J Physiol* 1993, 264:F1–F8.

55. Kuznetsov G, Bush KT, Zhang PL, Nigam SK: Perturbations in maturation of secretory proteins and their association with endoplasmic reticulum chaperones in a cell culture model for epithelial ischemia. *Proc Natl Acad Sci USA* 1996, 93:8584–8589.

56. Tsukamoto T, Nigam SK: Tight junction proteins become insoluble, form large complexes and associate with fodrin in an ATP depletion model for reversible junction disassembly. *J Biol Chem* 1997, 272:16133–16139.

57. Gething M-J, Sambrook J: Protein folding in the cell. *Nature* 1992, 355:33–45.

58. Braakman I, Helenius J, Helenius A: Role of ATP and disulphide bonds during protein folding in the endoplasmic reticulum. *Nature* 1992, 356:260–262.

59. Bush KT, Hendrickson BA, Nigam SK: Induction of the FK506–binding protein, FKBP13, under conditions which misfold proteins in the endoplasmic reticulum. *Biochem J* 1994, 303:705–708.

60. Kuznetsov G, Chen LB, Nigam SK: Several endoplasmic reticulum stress proteins, including ERp72, interact with thyroglobulin during its maturation. *J Biol Chem* 1994, 269:22990–22995.

61. Nigam SK, Goldberg AL, Ho S, *et al.*: A set of ER proteins with properties of molecular chaperones includes calcium binding proteins and members of the thioredoxin superfamily. *J Biol Chem* 1994, 269:1744–1749.

62. Knittler MR, Haas IG: Interaction of BIP with newly synthesized immunoglobulin light chain molecules: cycles of sequential binding and release. *EMBO J* 1992, 11:1573–1581.

63. Pelham H: Speculations on the functions of the major heat shock and glucose regulated proteins. *Cell* 1986, 46:959–961.

64. Pelham HR: Heat shock and the sorting of luminal ER proteins. *Embo J* 1989, 8:3171–3176.

65. Ellis R, Van Der Vies S: Molecular chaperones. *Annu Rev Biochem* 1991, 60:321–347.

66. Fra A, Sitia R: The endoplasmic reticulum as a site of protein degradation. *Subcell Biochem* 1993, 21:143–168.

67. Matsumoto K, Nakamura T: Emerging multipotent aspects of hepatocyte growth factor. *J Biochem* 1996, 119:591–600.

68. Igawa T, Matsumoto K, Kanda S, *et al.*: Hepatocyte growth factor may function as a renotropic factor for regeneration in rats with acute renal injury. *Am J Physiol* 1993, 265:F61–F69.

69. Schaudies RP, Johnson JP: Increased soluble EGF after ischemia is accompanied by a decrease in membrane-associated precursors. *Am J Physiol* 1993, 264:F523–F531.

70. Salido EC, Lakshmanan J, Fisher DA, *et al.*: Expression of epidermal growth factor in the rat kidney. An immunocytochemical and in situ hybridization study. *Histochemistry* 1991, 96:65–72.

71. Homma T, Sakai M, Cheng HF, *et al.*: Induction of heparin-binding epidermal growth factor-like growth factor mRNA in rat kidney after acute injury. *J Clin Invest* 1995, 96:1018–1025.

72. Metejka GL, Jennische E: IGF-I binding and IGF-I mRNA expression in the post-ischemic regenerating rat kidney. *Kidney Int* 1992, 42:1113–1123.

73. Ichimura T, Finch PW, Zhang G, *et al.*: Induction of FGF-7 after kidney damage: a possible paracrine mechanism for tubule repair. *Am J Physiol* 1996, 271:F967–F976.

74. Kawaida K, Matsumoto K, Shimazu H, Nakamura T: Hepatocyte growth factor prevents acute renal failure and accelerates renal regeneration in mice. *Proc Natl Acad Sci USA* 1994, 91:4357–4361.

75. Humes HD, Cielski DA, Coimbra T, *et al.*: Epidermal growth factor enhances renal tubule cell regeneration and repair and accelerates the recovery of renal function in postischemic acute renal failure. *J Clin Invest* 1989, 84:1757–1761.

76. Coimbra T, Cielinski DA, Humes HD: Epidermal growth factor accelerates renal repair in mercuric chloride nephrotoxicity. *Am J Physiol* 1990, 259:F438–F443.

77. Reiss R, Cielinski DA, Humes HD: *Kidney Int* 1990, 37:1515–1521.

78. Miller SB, Martin DR, Kissane J, Hammerman MR: Insulin-like growth factor I accelerates recovery from ischemic acute tubular necrosis in the rat. *Proc Natl Acad Sci USA* 1992, 89:11876–11880.

79. Rabkin R, Sorenson A, Mortensen D, Clark R: *J Am Soc Nephrol* 1992, 3:713.

80. Montesano R, Schaller G, Orci L: Induction of epithelial tubular morphogenesis in vitro by fibroblast-derived soluable factors. *Cell* 1991, 66:697–711.

81. Santos OFP, Nigam SK: Modulation of HGF-induced tubulogenesis and branching by multiple phosphorylation mechanisms. *Dev Biol* 1993, 159:535–548.

82. Sakurai H, Tsukamoto T, Kjelsberg CA, *et al.*: EGF receptor ligands are a large fraction of in vitro branching morphogens secreted by embryonic kidney. *Am J Physiol* 1997, 273:F463–F472.

83. Sakurai H, Barros EJG, Tsukamoto T, *et al.*: An in vitro tubulogenesis system using cell lines derived from the embrionic kidney shows dependence on multiple soluble growth factors. *Proc Natl Acad Sci USA* 1997, 94:6297–6284.

84. Rogers SA, Ryan G, Hammerman MR: *Cell Biol* 113:1447–1453.

85. Vega QC, Worby CA, Lechner MS, *et al.*: Glial cell line-derived neurotrophic factor activates the receptor tyrosine kinase RET and promotes kidney morphogenesis. *Proc Natl Acad Sci USA* 1996, 93:10657–10661.

86. Sakurai H, Nigam SK: Transforming growth factor-beta selectively inhibits branching morphogenesis but not tubulogenesis. *Am J Physiol* 1997, 272:F139–F146.

87. Miller SB, Martin DR, Kissane J, Hammerman, MR: Insulin-like growth factor I accelerates recovery from ischemic acute tubular necrosis in the rat. *Proc Natl Acad Sci USA* 1992, 89:11876–11880.

88. Bardella L, Comolli R: Differential expression of c-jun, c-fos and hsp 70 mRNAs after folic acid and ischemia reperfusion injury: effect of antioxidant treatment. *Exp Nephrol* 1994, 2:158–165.

89. Ouellette AJ, *et al.*: Expression of two "immediate early" genes, Egr-1 and c-fos, in response to renal ischemia and during compensatory renal hypertrophy in mice. *J Clin Invest* 1990, 85:766–771.

90. Bonventre JV, *et al.*: Localization of the protein product of the immediate early growth response gene, Egr-1, in the kidney after ischemia and reperfusion. *Cell Regulation* 1991, 2:251–60.

91. Witzgall R, *et al.*: Kid-1, a putative renal transcription factor: regulation during ontogeny and in response to ischemia and toxic injury. *Mol Cell Biol* 1993, 13:1933–1942.

92. Safirstein R, *et al.*: Expression of cytokine-like genes JE and KC is increased during renal ischemia. *Amer J Physiol* 1991, 261:F1095–F1101.

93. Goes N, *et al.*: Ischemic acute tubular necrosis induces an extensive local cytokine response. Evidence for induction of interferon-gamma, transforming growth factor-beta 1, granulocyte-macrophage colony–stimulating factor, interleukin-2, and interleukin-10. *Transplantation* 1995, 59:565–572.

94. Singh AK, *et al.*: Prominent and sustained upregulation of MIP-2 and gp130 signaling cytokines in murine renal ischemic-reperfusion injury. *J Am Soc Nephrol* 1997, 8:595A.

95. Soifer NE, *et al.*: Expression of parathyroid hormone–related protein in the rat glomerulus and tubule during recovery from renal ischemia. *J Clin Invest* 1993, 92:2850–2857.

96. Firth JD, Ratcliffe PJ: Organ distribution of the three rat endothelin messenger RNAs and the effects of ischemia on renal gene expression. *J Clin Invest* 1992, 90:1023–1031.

97. Witzgall R, *et al.*: Localization of proliferating cell nuclear antigen, vimentin, c-Fos, and clusterin in the postischemic kidney. Evidence for a heterogeneous genetic response among nephron segments, and a large pool of mitotically active and dedifferentiated cells. *J Clin Invest* 1994, 93:2175–2188.

98. Basile DP, Liapis H, Hammerman MR: Expression of bcl-2 and bax in regenerating rat renal tubules following ischemic injury. *Am J Physiol* 1997, 272:F640–F647.

99. Matejka GL, Jennische E: IGF-I binding and IGF-1 mRNA expression in the post-ischemic regenerating rat kidney. *Kidney Int* 1992, 42(5):1113–1123.

100. Ishibashi K, *et al.*: Expressions of receptor for hepatocyte growth factor in kidney after unilateral nephrectomy and renal injury. *Biochem Biophys Res Commun* 1993, 187:1454–1459.

101. Safirstein R, *et al.*: Changes in gene expression after temporary renal ischemia. *Kidney Int* 1990, 37:1515–1521.

102. Basile DP, *et al.*: Increased transforming growth factor-beta 1 expression in regenerating rat renal tubules following ischemic injury. *Am J Physiol* 1996, 270:F500–F509.

103. Padanilam BJ, Hammerman MR: Ischemia-induced receptor for activated C kinase (RACK1) expression in rat kidneys. *Amer J Physiol* 1997, 272:F160–F166.

104. Pombo CM, *et al.*: The stress-activated protein kinases are major c-Jun amino-terminal kinases activated by ischemia and reperfusion. *J Biol Chem* 1994, 269:26546–26551.

105. Safirstein R: Gene expression in nephrotoxic and ischemic acute renal failure [editorial]. *J Am Soc Nephrol* 1994, 4:1387–1395.

106. Safirstein R, Zelent AZ, Price PM: Reduced renal prepro-epidermal growth factor mRNA and decreased EGF excretion in ARF. *Kid Int* 1989, 36:810–815.

107. Raju VS, Maines, MD: Renal ischemia/reperfusion up-regulates heme oxygenase-1 (HSP32) expression and increases cGMP in rat heart. *J Pharmacol Exp Ther* 1996, 277:1814–1822.

108. Van Why SK, *et al.*: Induction and intracellular localization of HSP-72 after renal ischemia. *Am J Physiol* 1992, 263:F769–F775.

109. Padanilam BJ, Martin DR, Hammerman MR: Insulin-like growth factor I–enhanced renal expression of osteopontin after acute ischemic injury in rats. *Endocrinology* 1996, 137:2133–2140.

110. Walker PD: Alterations in renal tubular extracellular matrix components after ischemia-reperfusion injury to the kidney. *Lab Invest* 1994, 70:339–345.

111. Van Why SK, *et al.*: Expression and molecular regulation of Na+-K+-ATPase after renal ischemia. *Am J Physiol* 1994, 267:F75–F85.

112. Wang Z, *et al.*: Ischemic-reperfusion injury in the kidney: overexpression of colonic H+-K+-ATPase and suppression of NHE-3. *Kidney Int* 1997, 51:1106–1115.

113. McKanna JA, *et al.*: Localization of p35 (annexin I, lipocortin I) in normal adult rat kidney and during recovery from ischemia. *J Cell Physiol* 1992, 153:467–76.

114. Nakamura H, *et al.*: Subcellular characteristics of phospholipase A2 activity in the rat kidney. Enhanced cytosolic, mitochondrial, and microsomal phospholipase A2 enzymatic activity after renal ischemia and reperfusion. *J Clin Invest* 1991, 87:1810–1818.

115. Lewington AJP, Padanilam BJ, Hammerman MR: Induction of calcyclin after ischemic injury to rat kidney. *Am J Physiol* 1997, 273(42):F380–F385.

116. Om P, Hohenegger M: Energy metabolism in acute uremic rats. *Nephron* 1980, 25:249–253.

117. Schneeweiss B, Graninger W, Stockenhuber F, *et al.*: Energy metabolism in acute and chronic renal failure. *Am J Clin Nutr* 1990, 52:596–601.

118. Soop M, Forsberg E, Thörne A, Alvestrand A: Energy expenditure in postoperative multiple organ failure with acute renal failure. *Clin Nephrol* 1989, 31:139–145.

119. Spreiter SC, Myers BD, Swenson RS: Protein-energy requirements in subjects with acute renal failure receiving intermittent hemodialysis. *Am J Clin Nutr* 1980, 33:1433–1437.

120. Druml W: Nutritional support in acute renal failure. In *Nutrition and the Kidney*. Edited by Mitch WE, Klahr S. Philadelphia: Lippincott-Raven, 1998.

121. Clark AS, Mitch WE: Muscle protein turnover and glucose uptake in acutely uremic rats. *J Clin Invest* 1983, 72:836–845.

122. May RC, Kelly RA, Mitch WE: Mechanisms for defects in muscle protein metabolism in rats with chronic uremia: The influence of metabolic acidosis. *J Clin Invest* 1987; 79:1099–1103.

123. Kuhlmann MK, Shahmir E, Maasarani E, *et al.*: New experimental model of acute renal failure and sepsis in rats. *JPEN* 1994, 18:477–485.

124. Druml W, Mitch WE: Metabolism in acute renal failure. *Sem Dial* 1996, 9:484–490.

125. Bergström J: Factors causing catabolism in maintenance hemodialysis patients. *Miner Electrolyte Metab* 1992, 18:280–283.

126. Mitch WE: Amino acid release from the hindquarter and urea appearance in acute uremia. *Am J Physiol* 1981, 241:E415–E419.

127. Dobyan DC, Bulger RE, Eknoyan G: The role of phosphate in the potentiation and amelioration of acute renal failure. *Miner Electrolyte Metab* 1991, 17:112–115.

128. Druml W, Schwarzenhofer M, Apsner R, Horl WH: Fat soluble vitamins in acute renal failure. *Miner Electrolyte Metab* 1998, 24:220–226.

129. Mehta RL: Therapeutic alternatives to renal replacement therapy for critically ill patients in acute renal failure. *Semin Nephrol* 1994, 14:64–82.

130. Botella J, Ghezzi P, Sanz-Moreno C, *et al.*: Multicentric study on paired filtration dialysis as a short, highly efficient dialysis technique. *Nephrol Dial Transplant* 1991, 6:715–721.

131. Steiner RW: Continuous equilibration peritoneal dialysis in acute renal failure. *Perit Dial Intensive* 1989, 9:5–7.

132. Bellomo R, Ronco C, Mehta RL: Nomenclature for continuous renal replacement therapies. *Am J Kidney Dis* 1996, 28(5)S3:2–7.

133. Henderson LW: Hemofiltration: From the origin to the new wave. *Am J Kidney Dis* 1996, 28(5)S3:100–104.

134. Mehta RL: Renal replacement therapy for acute renal failure: Matching the method to the patient. *Semin Dial* 1993, 6:253–259.

135. Ronco C, Brendolan A, Crepaldi C, *et al*.: Importance of hollow fiber geometry in CAVH. *Contrib Nephrol* 1991, 15:175–178.

136. Mehta RL, McDonald BR, Aguilar MM, Ward DM: Regional citrate anticoagulation for continuous arteriovenous hemodialysis in critically ill patients. *Kidney Int* 1990, 38:976–981.

137. Grootendorst AF, Bouman C, Hoeben K, *et al*.: The role of continuous renal replacement therapy in sepsis multiorgan failure. *Am J Kidney Dis* 1996, 28(5) S3:S50–S57.

138. Wilkins RG, Faragher EB: Acute renal failure in an intensive care unit: Incidence, prediction and outcome. *Anesthesiology* 1983, 38:638.

139. Firth JD: Renal replacement therapy on the intensive care unit. *Q J Med* 1993, 86:75–77.

140. Bosworth C, Paganini EP, Cosentino F, *et al*.: Long term experience with continuous renal replacement therapy in intensive care unit acute renal failure. *Contrib Nephrol* 1991, 93:13–16.

141. Kierdorf H: Continuous versus intermittent treatment: Clinical results in acute renal failure. *Contrib Nephrol* 1991, 93:1–12.

142. Jakob SM, Frey FJ, Uhlinger DE: Does continuous renal replacement therapy favorably influence the outcome of patients? *Nephrol Dial Transplant* 1996, 11:1250–1235.

143. Mehta RL: Acute renal failure in the intensive care unit: Which outcomes should we measure? *Am J Kidney Dis* 1996, 28(5)S3:74–79.

144. Mauritz W, Sporn P, Schindler I, *et al*.: Acute renal failure in abdominal infection: comparison of hemodialysis and continuous arteriovenous hemofiltration. *Anasth Intensivther Notfallmed* 1986, 21:212–217.

145. Alarabi AA, Danielson BG, Wikstrom B, Wahlberg J: Outcome of continuous arteriovenous hemofiltration (CAVH) in one centre. *Ups J Med Sci* 1989, 94:299–303.

146. McDonald BR, Mehta RL: Decreased mortality in patients with acute renal failure undergoing continuous arteriovenous hemodialysis. *Contrib Nephrol* 1991, 93:51–56.

147. Kierdorf H: Continuous versus intermittent treatment: clinical results in acute renal failure. *Contrib Nephrol* 1991, 93:1–12.

148. Bellomo R, Mansfield D, Rumble S, *et al*.: Acute renal failure in critical illness. Conventional dialysis versus acute continuous hemodiafiltration. *Am Soc Artif Intern Organs J* 1992, 38:654–657.

149. Bellomo R, Boyce N: Continuous venovenous hemodiafiltration compared with conventional dialysis in critically ill patients with acute renal failure. *Am Soc Artif Intern Organs J* 1993, 39:794–797.

150. Kruczynski K, Irvine-Bird K, Toffelmire EB, Morton AR: A comparison of continuous arteriovenous hemofiltration and intermittent hemodialysis in acute renal failure patients in the intensive care unit. *Am Soc Artif Intern Organs J* 1993, 39:778–781.

151. Simpson K, Allison MEM: Dialysis and acute renal failure: can mortality be improved? *Nephrol Dial Transplant* 1993, 8:946.

152. Kierdorf H: Einfuss der kontinuierlichen Hamofiltration auf Proteinkatabolismus, Mediatorsubstanzen und Prognose des akuten Nierenversagens [Habilitation-Thesis], Medical Faculty Technical University of Aachen, 1994.

153. Mehta RL, McDonald B, Pahl M, *et al*.: Continuous vs. intermittent dialysis for acute renal failure (ARF) in the ICU: Results from a randomized multicenter trial. Abstract A1044. *JASN* 1996, 7(9):1456.

Glomerulonephritis and Vasculitis

Arthur H. Cohen
Richard J. Glassock

CHAPTER

3

Normal Vascular and Glomerular Anatomy

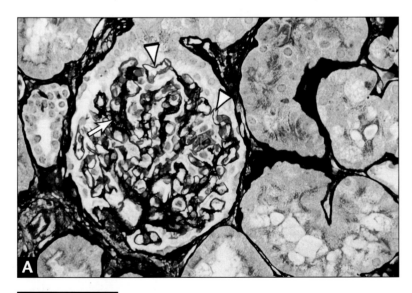
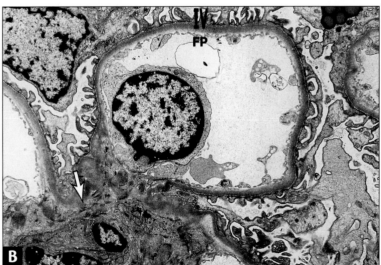

FIGURE 3-1

Microscopic view of the glomeruli. Glomeruli are spherical "bags" of capillaries emanating from afferent arterioles and confined within the urinary space, which is continuous with the proximal tubule. The capillaries are partially attached to the mesangium, a continuation of the arteriolar wall consisting of mesangial cells (**A**, *arrow*) and the matrix (**B**, *arrow*). The free wall of glomerular capillaries, across which filtration takes place, consists of a basement membrane (*arrowheads*) covered by visceral epithelial cells with individual foot processes (FP) and lined by endothelial cells.

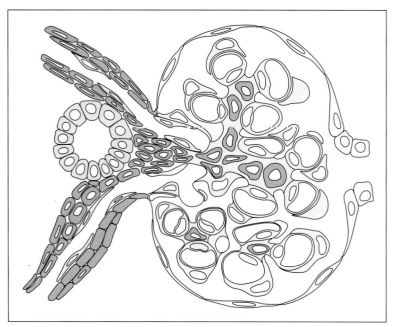

Schematic illustration of a glomerulus and adjacent hilar structure. Note the relationship of mesangial cells to the juxtaglomerular apparatus and distal tubule (macula densa).

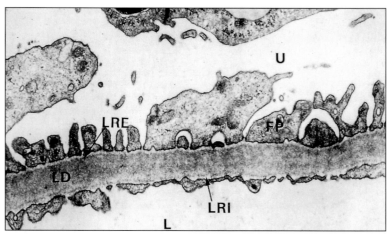

Electron photomicrograph illustrating a portion of the ultrastructure of the glomerular capillary wall. The normal width of the lamina rara externa (LRE) plus the lamina densa (LD) plus the lamina rara interna (LRI) equals about 250 to 300 nm. The spaces between the foot processes (FP), having diameters of 20 to 60 nm, are called *filtration slit pores*. It is believed they are the path by which filtered fluid reaches the urinary space (U). The endothelial cells on the luminal aspect of the basement membrane (BM) are fenestrated, having diameters from 70 to 100 nm. The BM (LRE plus LD plus LRI) is composed of type IV collagen and negativity charged proteoglycans (heparan sulfate). L—lumen. (*From* Churg *et al.* [1]; with permission.)

The Primary Glomerulopathies

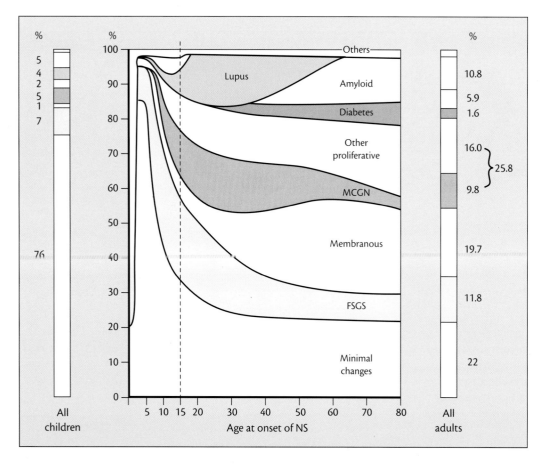

Age-associated prevalence of various glomerular lesions in nephrotic syndrome (NS). This schematic illustrates the age-associated prevalence of various diseases and glomerular lesions among children and adults undergoing renal biopsy for evaluation of nephrotic syndrome (Guy's Hospital and the International Study of Kidney Disease in Children) [2]. Both the systemic and primary causes of nephrotic syndrome are included. (Diabetes mellitus with nephropathy is underrepresented because renal biopsy is seldom needed for diagnosis.) The bar on the left summarizes the prevalence of various lesions in children aged 0 to 16 years; the bar on the right summarizes the prevalence of various lesions in adults aged 16 to 80 years. Note the high prevalence of minimal change disease in children and the increasing prevalence of membranous glomerulonephritis in the age group of 16 to 60 years. FSGS—focal segmental glomerulosclerosis; MCGN—mesangiocapillary glomerulonephritis. (*Adapted from* Cameron and Glassock [2].)

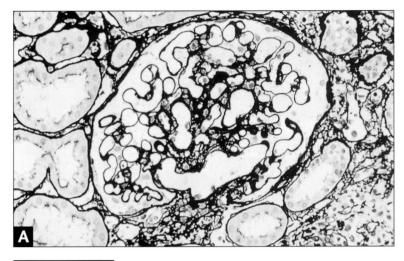

FIGURE 3-5

Light and electron microscopy in minimal change disease (lipoid nephrosis). **A,** This glomerulopathy, one of many associated with nephrotic syndrome, has a normal appearance on light microscopy. No evidence of antibody (immune) deposits is seen on immunoflu-orescence. **B,** Effacement (loss) of foot processes of visceral epithelial cells is observed on electron microscopy. This last feature is the major morphologic lesion indicative of massive proteinuria.

Minimal change disease is considered to be the result of glomerular capillary wall damage by lymphokines produced by abnormal T cells. This glomerulopathy is the most common cause of nephrotic syndrome in children (>70%) and also accounts for approximately 20% of adult patients with nephrotic syndrome. This glomerulopathy typically is a corticosteroid-responsive lesion, and usually has a benign outcome with respect to renal failure.

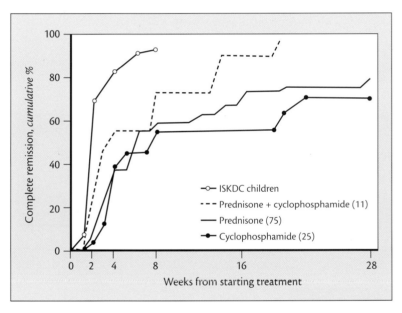

FIGURE 3-6

Therapeutic response in minimal change disease. This graph illustrates the cumulative complete response rate (absence of abnormal proteinuria) in patients of varying ages in relation to type and duration of therapy [2]. Note that most children with minimal change disease respond to treatment within 8 weeks. Adults require prolonged therapy to reach equivalent response rates. Numbers of patients are indicated in parentheses. (*Adapted from* Cameron [3].)

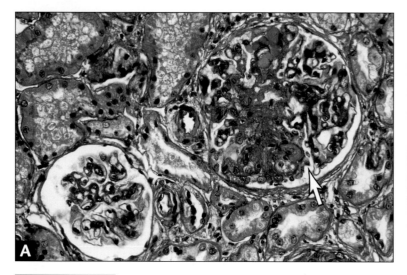
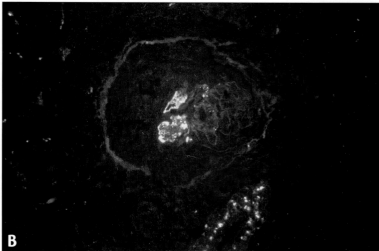

FIGURE 3-7

Light and immunofluorescent microscopy in focal segmental glomerulosclerosis (FSGS). Patients with FSGS exhibit massive proteinuria (usually nonselective), hypertension, hematuria, and renal functional impairment. Patients with nephrotic syndrome often are not responsive to corticosteroid therapy. Progression to chronic renal failure occurs over many years, although in some patients renal failure may occur in only a few years. **A,** This glomerulopathy is defined primarily by its appearance on light microscopy. Only a portion of the glomerular population, initially in the deep cortex, is affected. The abnormal glomeruli exhibit segmental obliteration of capillaries by increased extracellular matrix–basement membrane material, collapsed capillary walls, or large insudative lesions. These lesions are called hyalinosis (*arrow*) and are composed of immunoglobulin M and complement C3 (**B,** IgM immunofluorescence). The other glomeruli usually are enlarged but may be of normal size. In some patients, mesangial hypercellularity may be a feature. Focal tubular atrophy with interstitial fibrosis invariably is present.

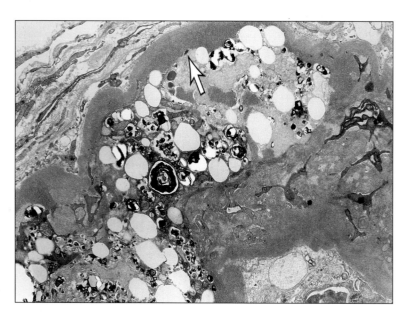

FIGURE 3-8

Electron microscopy of focal segmental glomerulosclerosis. The electron microscopic findings in the involved glomeruli mirror the light microscopic features, with capillary obliteration by dense hyaline "deposits" (*arrow*) and lipids. The other glomeruli exhibit primarily foot process effacement, occasionally in a patchy distribution.

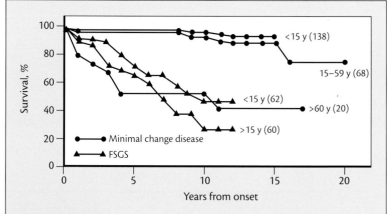

FIGURE 3-9

Evolution of focal segmental glomerulosclerosis (FSGS). This graph compares the renal functional survival rate of patients with FSGS to that seen in patients with minimal change disease (in adults and children). Note the poor prognosis, with about a 50% rate of renal survival at 10 years. (*Adapted from* Cameron [3].)

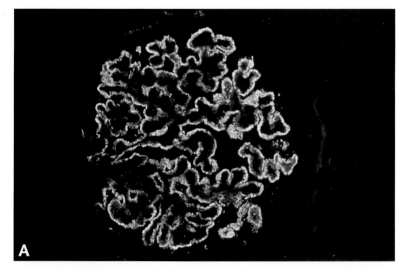

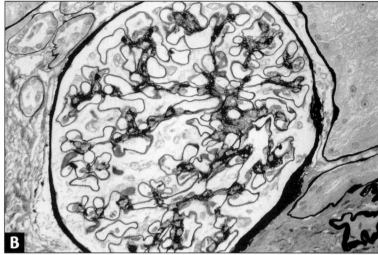

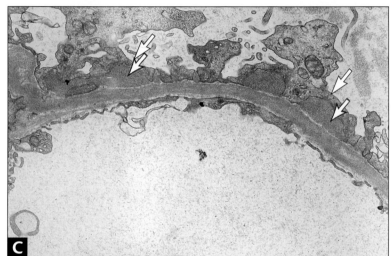

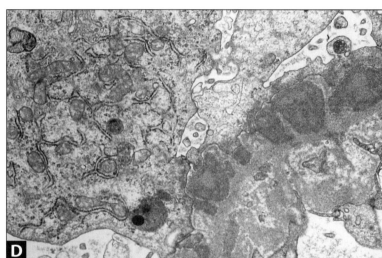

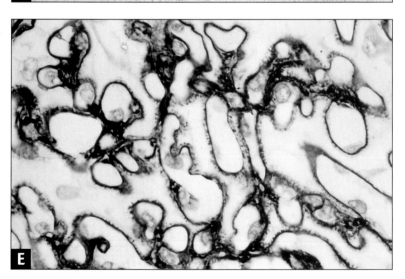

FIGURE 3-10

Light, immunofluorescent, and electron microscopy in membranous glomerulonephritis. Membranous glomerulonephritis is an immune complex–mediated glomerulonephritis, with the immune deposits localized to subepithelial aspects of almost all glomerular capillary walls. Membranous glomerulonephritis is the most common cause of nephrotic syndrome in adults in developed countries. In most instances (75%), the disease is idiopathic and the

antigen(s) of the immune complexes are unknown. In the remainder, membranous glomerulonephritis is associated with well-defined diseases that often have an immunologic basis (eg, systemic lupus erythematosus and hepatitis B or C virus infection); some solid malignancies (especially carcinomas); or drug therapy, such as gold, penicillamine, captopril, and some nonsteroidal anti-inflammatory reagents. Treatment is controversial.

The changes by light and electron microscopy mirror one another quite well and represent morphologic progression that is likely dependent on duration of the disease. **A,** At all stages immunofluorescence discloses the presence of uniform granular capillary wall deposits of immunoglobulin G and complement C3. **B,** In the early stage the deposits are small and without other capillary wall changes; hence, on light microscopy, glomeruli often are normal in appearance.

C, On electron microscopy, small electron-dense deposits (*arrows*) are observed in the subepithelial aspects of capillary walls. **D,** In the intermediate stage the deposits are partially encircled by basement membrane material. **E,** When viewed with periodic acid-methenamine stained sections, this abnormality appears as spikes of basement membrane perpendicular to the basement membrane, with adjacent nonstaining deposits. Similar features are evident on electron microscopy, with dense deposits and intervening basement membrane (**D**). Late in the disease the deposits are completely surrounded by basement membranes and are undergoing resorption.

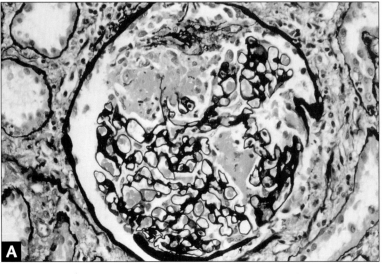
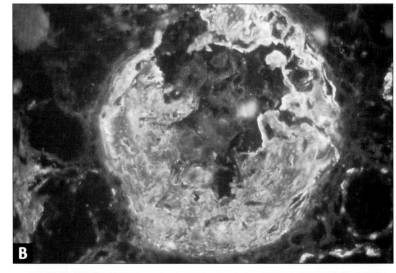
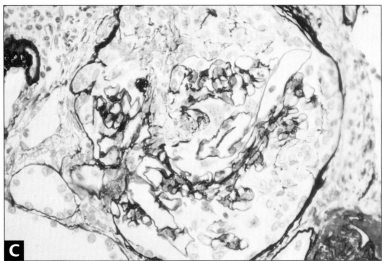
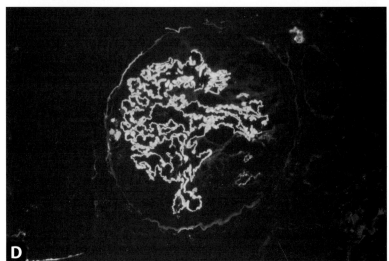

FIGURE 3-11 (*see* Color Plate)

Crescentic glomerulonephritis. A crescent is the accumulation of cells and extracellular material in the urinary space of a glomerulus. The cells are parietal and visceral epithelia as well as monocytes and other blood cells. The extracellular material is fibrin, collagen, and basement membrane material. In the early stages of the disease, the crescents consist of cells and fibrin. In the later stages the crescents undergo organization, with disappearance of fibrin and replacement by collagen. Crescents represent morphologic consequences of severe capillary wall damage. **A,** In most instances, small or large areas of destruction of capillary walls (cells and basement membranes) are observed (*arrow*), thereby allowing fibrin, other high molecular weight substances, and blood cells to pass readily from capillary lumina into the urinary space. **B,** Immunofluorescence frequently discloses fibrin in the urinary space. **C,** The proliferating cells in Bowman's space ultimately give rise to the typical crescent shape (*see* Color Plate). Whereas crescents may complicate many forms of glomerulonephritis, they are most commonly associated with either antiglomerular basement membrane (AGBM) antibodies or antineutrophil cytoplasmic

antibodies (ANCAs). The clinical manifestations are typically of rapidly progressive glomerulonephritis with moderate proteinuria, hematuria, oliguria, and uremia. The immunomorphologic features depend on the basic disease process. On light microscopy in both AGBM antibody–induced disease and ANCA–associated crescentic glomerulonephritis, the glomeruli without crescents often have a normal appearance. It is the remaining glomeruli that are involved with crescents. **D,** Anti-GBM disease is characterized by linear deposits of immunoglobulin G and often complement C3 in all capillary basement membranes, and in approximately two thirds of affected patients in tubular basement membranes (*see* Color Plate). The ANCA-associated lesion typically has little or no immune deposits on immunofluorescence; hence the term *pauci-immune crescentic glomerulonephritis* is used. By electron microscopy, as on light microscopy, defects in capillary wall continuity are easily identified. Both AGBM- and ANCA-associated crescentic glomerulonephritis can be complicated by pulmonary hemorrhage.

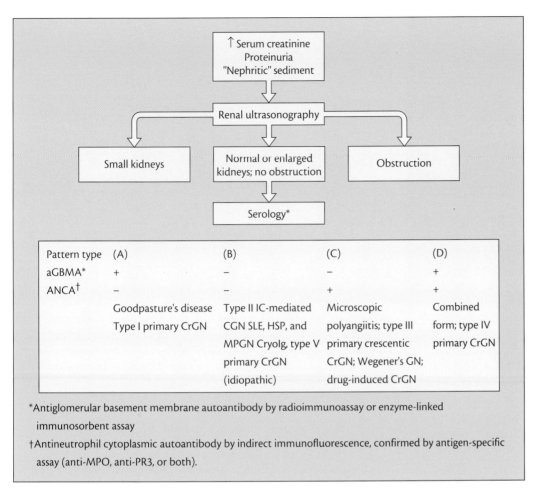

FIGURE 3-12

Evaluation of rapidly progressive glomeru-lonephritis. This algorithm schematically illustrates a diagnostic approach to the various causes of rapidly progressive glomerulonephritis. Serologic studies, especially measurement of circulating antiglomerular basement membrane anti-bodies, antineutrophil cytoplasmic anti-bodies, antinuclear antibodies, and serum complement component concentrations, are used for diagnosis. Serologic patterns (*A* through *D*) permit categorization of probable disease entities.

*Antiglomerular basement membrane autoantibody by radioimmunoassay or enzyme-linked immunosorbent assay

†Antineutrophil cytoplasmic autoantibody by indirect immunofluorescence, confirmed by antigen-specific assay (anti-MPO, anti-PR3, or both).

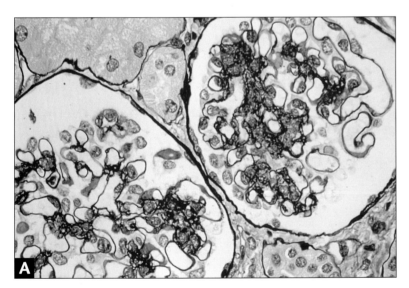

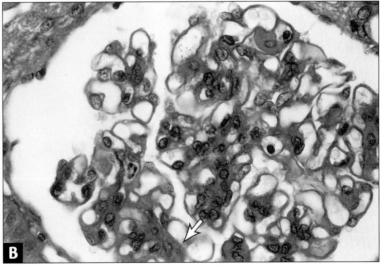

FIGURE 3-13

Light, immunofluorescence, and electron microscopy in immuno-globulin A (IgA) nephropathy. IgA nephropathy is a chronic glomerular disease in which IgA is the dominant or sole component of deposits that localize in the mesangial regions of all glomeruli. In severe or acute cases, these deposits also are observed in the capillary walls. This disorder may have a variety of clinical presenta-tions. Typically, the presenting features are recurrent macroscopic hematuria, often coincident with or immediately after an upper respi-ratory infection, along with persistent microscopic hematuria and low-grade proteinuria between episodes of gross hematuria.

Approximately 20% to 25% of patients develop end-stage renal disease over the 20 years after onset. **A,** On light microscopy, widening and often an increase in cellularity in the mesangial regions are observed, a process that affects the lobules of some glomeruli to a greater degree than others. This feature gives rise to the term *focal proliferative glomerulonephritis.* In advanced cases, segmental sclerosis often is present and associated with mas-sive proteinuria. During acute episodes, crescents may be present. **B,** Large round paramesangial fuchsinophilic deposits often are identified with Masson's trichrome or other similar stains (*arrows*).

(*Continued on next page*)

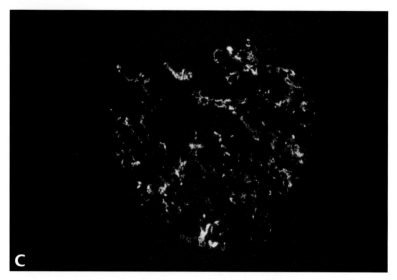

FIGURE 3-13 *(see* Color Plate) *(continued)*

C, Immunofluorescence defines the disease; granular mesangial deposits of IgA are seen with associated complement C3, and IgG or IgM, or both. IgG and IgM often are seen in lesser degrees of intensity than is IgA. **D,** On electron microscopy the abnormalities typically are those of large, rounded electron-dense deposits in paramesangial zones of most if not all lobules (*see* Color Plate). Capillary wall deposits (subepithelial, subendothelial, or both) may be present, especially in association with acute episodes. In addition, capillary basement membranes may show segmental thinning and rarefaction.

Heredofamilial and Congenital Glomerular Disorders

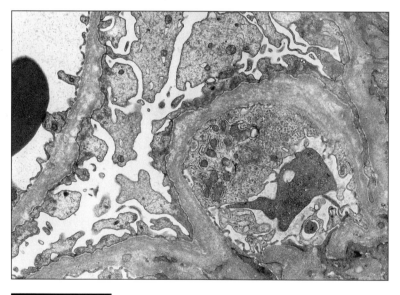

FIGURE 3-14

Alport's syndrome. Alport's syndrome (hereditary nephritis) is a hereditary disorder in which glomerular and other basement membrane collagen is abnormal. This disorder is characterized clinically by hematuria with progressive renal insufficiency and proteinuria. Many patients have neurosensory hearing loss and abnormalities of the eyes. The disease is inherited as an X-linked trait; in some families, however, autosomal recessive and perhaps autosomal dominant forms exist. Clinically, the disease is more severe in males than in females. End-stage renal disease develops in persons 20 to 40 years of age. In some families, ocular manifestations, thrombocytopenia with giant platelets, esophageal leiomyomata, or all of these also occur. In the X-linked form of Alport's syndrome, mutations occur in genes encoding the α-5 chain of type IV collagen (COL4A5). In the autosomal recessive form of this syndrome, mutations of either α-3 or α-4 chain genes have been described. On light microscopy, in the early stages of the disease the glomeruli appear normal. With progression of the disease, however, an increase in the mesangial matrix and segmental sclerosis develop. Interstitial foam cells are common but are not used to make a diagnosis. Results of immunofluorescence typically are negative, except in glomeruli with segmental sclerosis in which segmental immunoglobulin M and complement (C3) are in the sclerotic lesions. Ultrastructural findings are diagnostic and consist of profound abnormalities of glomerular basement membranes. These abnormalities range from extremely thin and attenuated to considerably thickened membranes. The thickened glomerular basement membranes have multiple layers of alternating medium and pale staining strata of basement membrane material, often with incorporated dense granules. The subepithelial contour of the basement membrane typically is scalloped.

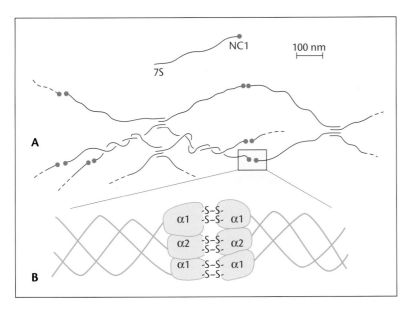

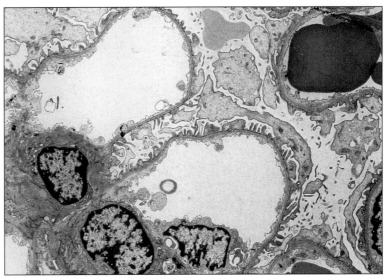

FIGURE 3-15

Basement membrane collagen type IV. The postulated arrangement of type IV collagen chains in a normal glomerular basement membrane is illustrated. The joining of noncollagen (NC-1) and 7S domains creates a lattice (chicken wire) arrangement (**A**). In the glomerular basement membrane, α1 and α2 chains predominate in the triple helix (**B**), but α3, 4, 5, and 6 chains are also found (not shown). Disruption of synthesis of any of these chains may lead to anatomic and pathologic alterations, such as those seen in Alport's syndrome. *Arrows* indicate fibrils. (*Adapted from* Abrahamson *et al.* [4].)

FIGURE 3-16

Thin basement membrane nephropathy. Glomeruli with abnormally thin basement membranes may be a manifestation of benign familial hematuria. Glomeruli with thin basement membranes may also occur in persons who do not have a family history of renal disease but who have hematuria, low-grade proteinuria, or both. Although the ultrastructural abnormalities have some similarities in common with the capillary basement membranes of Alport's syndrome, these two glomerulopathies are not directly related. Clinically, persistent microscopic hematuria and occasional episodic gross hematuria are important features. Nonrenal abnormalities are absent. On light microscopy, the glomeruli are normal; no deposits are seen on immunofluorescence. Here, the electron microscopic abnormalities are diagnostic; all or virtually all glomerular basement membranes are markedly thin (<200 nm in adults) without other features such as splitting, layering, or abnormal subepithelial contours.

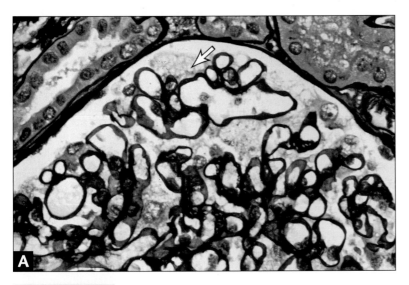

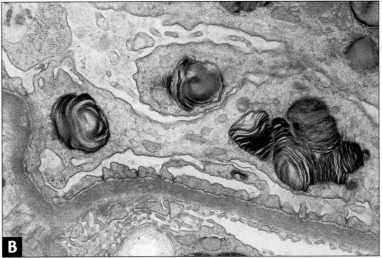

FIGURE 3-17

Fabry's disease. Fabry's disease, also known as *angiokeratoma corporis diffusum* or Anderson-Fabry's disease, is the result of deficiency of the enzyme α-galactosidase with accumulation of sphingolipids in many cells. In the kidney, accumulation of sphingolipids especially affects glomerular visceral epithelial cells. Deposition of sphingolipids in the vascular tree may lead to premature coronary artery occlusion (angina or myocardial infarction) or cerebrovascular insufficiency (stroke). Involvement of nerves leads to painful acroparesthesias and decreased perspiration (anhidrosis). The most common renal manifestation is that of proteinuria with progressive renal insufficiency. On light microscopy, the morphologic abnormalities of the glomeruli primarily consist of enlargement of visceral epithelial cells and accumulation of multiple uniform small vacuoles in the cytoplasm (*arrow* in **A**). Ultrastructurally, the inclusions are those of whorled concentric layers appearing as "zebra bodies" or myeloid bodies representing sphingolipids (**B**). These structures also may be observed in mesangial and endothelial cells and in arterial and arteriolar smooth muscle cells and tubular epithelia.

(*Continued on next page*)

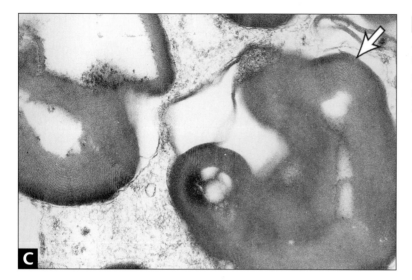

C

FIGURE 3-17 (continued)
At considerably higher magnification, the inclusions are observed to consist of multiple concentric alternating clear and dark layers, with a periodicity ranging from 3.9 to 9.8 nm. This fine structural appearance (best appreciated at the *arrow*) is characteristic of stored glycolipids (C).

Infection-Associated Glomerulopathies

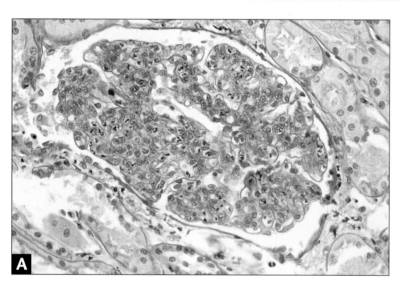

A

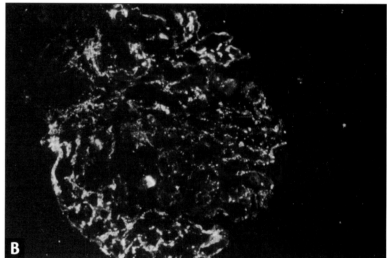

B

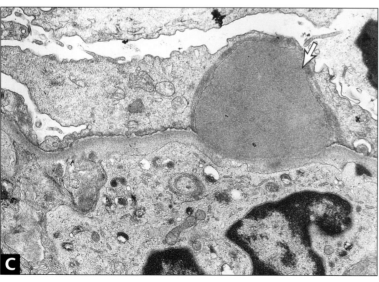

C

FIGURE 3-18 (*see* Color Plate)

Light, immunofluorescent, and electron microscopy of poststreptococcal (postinfectious) glomerulonephritis. Glomerulonephritis may follow in the wake of cutaneous or pharyngeal infection with a limited number of "nephritogenic" serotypes of group A β-hemolytic streptococcus. Typically, patients with glomerulonephritis exhibit hematuria, edema, proteinuria, and hypertension. Renal function frequently is depressed, sometimes severely. Most patients recover spontaneously, and a few go on to rapidly progressive or chronic indolent disease. **A,** On light microscopy the glomeruli are enlarged and hypercellular, with numerous leukocytes in the capillary lumina and a variable increase in mesangial cellularity. The leukocytes are neutrophils and monocytes. The capillary walls are single-contoured, and crescents may be present. **B,** On immunofluorescence, granular capillary wall and mesangial deposits of immunoglobulin G and complement C3 are observed (starry-sky pattern) (*see* Color Plate). Three predominant patterns occur depending on the location of the deposits; these include garlandlike, mesangial, and starry-sky patterns. **C,** The ultrastructural findings are those of electron-dense deposits, characteristically but not solely in the subepithelial aspects of the capillary walls, in the form of large gumdrop or humpshaped deposits (*arrow*). However, electron-dense deposits also are found in the mesangial regions and occasionally subendothelial locations. Endothelial cells often are swollen, and leukocytes are not only found in the capillary lumina but occasionally in direct contact with basement membranes in capillary walls with deposits. Similar findings may be observed in glomerulonephritis after infectious diseases other than certain strains of *Streptococci*.

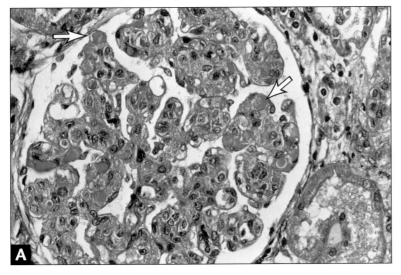

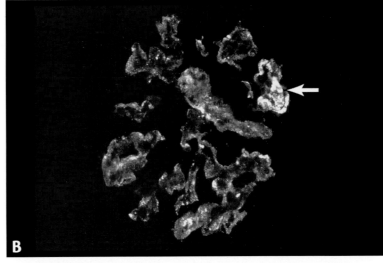

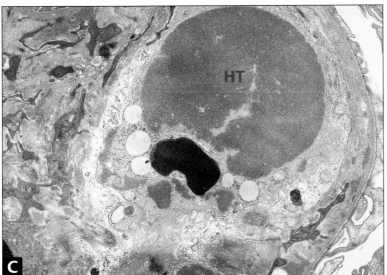

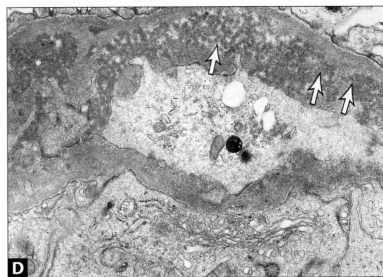

FIGURE 3-19

Hepatitis C virus infection. The most common glomerulonephritis in patients infected with the hepatitis C virus is membranoproliferative glomerulonephritis with, in some instances, cryoglobulinemia and cryoglobulin precipitates in glomerular capillaries. Thus, the morphology is basically the same as in membranoproliferative glomerulonephritis type I. **A,** With cryoglobulins, precipitates of protein representing cryoglobulin in the capillary lumina and appearing as hyaline thrombi (HT) are observed (*arrows*), often with numerous monocytes in most capillaries. **B,** Immunofluorescence microscopy discloses peripheral granular to confluent granular capillary wall deposits of immunoglobulin M (IgM) and complement C3; the same immune proteins are in the luminal masses corresponding to hyaline thrombi (*arrow*). **C,** Electron microscopy indicates the luminal masses (HT). **D,** On electron microscopy, the deposits also appear to be composed of curvilinear or annular structures (*arrows*). Hepatitis C viral antigen has been documented in the circulating cryoglobulins. Membranous glomerulonephritis with a mesangial component also has been infrequently described in patients infected with the hepatitis C virus.

Vascular Disorders

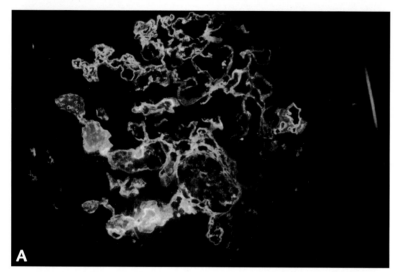

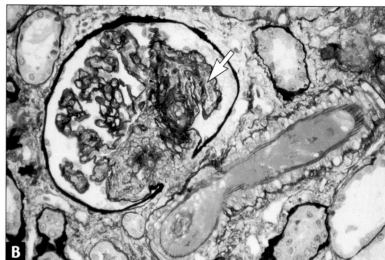

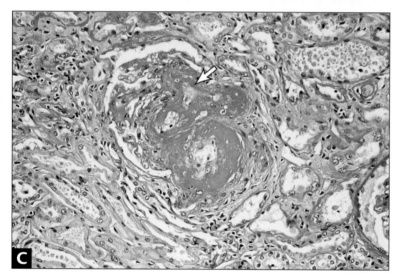

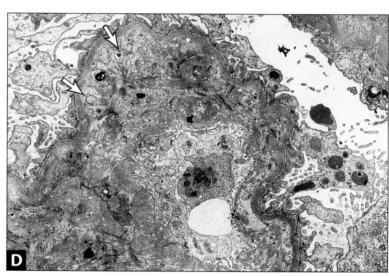

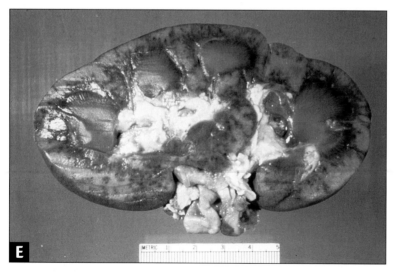

FIGURE 3-20

Light microscopy of thrombotic microangiopathies. This group of disorders includes hemolytic-uremic syndrome and thrombotic thrombocytopenic purpura, malignant hypertension, and renal disease in progressive systemic sclerosis (scleroderma renal crises). **A,** These lesions are characterized primarily by fibrin deposition in the walls of the glomeruli (fibrin). **B,** This fibrin deposition is associated with endothelial cell swelling (*arrow*) and thickened capillary walls, sometimes with a double contour. Variable capillary wall wrinkling and luminal narrowing occur. Mesangiolysis (dissolution of the mesangial matrix and cells) is not uncommon and may be associated with microaneurysm formation. With further endothelial cell damage, capillary thrombi ensue. **C,** Arteriolar thrombi also may be present. In arterioles, fibrin deposits in the walls and lumina are known as thrombonecrotic lesions, with extension of this process into the glomeruli on occasion (*arrow*). The arterial walls are thickened, with loose concentric intimal proliferation. **D,** On electron microscopy, the subendothelial zones of the glomerular capillary wall are widened (*arrows*). Flocculent material accumulates, corresponding to mural fibrin, with associated endothelial cell swelling. **E,** With widespread arterial thrombosis, cortical necrosis is a common complicating feature. The necrotic cortex consists of pale confluent multifocal zones throughout the cortex.

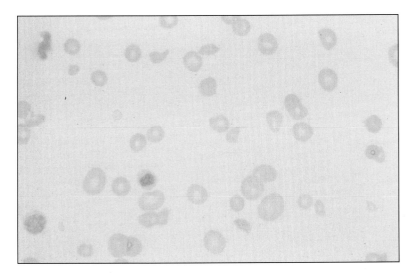

FIGURE 3-21 (*see* Color Plate)

Microangiopathic hemolytic anemia. Bizarrely shaped and fragmented erythrocytes are commonly seen in Wright's stained peripheral blood smears from patients with active lesions of thrombotic microangiopathy. These abnormally shaped erythrocytes presumably arise when the fibrin strands within small blood vessels shear the cell membrane, with imperfect resolution of the biconcave disk shape. The resultant intravascular hemolysis causes anemia, reticulocytosis, and reduced plasma haptoglobin level.

References

1. Churg J, Bernstein J, Glassock RJ: *Renal Disease. Classification and Atlas of Glomerular Diseases*, edn 2. New York: Igaku-Shoin; 1995.

2. Cameron JS, Glassock RJ: The natural history and outcome of the nephrotic syndrome. In *The Nephrotic Syndrome*. Edited by Cameron JS and Glassock RJ. New York: Marcel Dekker, 1987.

3. Cameron JS: The long-term outcome of glomerular diseases. In *Diseases of the Kidney* Vol II, edn 6. Edited by Schrier RW, Gottschalk CW. Boston: Little Brown; 1996.

4. Abrahamson D, Van der Heurel GB, Clapp WL, *et al.*: Nephritogenic antigens in the glomerular basement membrane. In *Immunologic Renal Diseases*. Edited by Nielson EG, Couser WG. Philadelphia: Lippincott-Raven, 1997.

Tubulointerstitial Disease

Jean-Pierre Grünfeld

Dominique Chauveau, Arthur H. Cohen, Garaben Eknoyan,
Richard J. Glassock, James M. Gloor, Lisa M. Guay-Woodford,
Alain Meyrier, Yves Pirson, Steven J. Scheinman, Vicente E. Torres,
Luan D. Truong, Jean-Louis Vanherweghem

CHAPTER

4

Renal Interstitium and Major Features of Chronic Tubulointerstitial Nephritis

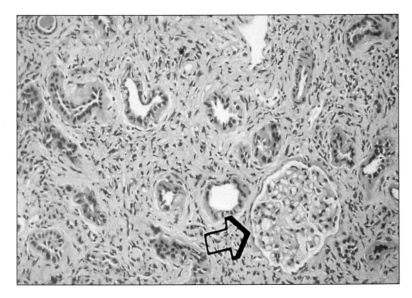

FIGURE 4-1

Primary chronic tubulointerstitial nephritis (TIN). The *arrow* indicates a normal glomerulus. Apart from providing structural support, the interstitium serves as a conduit for solute transport and is the site of production of several cytokines and hormones (erythropoietin and prostaglandins). For the exchange processes to occur between the tubules and vascular compartment, the absorbed or secreted substances must traverse the interstitial space. The structure, composition, and permeability characteristics of the interstitial space must, of necessity, exert an effect on any such exchange. Although the normal structural and functional correlates of the interstitial space are poorly defined, changes in its composition and structure in chronic TIN are closely linked to changes in tubular function. In addition, replacement of the normal delicate interstitial structures by fibrosclerotic changes of chronic TIN would affect the vascular perfusion of the adjacent tubule, thereby contributing to tubular dysfunction and progressive ischemic injury.

CONDITIONS ASSOCIATED WITH PRIMARY CHRONIC TUBULOINTERSTITIAL NEPHROPATHY

Immunologic diseases	Urinary tract obstructions	Hematologic diseases	Miscellaneous	Hereditary diseases	Endemic diseases
Systemic lupus erythematosus	Vesicoureteral reflux	Sickle hemoglobinopathies	Vascular diseases	Medullary cystic disease	Balkan nephropathy
Sjögren syndrome	Mechanical	Multiple myeloma	Nephrosclerosis	Hereditary nephritis	Nephropathia epidemica
Transplanted kidney		Lymphoproliferative disorders	Atheroembolic disease	Medullary sponge kidney	
Cryoglobulinemia		Aplastic anemia	Radiation nephritis	Polycystic kidney disease	
Goodpasture's syndrome			Diabetes mellitus		
Immunoglobulin A nephropathy			Sickle hemoglobinopathies		
Amyloidosis			Vasculitis		
Pyelonephritis					

Infections	Drugs	Heavy metals	Metabolic disorders	Granulomatous disease	Idiopathic TIN
Systemic	Analgesics	Lead	Hyperuricemia-hyperuricosuria	Sarcoidosis	
Renal	Cyclosporine	Cadmium	Hypercalcemia-hypercalciuria	Tuberculosis	
Bacterial	Nitrosourea		Hyperoxaluria	Wegener's granulomatosis	
Viral	Cisplatin		Potassium depletion		
Fungal	Lithium		Cystinosis		
Mycobacterial	Miscellaneous				

FIGURE 4-2

Tubulointerstitial nephropathy (TIN) occurs in a motley group of diseases of varied and diverse causes. These diseases are arbitrarily grouped together because of the unifying structural changes associated with TIN noted on morphologic examination of the kidneys.

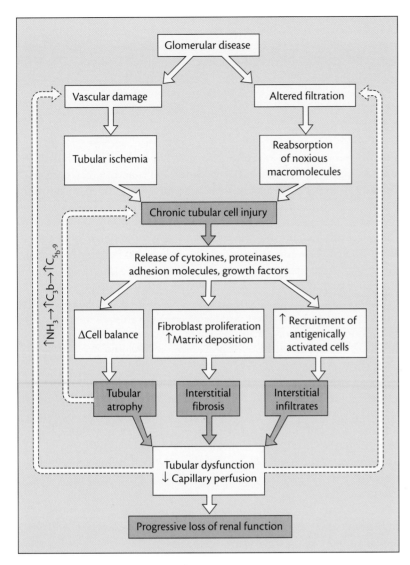

FIGURE 4-3

Schematic presentation of the potential pathways incriminated in the pathogenesis of chronic tubulointerstitial nephritis (TIN) caused by primary tubular injury (*dark boxes*) or secondary to glomerular disease (*light boxes*). The mechanism by which TIN is mediated remains to be elucidated. Chronic tubular epithelial cell injury appears to be pivotal in the process. The injury may be direct through cytotoxicity or indirect by the induction of an inflammatory or immunologic reaction. Studies in experimental models and humans provide compelling evidence for a role of immune mechanisms. The infiltrating lymphocytes have been shown to be activated immunologically. It is the inappropriate release of cytokines by the infiltrating cells and loss of regulatory balance of normal cellular regeneration that results in increased fibrous tissue deposition and tubular atrophy. Another potential mechanism of injury is that of increased tubular ammoniagenesis by the residual functioning but hypertrophic tubules. Increased tubular ammoniagenesis contributes to the immunologic injury by activating the alternate complement pathway.

Altered glomerular permeability with consequent proteinuria appears to be important in the development of TIN in primary glomerular diseases. By the same token, the proteinuria that develops late in the course of primary TIN may contribute to the tubular cell injury and aggravate the course of the disease.

In primary vascular diseases, TIN has been attributed to ischemic injury. In fact, hypertension is probably the most common cause of TIN. The vascular lesions that develop late in the course of primary TIN, in turn, can contribute to the progression of TIN. (*Adapted from* Eknoyan [1].)

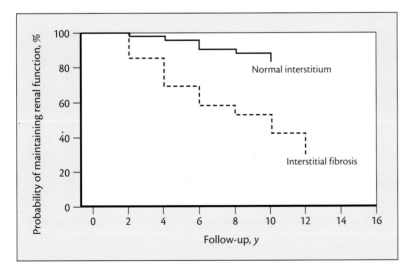

FIGURE 4-4

Effect on long-term prognosis of the presence of cortical chronic tubulointerstitial nephritis in patients with mesangioproliferative glomerulonephritis (n=455), membranous nephropathy (n = 334), and membranoproliferative glomerulonephritis (n = 220). The extent of tubulointerstitial nephritis correlates not only with altered glomerular and tubular dysfunction at the time of kidney biopsy but also provides a prognostic index of the progression rate to end-stage renal disease. As shown, the presence of interstitial fibrosis on the initial biopsy exerts a significant detrimental effect on the progression rate of renal failure in a variety of glomerular diseases. (*Adapted from* Eknoyan [1].)

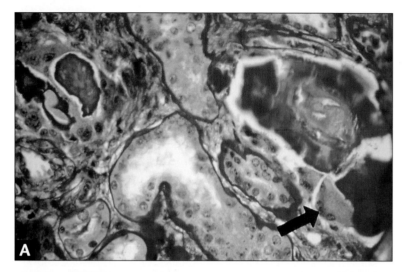

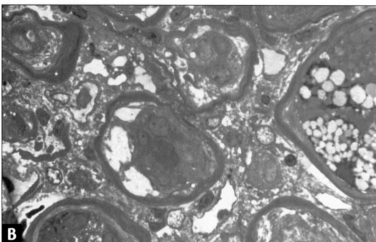

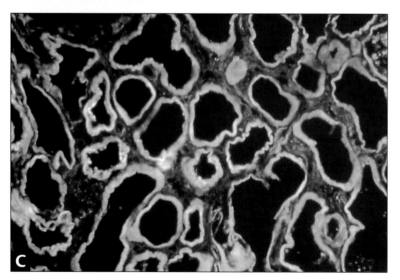

FIGURE 4-5 (see Color Plate)

A, Myeloma cast nephropathy. The *arrow* indicates a multinucleated giant cell (*see* Color Plate). **B,** Light chain deposition disease. Note the changes indicative of chronic tubulointerstitial nephritis (TIN) and light chain deposition along the tubular basement membrane (*dark purple*) (*see* Color Plate). **C,** Immunofluorescent stain for κ light chain deposition along the tubular basement membrane. The renal complications of multiple myeloma are a major risk factor in the morbidity and mortality of this neoplastic disorder. Whereas the pathogenesis of renal involvement is multifactorial (hypercalcemia and hyperuricemia), it is the lesions that result from the excessive production of light chains that cause chronic TIN. These lesions are initiated by the precipitation of the light chain dimers in the distal tubules and result in what has been termed *myeloma cast nephropathy*. The affected tubules are surrounded by multinucleated giant cells. Adjoining tubules show varying degrees of atrophy. The propensity of light chains to lead to myeloma cast nephropathy appears to be related to their concentration in the tubular fluid, the tubular fluid pH, and their structural configuration. This propensity accounts for the observation that increasing the flow rate of urine or its alkalinization will prevent or reverse the casts in their early stages of formation.

Direct tubular toxicity of light chains also may contribute to tubular injury. λ Light chains appear to be more injurious than are κ light chains. Binding of human κ and λ light chains to human and rat proximal tubule epithelial cell brush-border membrane has been demonstrated. Epithelial cell injury associated with the absorption of these light chains in the proximal tubules has been implicated in the pathogenesis of cortical TIN. Another mechanism relates to the perivascular deposition of paraproteins, either as amyloid fibrils that are derived from λ chains or as fragments of light chains that are derived from kappa chains, and produce the so-called light chain deposition disease.

Of the various lesions, myeloma cast nephropathy appears to be the most common, being observed at autopsy in one third of cases, followed by amyloid deposition, which is present in 10% of cases. Light chain deposition is relatively rare, being present in less than 5% of cases.

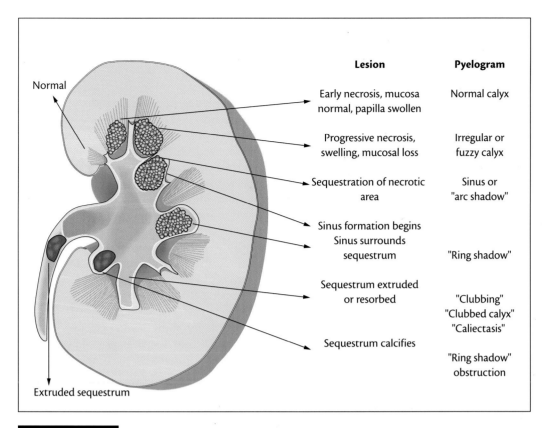

Lesion	Pyelogram
Early necrosis, mucosa normal, papilla swollen	Normal calyx
Progressive necrosis, swelling, mucosal loss	Irregular or fuzzy calyx
Sequestration of necrotic area	Sinus or "arc shadow"
Sinus formation begins Sinus surrounds sequestrum	"Ring shadow"
Sequestrum extruded or resorbed	"Clubbing" "Clubbed calyx" "Caliectasis"
Sequestrum calcifies	"Ring shadow" obstruction

Normal

Extruded sequestrum

FIGURE 4-6

The progressive stages of the papillary form of renal papillary necrosis and their associated radiologic changes seen on intravenous pyelography. Papillary necrosis occurs in one of two forms. In the medullary form, also termed *partial papillary necrosis*, the inner medulla is affected; however, the papillary tip and fornices remain intact. In the papillary form, also termed *total papillary necrosis*, the calyceal fornices and entire papillary tip are necrotic. In total papillary necrosis (shown here), the lesion is characterized from the outset by necrosis, demarcation, and sequestration of the papillae, which ultimately slough into the pelvis and may be recovered in the urine. In most of these cases, however, the necrotic papillae are not sloughed but are either resorbed or remain *in situ*, where they become calcified or form the nidus of a calculus. In these patients, excretory radiologic examination and computed tomography scanning are diagnostic. Unfortunately, these changes may not be evident until the late stages of RPN, when the papillae already are shrunken and sequestered. In fact, even when the papillae are sloughed out, excretory radiography can be negative.

The passage of sloughed papillae is associated with lumbar pain, which is indistinguishable from ureteral colic of any cause and is present in about half of patients. Oliguria occurs in less than 10% of patients. A definitive diagnosis of RPN can be made by finding portions of necrotic papillae in the urine. A deliberate search should be made for papillary fragments in urine collected during or after attacks of colicky pain of all suspected cases, by straining the urine through filter paper or a piece of gauze. The separation and passage of papillary tissue may be associated with hematuria, which is microscopic in some 40% to 45% of patients and gross in 20%. The hematuria can be massive, and occasionally, instances of exsanguinating hemorrhage requiring nephrectomy have been reported. (*Adapted from* Eknoyan *et al.* [2].

CONDITIONS ASSOCIATED WITH RENAL PAPILLARY NECROSIS

Diabetes mellitus
Urinary tract obstruction
Pyelonephritis
Analgesic nephropathy
Sickle hemoglobinopathy
Rejection of transplanted kidney
Vasculitis
Miscellaneous

FIGURE 4-7

Diabetes mellitus is the most common condition associated with papillary necrosis. The occurrence of capillary necrosis is likely more common than is generally appreciated, because pyelography (the best diagnostic tool for detection of papillary necrosis) is avoided in these patients because of dye-induced nephrotoxicity. When sought, papillary necrosis has been reported in as many as 25% of cases. Analgesic nephropathy accounts for 15% to 25% of papillary necrosis in the United States but accounts for as much as 70% of cases in countries in which analgesic abuse is common. Papillary necrosis also has been reported in patients receiving nonsteroidal anti-inflammatory drugs.

Sickle hemoglobinopathy is another common cause of papillary necrosis, which, when sought by intravenous pyelography, is detected in well over half of cases.

Infection is usually but not invariably a concomitant finding in most cases of RPN. In fact, with few exceptions, most patients with RPN ultimately develop a urinary tract infection, which represents a complication of papillary necrosis: that is, the infection develops after the primary underlying disease has initiated local injury to the renal medulla, with foci of impaired blood flow and poor tubular drainage. Infection contributes significantly to the symptomatology of RPN, because fever and chills are the presenting symptoms in two thirds of patients and a positive urine culture is obtained in 70%. However, RPN is not an extension of severe pyelonephritis. In most patients with florid acute pyelonephritis, RPN does not occur.

Urinary Tract Infection

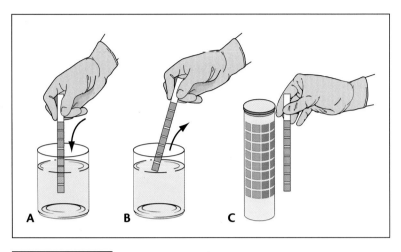

Urine testing. **Parts A through C** illustrate the testing process. Normal urine is sterile, but suprapubic aspiration of the bladder,

which is by no means a routine procedure, would be the only way of proving it. Urinary tract infection (UTI) cannot be identified simply by the presence of bacteria in a voided specimen, because micturition flushes saprophytic urethral organisms along with the urine. Thus, a certain number of colony-forming units of uropathogens are to be expected in the urine sample. Midstream collection is the most common method of urine sampling used in adults. When urine cannot be studied without delay, it must be stored at 4°C until it is sent to the bacteriology laboratory. The urine test strip is the easiest means of diagnosing UTI qualitatively. This test detects leukocytes and nitrites. Simultaneous detection of the two is highly suggestive of UTI. This test is 95% sensitive and 75% specific, and its negative predictive value is close to 96% [3]. The test does not, however, detect such bacteria as *Staphyloccocus saprophyticus*, a strain responsible for some 3% to 7% of UTIs. Thus, treating UTI solely on the basis of test strip risks failure in about 15% of simple community-acquired infections and a much larger proportion of UTIs acquired in a hospital.

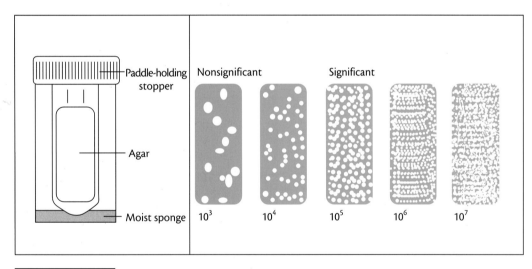

Culture interpretation. Urinalysis must examine bacterial and leukocyte counts (per milliliter). An approximate way of estimating bacterial counts in the urine uses a dip-slide method (*left*): a plastic paddle covered on both sides with culture medium is

immersed in the urine, shaken, and incubated overnight at 37°C (*right*).

The most specific results, however, are provided by laboratory analysis, which allows precise counting of bacteria and leukocytes. Normal values for a midstream specimen are less than or equal to 10^5 *Escherichia coli* organisms and 10^4 leukocytes per milliliter. These classic "Kass criteria," however, are not always reliable. In some cases of incipient cystitis, the number of *E. coli* per milliliter can be lower, on the order of 10^2 to 10^4 [4]. When fecal contamination has been ruled out, growth of bacteria that are not normally urethral saprophytes indicates infection. This is the case for *Pseudomonas, Klebsiella, Enterobacter, Serratia*, and *Moraxella*, among others, especially in a hospital setting or after urologic procedures.

A. MAIN MICROBIAL STRAINS RESPONSIBLE FOR URINARY TRACT INFECTION

Microbial Strain	First Episode or Delayed Relapse, %	Relapse Due to Early Reinfection, %
Escherichia coli	71–79	60
Proteus mirabilis	1.1–9.7	15
Klebsiella	—	20
Enterobacter	1.0–9.2	—
Enterococcus	1.0–3.2	—
Staphylococcus saprophyticus	3–7	—
Other species	2–6	5

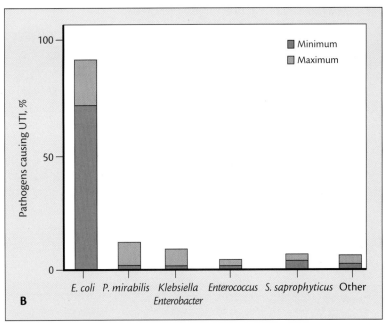

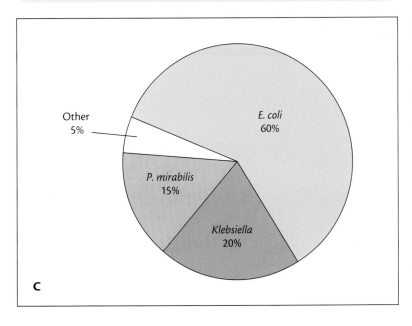

FIGURE 4-10

Principal pathogens of urinary tract infection (UTI). **A** and **B,** Most pathogens responsible for UTI are enterobacteriaceae with a high predominance of *Escherichia coli*. This is especially true of spontaneous UTI in females (cystitis and pyelonephritis). Other strains are less common, including *Proteus mirabilis* and more rarely gram-positive microbes. Among the latter, *Staphylococcus saprophyticus* deserves special mention because this gram-positive pathogen is responsible for 5% to 15% of such primary infections, is not detected by the leukocyte esterase dipstick, and is resistant to antimicrobial agents that are active on gram-negative rods.

C, Acute simple pyelonephritis is a common form of upper UTI in females and results from the encounter of a parasite and a host. In the absence of urologic abnormality, this renal infection is mostly due to uropathogenic strains of bacteria [5,6], and a majority of cases to community-acquired *E. coli*. The clinical picture consists of fever, chills, renal pain, and general discomfort. Tissue invasion is associated with a high erythrocyte sedimentation rate and C-reactive protein level well above 2 mg/dL.

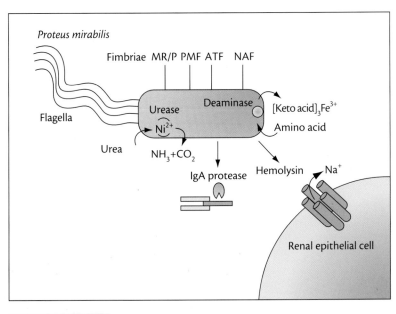

FIGURE 4-11

Proteus mirabilis is endowed with other nonfimbrial virulence factors, including the property of secreting urease, which splits urea into NH_3 and CO_2.

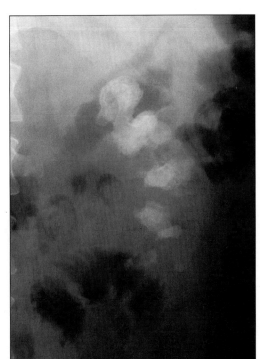

FIGURE 4-12

Staghorn calculi. Ammonium generation alkalinizes the urine, creating conditions favorable for build-up of voluminous struvite stones. These stones can progressively invade the entire pyelocalyceal system, forming staghorn calculi. These stones are an endless source of microbes, and the urinary tract obstruction perpetuates infection.

APPROPRIATE ANTIBIOTICS FOR URINARY TRACT INFECTIONS

Antibiotics	General Indications	Pregnancy	Prophylaxis
Aminoglycosides	+	+*	-
Aminopenicillins	+†	+	-
Carboxypenicillins	+	+	-
Ureidopenicillins	+	+	-
Quinolones	+‡	-	+
Fluoroquinolones	+§	-	+
Cephalosporins			
First generation	+¶	+	+†
Second generation	+	+	-
Third generation	+	+	-
Monobactams	+	+	-
Carbapenem	+	+	-
Cotrimoxazole	+	-	+†
Fosfomycin trometamole	+**	-	-
Nitrofurantoin	+††	-	+

* Aminoglycosides should not be prescribed during pregnancy except for very severe infection and for the shortest possible duration.

With the exception of amoxicillin plus clavulanic acid, aminopenicillins should not be prescribed as first-line treatment, owing to the frequency of primary resistance to this class of antibiotics.

† According to antibiotic sensitivity tests.

§ Fluoroquinolones carry a risk of tendon rupture (especially Achilles tendon).

¶ Oral administration only.

** Single-dose treatment of cystitis.

†† Simple cystitis; not pyelonephritis or prostatitis.

FIGURE 4-13

Appropriate antibiotics for urinary tract infections (UTI). An appropriate antibiotic for treating UTI must be bactericidal and conform to the following general specifications: 1) its pharmacology must include, in case of oral administration, rapid absorption and attainment of peak serum concentrations, 2) its excretion must be predominantly renal, 3) it must achieve high concentrations in the renal or prostate tissue, and 4) it must cover the usual spectrum of enterobacteria with reasonable chance of being effective on an empirical basis. Excluding special considerations for childhood and pregnancy, several classes of antibiotics fulfill these specifications and can be used alone or in combination. The choice also depends on market availability, cost, patient tolerance, and potential for inducing emergence of resistant strains.

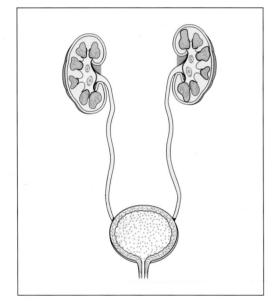

FIGURE 4-14

Cystitis in a female patient. In case of urinary tract infection (UTI), distinguishing between lower and upper tract infection is classic, but also beside the point. The real goal is to determine whether infection is confined to the bladder mucosa, which is the case in simple cystitis in females, or whether it involves solid organs (ie, prostatitis or pyelonephritis). The *dots* in this figure symbolize the presence of bacteria and leukocytes (ie, infection) in the relevant organ. Here, infection is confined to the bladder mucosa, which can be severely inflamed and edematous. This could be reflected radiographically by mucosal wrinkling on the cystogram. In some cases inflammation is severe enough to be accompanied by bladder purpura, which induces macroscopic hematuria but is not a particular grave sign.

FIGURE 4-15

Criteria for tissue invasion.

CRITERIA FOR TISSUE INVASION

Clinical

Kidney or prostate infection is marked by fever over 38°C, chills, and pain. The patient appears acutely ill.

Laboratory

Tissue invasion is invariably accompanied by an erythrocyte sedimentation rate over 20 mm/h and serum C-reactive protein levels over 2.0 mg/dL. Blood cultures grow in 30%–50% of cases, which in an immunocompetent host indicates simply bacteremia, not septicemia. This reflects easy permeability between the urinary and the venous compartments of the kidney.

Imaging

When indicated, ultrasound imaging, tomodensitometry, and scintigraphy provide objective evidence of pyelonephritis. In case of vesicoureteral reflux, urinary tract infection necessarily involves the upper urinary tract.

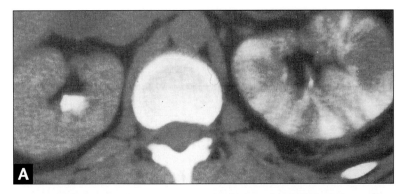

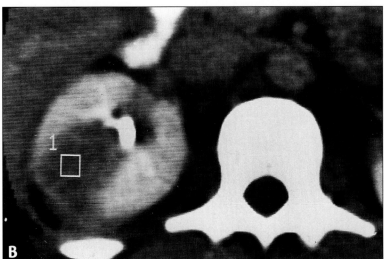

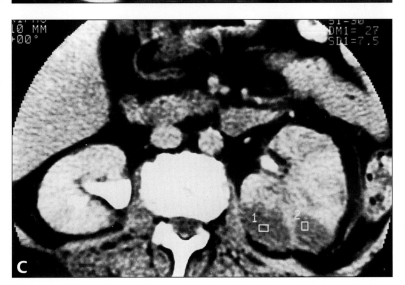

FIGURE 4-16

Computed tomodensitometry. Simple pyelonephritis does not require much imaging; however, it should be remembered that there is no correlation between the severity of the clinical picture and the renal lesions. Therefore, a diagnosis of "simple" pyelonephritis at first contact can be questioned when response to treatment is not clear after 3 or 4 days. This is an indication for uroradiologic imaging, such as renal tomodensitometry followed by radiography of the urinary tract while it is still opacified by the contrast medium.

The typical picture of acute pyelonephritis observed after contrast medium injection [7] consists of hypodensities of the infected areas in an edematous, swollen kidney. The pathophysiology of hypodense images has been elucidated by animal experiments in primates [8], which have shown that renal infection with uropathogenic *Escherichia coli* induces intense vasoconstriction.

Computed tomodensitometric images of acute pyelonephritis can take various appearances. **A,** The most common findings consist of one or several wedge-shaped or streaky zones of low attenuation extending from papilla to cortex. **B,** Hypodense images can be round. On this figure, the infected zone reaches the renal cortex and is accompanied with adjacent perirenal edema. **C,** Several such images can coexist in the same kidney.

(*Continued on next page*)

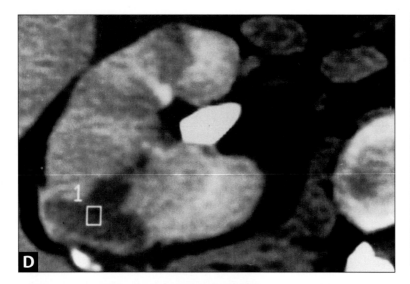

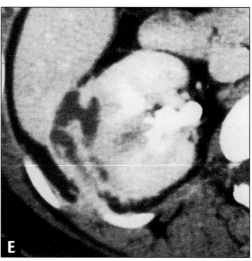

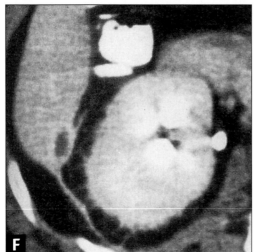

FIGURE 4-16 *(continued)*

E, Marked juxtacortical, circumscribed hypodense zones, bulging under the renal capsule usually correspond to lesions close to lique-faction and should be closely followed, as they can lead to abscess formation and opening into the perinephric space (E and F). (Parts E and F *from* Talner *et al.* [7]; with permission.)

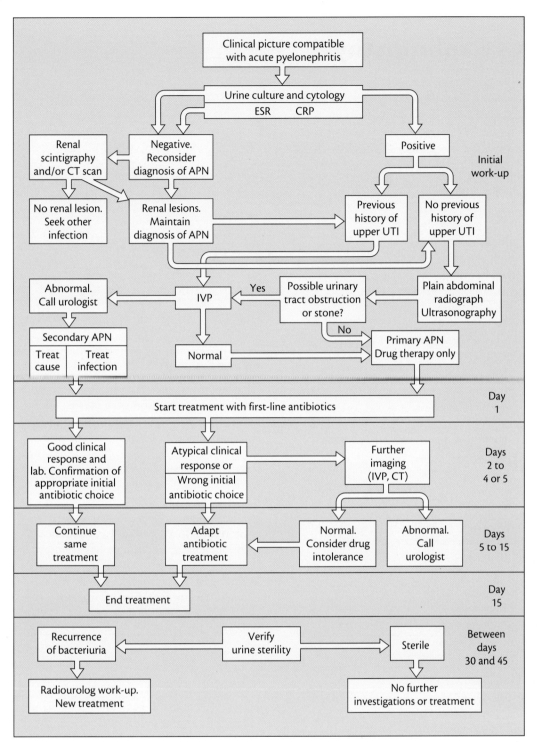

FIGURE 4-17

A general algorithm for the investigation and treatment of acute pyelonephritis (APN). Treatment of acute pyelonephritis is based on antibiotics selected from the list in Figure 4-13. Preferably, initial treatment is based on parenteral administration. It is debatable whether common forms of simple pyelonephritis initially require both an aminoglycoside and another antibiotic. Initial parenteral treatment for an average of 4 days should be followed by about 10 days of oral therapy based on bacterial sensitivity tests. It is strongly recommended that urine culture be carried out some 30 to 45 days after the end of treatment, to verify that bacteriuria has not recurred. APN—acute pyelonephritis; CRP—C-reactive protein; ESR—erythrocyte sedimentation rate; IVP—intravenous pyelography; UTI—urinary tract infection. (*Adapted from* Meyrier and Guibert [5].)

Reflux and Obstructive Nephropathy _____

CAUSES OF OBSTRUCTIVE NEPHROPATHY

Intraluminal
  Calculus, clot, renal papilla, fungus ball

Intrinsic
  Congenital
    Calyceal infundibular obstruction
    Ureteropelvic junction obstruction
    Ureteral stricture or valves
    Posterior urethral valves
    Anterior urethral valves
    Urethral stricture
    Meatal stenosis
    Prune-belly syndrome
  Neoplastic
    Carcinoma of the renal pelvis, ureter, or bladder
    Polyps

Extrinsic
  Congenital (aberrant vessels)
    Congenital hydrocalycosis
    Ureteropelvic junction obstruction
    Retrocaval ureter
  Neoplastic tumors
  Benign tumors
    Benign prostatic hypertrophy
    Pelvic lipomatosis
    Cysts
  Primary retroperitoneal tumors
    Mesodermal origin (*eg*, sarcoma)
    Neurogenic origin (*eg*, neurofibroma)
    Embryonic remnant (*eg*, teratoma)
  Retroperitoneal extension of pelvic or abdominal tumors
    Uterus, cervix
    Bladder, prostate
    Rectum, sigmoid colon
  Metastatic tumor
    Lymphoma
  Inflammatory
    Retroperitoneal fibrosis
    Inflammatory bowel disease
    Diverticulitis
    Infection or abscess
  Gynecologic
    Pregnancy
    Uterine prolapse
    Surgical disruption or ligation

Functional
  Neurogenic bladder
  Drugs (anticholinergics, antidepressants, calcium
    channel blockers)

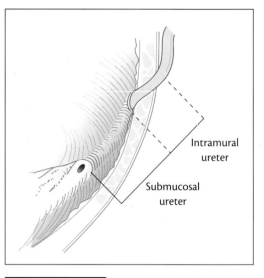

FIGURE 4-19

Anatomy of the ureterovesical junction. The ureterovesical junction permits free antegrade urine flow from the upper urinary tract into the bladder and prevents retrograde urinary reflux from the bladder into the ureter and kidney. Passive compression of the distal submucosal portion of the ureter against the detrusor muscle as a result of bladder filling impedes vesicoureteral reflux (VUR). An active mechanism preventing reflux also has been proposed in which contraction of longitudinally arranged distal ureteral muscle fibers occludes the ureteral lumen, impeding retrograde urine flow [9–11]. (*Adapted from* Politano [12].)

FIGURE 4-18

Obstructive nephropathy is responsible for end-stage renal failure in approximately 4% of persons. Obstruction to the flow of urine can occur anywhere in the urinary tract. Obstruction can be caused by luminal bodies; mural defects; extrinsic compression by vascular, neoplastic, inflammatory, or other processes; or dysfunction of the autonomic nervous system or smooth muscle of the urinary tract. The functional and clinical consequences of urinary tract obstruction depend on the developmental stage of the kidney at the time the obstruction occurs, severity of the obstruction, and whether the obstruction affects one or both kidneys.

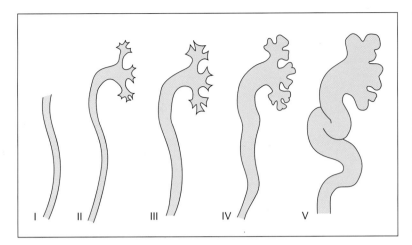

FIGURE 4-20

International system of radiographic grading of vesicoureteral reflux (VUR). The severity of VUR is most frequently classified according to the International Grading System of Vesicoureteral Reflux, using a standardized technique for performance of voiding cystourethrography. The definitions of this system are as follows. In grade I, reflux only into the ureter occurs. In grade II, reflux into the ureter, pelvis, and calyces occurs. No dilation occurs, and the calyceal fornices are normal. In grade III, mild or moderate dilation, tortuosity, or both of the ureter are observed, with mild or moderate dilation of the renal pelvis. No or only slight blunting of the fornices is seen. In grade IV, moderate dilation, tortuosity, or both of the ureter occur, with moderate dilation of the renal pelvis and calyces. Complete obliteration of the sharp angle of the fornices is observed; however, the papillary impressions are maintained in most calyces. In grade V, gross dilation and tortuosity of the ureter occur; gross dilation of the renal pelvis and calyces is seen. The papillary impressions are no longer visible in most calyces [13].

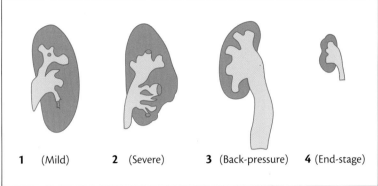

1   (Mild)   2   (Severe)   3   (Back-pressure)   4   (End-stage)

FIGURE 4-21

Grading of renal scarring associated with vesicoureteral reflux. Reflux renal parenchymal scarring detected on intravenous pyelography can be classified according to the system adopted by the International Reflux Study Committee consisting of four grades of severity. In grade 1, mild scarring in no more than two locations is seen. More severe and generalized scarring is seen in grade 2 but with normal areas of renal parenchyma between scars. In grade 3, or so-called "back-pressure" type, contraction of the whole kidney occurs and irregular thinning of the renal cortex is superimposed on widespread distortion of the calyceal anatomy, similar to changes seen in obstructive uropathy. Grade 4 is characterized by end-stage renal disease and a shrunken kidney having very little renal function [14].

Parenchymal scarring detected by radionuclide renal scintigraphy is classified similarly. In grade 1, no more than two scarred areas are detected. In grade 2, more than two affected areas are seen, with some areas of normal parenchyma between them. Grade 3 renal scarring is characterized by general damage to the entire kidney, similar to obstructive nephropathy. In grade 4, a contracted kidney in end-stage renal failure is seen, with less than 10% of total overall function [15].

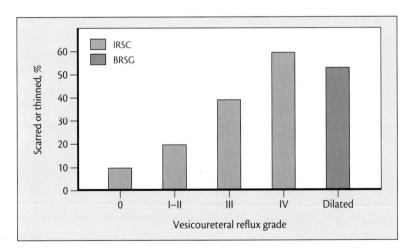

FIGURE 4-22

Frequency of parenchymal scarring at the time of diagnosis of vesicoureteral reflux (VUR). Many children in whom VUR is detected after a urinary tract infection already have evidence of renal parenchymal scarring. In two large prospective studies, the frequency of scars seen in persons with VUR increased with VUR severity. The International Reflux Study in Children (IRSC) studied 306 children under 11 years of age with grades III to V VUR [16]. The frequency of parenchymal scarring or thinning increased from 10% in children with nonrefluxing renal units (in children with contralateral VUR) to 60% in those with severely refluxing grade V kidneys. In another large prospective study, the Birmingham Reflux Study Group (BRSG) reported renal scarring in 54% of 161 children under 14 years of age with severe VUR resulting in ureteral dilation (greater than grade 3 using the classification system adopted by the International Reflux Study in Children group) at the time reflux was detected [17]. Participants in these studies were children previously diagnosed as having had urinary tract infection.

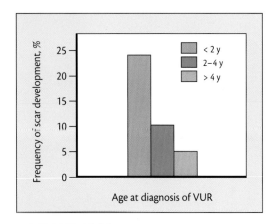

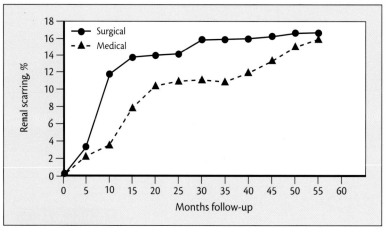

FIGURE 4-23

Development of new renal scars versus age at diagnosis of vesicoureteral reflux (VUR). The frequency of new scar formation appears to be inversely related to age. The International Reflux Study in Children (IRSC) examined children with high-grade VUR and found that new scars developed in 24% under 2 years of age, 10% from 2 to 4 years of age, and 5% over 4 years of age [18].

FIGURE 4-24

New scar formation at follow-up examinations over 5 years in children with high-grade vesicoureteral reflux (VUR). The International Reflux Study in Children (IRSC) (European group) was designed to compare the effectiveness of medical versus surgical therapy of VUR in children diagnosed after urinary tract infection. Surgery was successful in correcting VUR in 97.5% of 231 reimplanted ureters in 151 children randomized to surgical therapy. Medical therapy consisted of long-term antibiotic uroprophylaxis using nitrofurantoin, trimethoprim, or trimethoprim-sulfamethoxazole. No statistically significant advantage was demonstrable for either treatment modality with respect to new scar formation after 5 years of observation in either study. New scars were identified in 20 of the 116 children treated surgically (17%) and 19 of the 155 children treated medically (16%) at follow-up examinations over 5 years. Those children treated surgically who developed parenchymal scars generally did so within the first 2 years after ureteral repeat implantation, whereas scarring occurred throughout the observation period in the group that did not have surgery. VUR persisted in 80% of children randomized to medical treatment after follow-up examinations over 5 years.

The results of the IRSC paralleled the findings of the Birmingham Reflux Study Group (BRSG) investigation of medical versus surgical therapy for VUR in 161 children. After 2 years of observation, progressive or new scar formation was seen in 16% of children with refluxing ureters in the group treated surgically and 19% in the group treated medically. In contrast to the IRSC, however, new scar formation was rare after 2 years of observation in both groups [18,19].

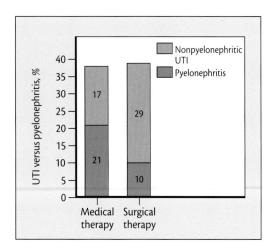

FIGURE 4-25

Incidence of urinary tract infection versus pyelonephritis in severe vesicoureteral reflux (VUR). Although the incidence of urinary tract infections (UTIs) is the same in surgically and medically treated children with VUR, the severity of infection is greater in those treated medically. The International Reflux Study in Children (IRSC) (European group) studied 306 children with VUR and observed them over 5 years; 155 were randomized to medical therapy, and 151 had surgical correction of their reflux. Although the incidence of UTI statistically was no different between the groups (38% in the medical group, 39% in the surgical group), children treated medically had an incidence of pyelonephritis twice as high (21%) as those treated surgically (10%) [20].

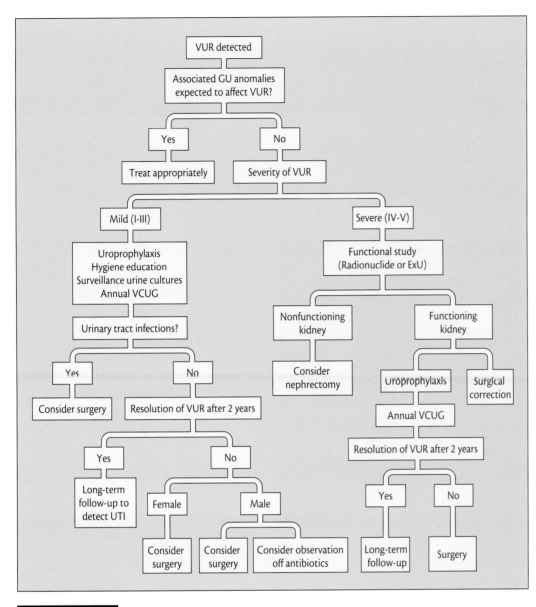

FIGURE 4-26

Proposed treatment of vesicoureteral reflux (VUR) in children. This algorithm provides an approach to evaluate and treat VUR in children. In VUR associated with other genitourinary anomalies, therapy for reflux should be part of a comprehensive treatment plan directed toward correcting the underlying urologic malformation. Children with mild VUR should be treated with prophylactic antibiotics, attention to perineal hygiene and regular bowel habits, surveillance urine cultures, and annual voiding cystourethrogram (VCUG). Children with recurrent urinary tract infection on this regimen should be considered for surgical correction. In children in whom VUR resolves spontaneously, a high index of suspicion for urinary tract infection should be maintained, and urine cultures should be obtained at times of febrile illness without ready clinical explanation.

In persons in whom mild VUR fails to resolve after 2 to 3 years of observation, consideration should be given to voiding pattern. A careful voiding history and an evaluation of urinary flow rate may reveal abnormalities in bladder function that impede resolution of reflux. Correction of dysfunctional voiding patterns may result in resolution of VUR. In the absence of dysfunctional voiding, it is controversial whether older women with persistent VUR are best served by surgical correction or close observation with uroprophylactic antibiotic therapy and surveillance urine cultures, especially during pregnancy. Male patients with persistent low-grade VUR may be candidates for close observation with surveillance urine cultures while not receiving antibiotic therapy, especially if they are over 4 years of age and circumcised. Circumcision lowers the incidence of urinary tract infection. In severe VUR the function of the affected kidney should be evaluated with a functional study (radionuclide renal scan). High-grade VUR in nonfunctioning kidneys is unlikely to resolve spontaneously, and nephrectomy may be indicated to decrease the risk of urinary tract infection and avoid the need for uroprophylactic antibiotic therapy. In patients with functioning kidneys who have high-grade VUR, the likelihood for resolution should be considered. Severe VUR, especially if bilateral, is unlikely to resolve spontaneously. Proceeding directly to repeat implantation may be indicated in some cases. Medical therapy with uroprophylactic antibiotics and serial VCUG may also be used, reserving surgical therapy for those in whom resolution fails to occur.

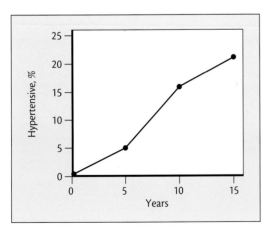

FIGURE 4-27

Development of hypertension in 55 normotensive subjects with reflux nephropathy at follow-up examinations over 15 years. The incidence of hypertension in persons with reflux nephropathy increases with age and appears to develop most commonly in young adults within 10 to 15 years of diagnosis. In a cohort of 55 normotensive persons with reflux nephropathy observed for 15 years, 5% became hypertensive after 5 years. This percentage increased to 16% at 10 years, and 21% at 15 years. The grading system for severity of scarring was different from the system adopted by the International Reflux Study Committee. Nevertheless, using this system, 78% of persons in the group could be classified as having reflux nephropathy severity scores between 1 and 4 [21].

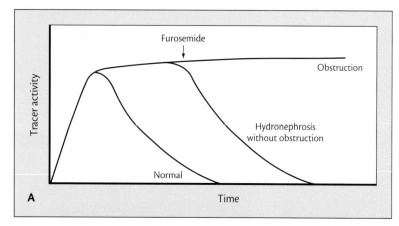

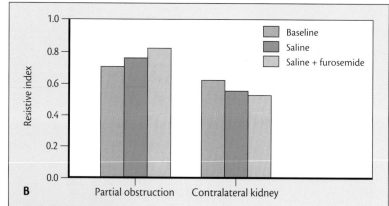

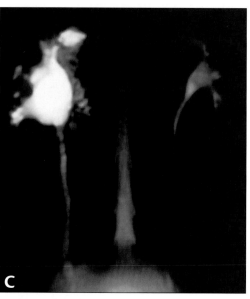

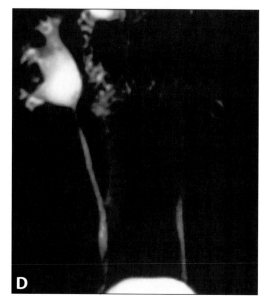

FIGURE 4-28

Diagnosis of obstructive nephropathy. **A,** Diuresis renography. **B,** Doppler ultrasonography. **C** and **D,** Magnetic resonance urogram utilizing a single-shot fast spin-echo technique with anterior-posterior projection (*part C*) and left posterior oblique projection (*part D*). Images demonstrate a widely patent right ureteropelvic junction in a patient with abdominal pain and suspected ureteropelvic junction obstruction. Administration of gadolinium is not required for this technique. Note also the urine in the bladder, cerebrospinal fluid in the spinal canal, and fluid in the small bowel.

Ultrasonography is the procedure of choice to determine the presence or absence of a dilated renal pelvis or calices and to assess the degree of associated parenchymal atrophy.

Nevertheless, obstruction rarely can occur without hydronephrosis, when the ureter and renal pelvis are encased in a fibrotic process and unable to expand. In contrast, mild dilation of the collecting system of no functional significance is not unusual. Even obvious hydronephrosis in some cases may not be associated with functional obstruction [22]. Diuresis renography is helpful when the functional significance of the dilation of the collecting system is in question [23,24]. Renal Doppler ultrasonography before and after administration of normal saline and furosemide also has been used to differentiate obstructive from nonobstructive pyelocaliectasis [25]. Other techniques such as excretory urography, computed tomography, and retrograde or antegrade ureteropyelography are helpful to determine the cause of the urinary tract obstruction. The utility of excretory urography is limited in patients with advanced renal insufficiency. In these cases, magnetic resonance urography can provide coronal imaging of the renal collecting systems and ureters similar to that of conventional urography without the use of iodinated contrast. (Parts **C** and **D** *courtesy of* B.F. King, MD.)

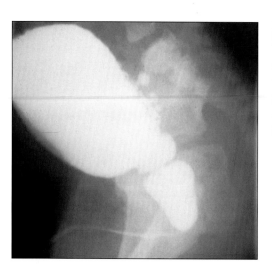

FIGURE 4-29

Voiding cystourethrogram (VCUG) demonstrating posterior urethral valves and dilation of the posterior urethra. Urethral valves are best detected by VCUG. The obstructing valves are seen as oblique or perpendicular folds with proximal urethral dilation and elongation. Distal to the valves the urinary stream is diminished. Alleviating the bladder outlet obstruction is indicated, either by lysis of the valves themselves or by way of vesicostomy, in small infants until sufficient growth occurs to make valve resection technically feasible.

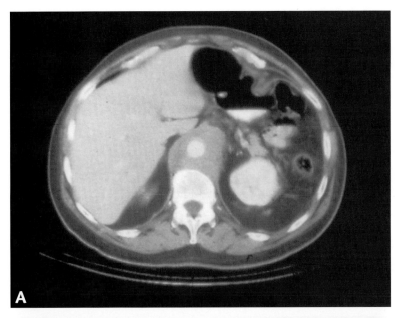

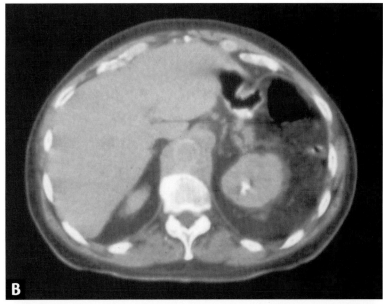

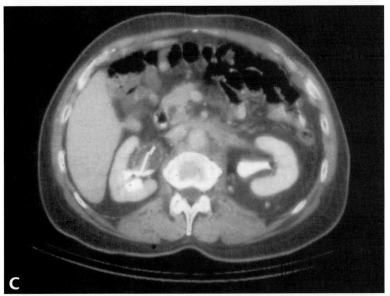

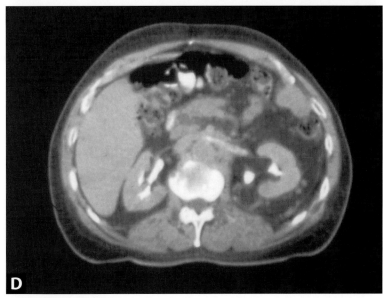

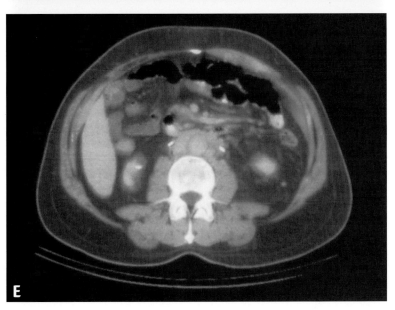

FIGURE 4-30

Idiopathic retroperitoneal fibrosis: computed tomography scans of the abdomen before (A,C,E,G; note right ureteral stent and mild left ureteropyelocaliectasis) and 7 years after ureterolysis (B,D,F,H; note omental interposition). Retroperitoneal fibrosis is characterized by the accumulation of inflammatory and fibrotic tissue around the aorta, between the renal hila and the pelvic brim. Most cases are idiopathic; the remainder are associated with immune-mediated connective tissue diseases, ingestion of drugs such as methysergide, abdominal aortic aneurysms, or malignancy. Idiopathic retroperitoneal fibrosis can be associated with mediastinal fibrosis, sclerosing cholangitis, Riedel's thyroiditis, and fibrous pseudotumor of the orbit. In the clinical setting, patients with idiopathic retroperitoneal fibrosis exhibit systemic symptoms such as malaise, anorexia and weight loss, and abdominal or flank pain. Renal insufficiency is often seen and is caused by bilateral ureteral obstruction. Laboratory test results usually demonstrate anemia and an elevated sedimentation rate.

(Continued on next page)

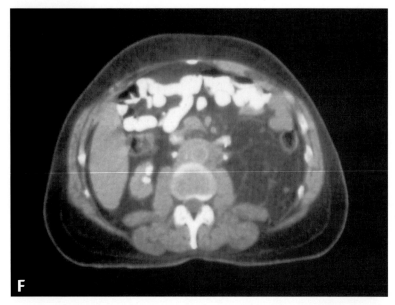

F

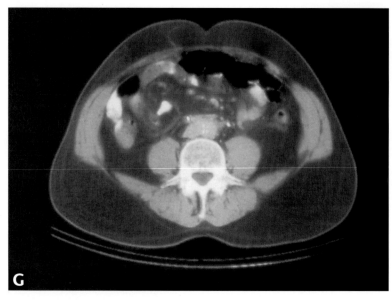

G

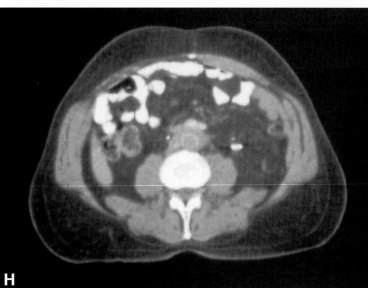

H

FIGURE 4-30 *(continued)*

The treatment is directed to the release of the ureteral obstruction, which initially can be achieved by placement of ureteral stents. Administration of corticosteroids is helpful to control the systemic manifestations of the disease and often to reduce the bulk of the tumor and relieve the ureteral obstruction. Administration of corticosteroids, however, should be considered only when malignancy and retroperitoneal infection can be ruled out. As in other chronic renal diseases, administration of corticosteroids should be kept at the minimal level capable of controlling symptoms. Surgical ureterolysis, which consists of freeing the ureters from the fibrotic mass, lateralizing them, and wrapping them in omentum to prevent repeat obstruction, is often necessary. Other immunosuppressive agents have been used rarely when the systemic manifestations of the disease cannot be controlled with safe doses of corticosteroids. In most cases the long-term outcome of idiopathic retroperitoneal fibrosis is satisfactory [26–28].

Cystic Diseases of the Kidney

PRINCIPAL CYSTIC DISEASES OF THE KIDNEY

Nongenetic	Genetic
Acquired disorders	Autosomal-dominant
Simple renal cysts (solitary or multiple)	**Autosomal-dominant polycystic kidney disease**
Cysts of the renal sinus (or peripelvic lymphangiectasis)	**Tuberous sclerosis complex**
Acquired cystic kidney disease (in patients with chronic renal impairment)	**von Hippel-Lindau disease**
	Medullary cystic disease
Multilocular cyst (or multilocular cystic nephroma)	Glomerulocystic kidney disease
Hypokalemia-related cysts	Autosomal-recessive
Developmental disorders	**Autosomal-recessive polycystic kidney disease**
Medullary sponge kidney	**Nephronophthisis**
Multicystic dysplastic kidney	X-linked
Pyelocalyceal cysts	Orofaciodigital syndrome, type I

FIGURE 4-31

Principal cystic diseases of the kidney. Classification of the renal cystic disorders, with the most common ones printed in bold type. (*Adapted from* Fick and Gabow [29], Welling and Grantham [30], and Pirson *et al.* [31].)

IMAGING CHARACTERISTICS OF THE MOST COMMON RENAL CYSTIC DISEASES

Disease	Kidney Size	Cyst Size	Cyst Location	Liver
Simple renal cysts	Normal	Variable (mm–10 cm)	All	Normal
Acquired renal cystic disease	Most often small, sometimes large	0.5–2 cm	All	Normal
Medullary sponge kidney	Normal or slightly enlarged	mm	Precalyceal	Normal (most often)
ADPKD	Enlarged	Variable (mm–10 cm)	All	Cysts (most often)
ARPKD	Enlarged	mm increase with age	All	CHF
NPH	Small	mm–2 cm (when present)	Medullary	Normal

FIGURE 4-32

Characteristics of the most common renal cystic diseases detectable by imaging techniques (ultrasonography, computed tomography, magnetic resonance). In the context of family history and clinical findings, these allow the clinician to establish a definitive diagnosis in the vast majority of patients. ADPKD—autosomal-dominant polycystic kidney disease; ARPKD—autosomal-recessive polycystic kidney disease; CHF—congenital hepatic fibrosis; NPH—nephronophthisis.

CLINICAL MANIFESTATIONS OF ADPKD

Manifestation	Prevalence, %	Reference
Renal		
Hypertension	Increased with age (80 at ESRD)	Parfrey and Barrett [32]
Pain (acute and chronic)	60	Pirson et al. [31] and Gabow [33]
Gross hematuria	50	Pirson et al. [31] and Gabow [33]
Urinary tract infection	Men 20; women 60	Pirson et al. [31]
Calculi	20	Torres et al. [34]
Renal failure	50 at 60 y	Choukroun et al. [35]
Hepatobiliary (see Fig. 4-35)		
Cardiovascular		
Cardiac valvular abnormality	20	Gabow [33]
Intracranial arteries		
Aneurysm	8	Pirson et al. [31]
Dolichoectasia	2	Schievink et al. [36]
? Ascending aorta dissection	Rare	
? Coronary arteries aneurysm	Rare	
Other		
Pancreatic cysts	9	Torra et al. [37]
Arachnoid cysts	8	Schievink et al. [38]
Hernia		
Inguinal	13	Gabow [39]
Umbilical	7	Gabow [39]
Spinal meningeal diverticula	0.2	Schievink and Torres [40]

FIGURE 4-33

Main clinical manifestations of autosomal-dominant polycystic kidney disease (ADPKD). Renal involvement may be totally asymptomatic at early stages. Arterial hypertension is the presenting clinical finding in about 20% of patients. Its frequency increases with age. Flank or abdominal pain is the presenting symptom in another 20%. Gross hematuria is most often due to bleeding into a cyst, and more rarely to stone. Renal infection, a frequent reason for hospital admission, can involve the upper collecting system, renal parenchyma or renal cyst. Diagnostic data are obtained by ultrasonography, excretory urography and CT. Frequently, stones are radiolucent or faintly opaque, because of their uric acid content. The main determinants of progression of renal failure are the genetic form of the disease and gender (more rapid progression in males). Hepatobiliary and intracranial manifestations are detailed in Figures 4-35 and 4-36, respectively. Pancreatic and arachnoid cysts are most usually asymptomatic. Spinal meningeal diverticula can cause postural headache. ESRD—end-stage renal disease.

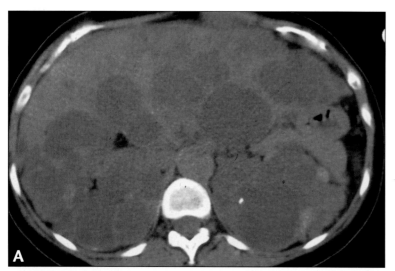

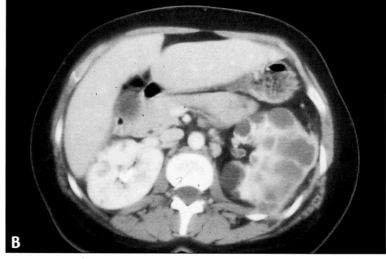

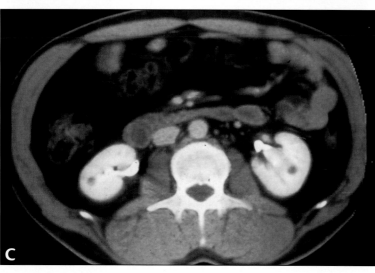

FIGURE 4-34

Kidney involvement in autosomal-dominant polycystic kidney disease (ADPKD). Examples of various cystic involvements of kidneys in ADPKD. The degree of involvement depends on age at presentation and disease severity. **A,** With advanced disease, as in this 54-year-old woman, renal parenchyma is almost completely replaced by innumerable cysts. Note also the cystic involvement of the liver. **B,** Marked asymmetry in the number and size of cysts between the two kidneys may be observed, as in this 36-year-old woman. In the early stage of the disease, making the diagnosis may be more difficult (see Fig. 4-37 for the minimal sonographic criteria to make a diagnosis of ADPKD in PKD1 families). **C and D,** Contrast-enhanced CT is more sensitive than ultrasonography in the detection of small cysts.

(*Continued on next page*)

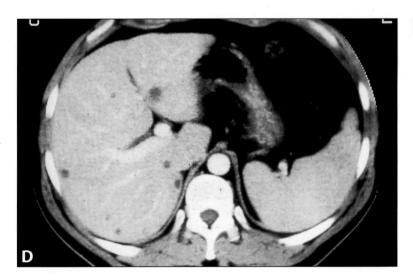

FIGURE 4-34 (*continued*)

The presence of liver cysts helps to establish the diagnosis, as in this 38-year-old man with PKD2 disease and mild kidney involvement.

HEPATOBILIARY MANIFESTATIONS OF ADPKD

Finding	Frequency
Asymptomatic liver cysts	Very common; increased prevalence with age (up to 80% at age 60)
Symptomatic polycystic liver disease	Uncommon (male/female ratio: 1/10)
Complicated cysts (hemorrhage, infection)	
Massive hepatomegaly	
Chronic pain/discomfort	
Early satiety	
Supine dyspnea	
Abdominal hernia	
Obstructive jaundice	
Hepatic venous outflow obstruction	
Congenital hepatic fibrosis	Rare (not dominantly transmitted)
Idiopathic dilatation of intrahepatic or extrahepatic biliary tract	Very rare
Cholangiocarcinoma	Very rare

FIGURE 4-35

Hepatobiliary manifestations of autosomal-dominant polycystic kidney disease (ADPKD). Liver cysts are the most frequent extrarenal manifestation of ADPKD. Their prevalence increases dramatically from the third to the sixth decade of life, reaching a plateau of 80% thereafter [41,42]. They are observed earlier and are more numerous and extensive in women than in men. Though usually mild and asymptomatic, cystic liver involvement occasionally is massive and symptomatic. Rare cases have been reported of congenital hepatic fibrosis or idiopathic dilatation of the intrahepatic or extrahepatic tract associated with ADPKD [41,42].

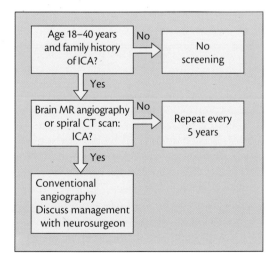

FIGURE 4-36

Intracranial aneuysm (ICA) screening in autosomal-dominant polycystic kidney disease (ADPKD). On the basis of decision analyses (taking into account ICA prevalence, annual risk of rupture, life expectancy, and risk of prophylactic treatment), it is currently proposed to screen for ICA in 18 to 40-year-old ADPKD patients with a family history of ICA [41,43]. Screening could also be offered to patients in high-risk occupations and those who want reassurance. Guidelines for prophylactic treatment are the same ones used in the general population: the neurosurgeon and the interventional radiologist opt for either surgical clipping or endovascular occlusion, depending on the site and size of ICA.

ULTRASONOGRAPHIC DIAGNOSTIC CRITERIA FOR ADPKD

Age	Cysts*
15–29	2, uni- or bilateral
30–59	2 in each kidney
≥60	4 in each kidney

*Minimal number of cysts to establish a diagnosis of ADPKD in PKD1 families at risk.

FIGURE 4-37

Ultrasonographic diagnostic criteria for autosomal-dominant poly-cystic kidney disease (ADPKD). These criteria are for the PKD1 form of ADPKD, as established by Ravine's group on the basis of both a sensitivity and specificity study [44,45]. Note that the absence of cyst before age 30 years does not rule out the diagnosis, the false-negative rate being inversely related to age. When ultra-sound diagnosis remains equivocal, the next step should be either contrast-enhanced CT (more sensitive than ultrasonography in the detection of small cysts) or gene linkage. A similar assessment is not yet available for the PKD2 form. (*Adapted from* Ravine *et al.* [45].)

FIGURE 4-38

Renal replacement therapy. Transplantation is considered in any autosomal-dominant polycystic kidney disease (ADPKD) patient with a life expectancy of more than 5 years and with no contraindi-cations to surgery or immunosuppression. Pretransplant work-up should include abdominal CT, echocardiography, myocardial stress scintigraphy, and, if needed (*see* Figure 4-36), screening for intracra-nial aneurysm. Pretransplant nephrectomy is advised for patients with a history of renal cyst infection, particularly if the infections were recent, recurrent, or severe. Patients not eligible for transplanta-tion may opt for hemodialysis or peritoneal dialysis. Although kid-ney size is rarely an impediment to peritoneal dialysis, this option is less desirable for patients with very large kidneys, because their vol-ume may reduce the exchangeable surface area and the tolerance for abdominal distension. Outcome for patients with ADPKD following renal replacement therapy is similar to that of matched patients with another primary renal disease [46,47].

CLINICAL FEATURES OF TSC

Finding	Frequency, %	Age at onset, y
Skin		
Hypomelanotic macules	90	Childhood
Facial angiofibromas	80	5–15
Forehead fibrous plaques	30	≥5
"Shagreen patches" (lower back)	30	≥10
Periungual fibromas	30	≥15
Central nervous system		
Cortical tubers	90	Birth
Subependymal tumors (may be calcified)	90	Birth
Focal or generalized seizures	80	0–1
Mental retardation/ behavioral disorder	50	0–5
Kidney		
Angiomyolipomas	60	Childhood
Cysts	30	Childhood
Renal cell carcinoma	2	Adulthood
Eye		
Retinal hamartoma	50	Childhood
Retinal pigmentary abnormality	10	Childhood
Liver (angiomyolipomas, cysts)	40	Childhood
Heart (rhabdomyoma)	2	Childhood
Lung (lymphangiomyomatosis; affects females)	1	≥20

FIGURE 4-39

Clinical features of tuberous sclerosis complex (TSC). TSC is an autosomal-dominant multisystem disorder with a minimal preva-lence of one in 10,000 [47,48]. It is characterized by the develop-ment of multiple hamartomas (benign tumors composed of abnor-mally arranged and differentiated tissues) in various organs. The most common manifestations are dermatologic (*see* Fig. 4-40) and neurologic. Renal involvement occurs in 60% of cases and includes cysts. Retinal involvement, occurring in 50% of cases, is almost always asymptomatic. Liver involvement, occurring in 40% of cases, includes angiomyolipomas and cysts. Involvement of other organs is much rarer [48,49].

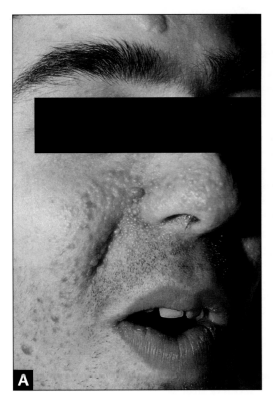

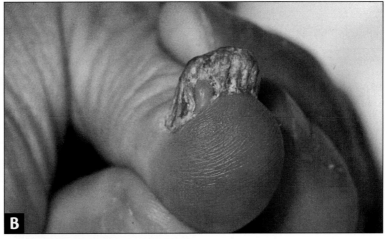

FIGURE 4-40 (*see* Color Plate)

Skin involvement in tuberous sclerosis complex (TSC). **A,** Facial angiofibromas and forehead plaque. **B,** Ungual fibroma. Previously (and inappropriately) called *adenoma sebaceum,* facial angiofibromas are pink to red papules or nodules, often concentrated in the nasolabial folds. Forehead fibrous plaques appear as raised, soft patches of red or yellow skin. Ungual fibromas appear as peri- or subungual pink tumors; they are found more often on the toes than on the fingers and are more common in female patients. Other skin lesions include hypomelanotic macules and "shagreen patches" (slightly elevated patches of brown or pink skin). (*Courtesy of* A. Bourloud and C. van Ypersele.)

ORGAN INVOLVEMENT IN VHL

Findings	Frequency, %	Mean age (range) at diagnosis, y
Central nervous system		30 (9–71)
Hemangioblastoma		
Cerebellar	60	
Spinal cord	20	
Endolymphatic sac tumor	Rare	
Eye/retinal hemangioblastoma	60	25 (8–70)
Kidney		
Clear cell carcinoma	40	40 (18–70)
Cysts	30	35 (15–60)
Adrenal glands/ pheochromocytoma	15	20 (5–60)
Pancreas		30 (13–70)
Cysts	40	
Microcystic adenoma	4	
Islet cell tumor	2	
Carcinoma	1	
Liver (cysts)	Rare	?

FIGURE 4-41

Organ involvement in Von Hippel-Lindau disease (VHL). VHL is an autosomal-dominant multisystem disorder with a prevalence rate of roughly one in 40,000 [49,50]. It is characterized by the development of tumors, benign and malignant, in various organs. VHL-associated tumors tend to arise at an earlier age and more often are multicentric than the sporadic varieties. Morbidity and mortality are mostly related to central nervous system hemangioblastoma and renal cell carcinoma. Involvement of cerebellum, retinas, kidneys, adrenal glands, and pancreas is illustrated.

The VHL gene is located on the short arm of chromosome 3 and exhibits characteristics of a tumor suppressor gene. Mutations are now identified in 70% of VHL families [51].

CLINICAL MANIFESTATIONS OF ARPKD

Renal
  Antenatal (ultrasonographic changes)
    Oligohydramnios with empty bladder
    Increased renal volume and echogenicity
  Neonatal period
    Dystocia and oligohydramnios
    Enlarged kidneys
    Renal failure
    Respiratory distress with pulmonary hypoplasia (possibly fatal)
  Infancy or childhood
    Nephromegaly (may regress with time)
    Hypertension (often severe in the first year of life)
    Chronic renal failure (slowly progressive, with a 60% probability of renal survival at
      15 years of age and 30% at 25 years of age)
Hepatic
  Portal fibrosis
  Intrahepatic biliary tract ectasia

FIGURE 4-42

Clinical manifestations of autosomal-recessive polycystic kidney disease (ARPKD). ARPKD is characterized by the development of cysts originating from collecting tubules and ducts, invariably associated with congenital hepatic fibrosis. Its prevalence is about one in 40,000 [52]. In the most severe cases, with marked oligohydramnios and an empty bladder, the diagnosis may be suspected as early as the 12th week of gestation. Some neonates die from either respiratory distress or renal failure. In most survivors, the disease is recognized during the first year of life. Excretory urography shows medullary striations owing to tubular ectasia. Kidney enlargement may regress with time. End-stage renal failure develops before age 25 in 70% of patients.

Liver involvement consists of portal fibrosis and intrahepatic biliary ectasia, frequently resulting in portal hypertension (leading to hypersplenism and esophageal varices) and less often in cholangitis, respectively. US may show dilatation of the biliary ducts, and even cysts. The respective severity of kidney and liver involvement vary widely between families and even in a single kindred.

A comparison of the diagnostic features of autosomal-dominant polycystic kidney disease (ADPKD) and ARPKD is summarized in Figure 4-32. Renal US of the parents of a child with ARPKD is, of course, normal. It should be noted that congenital hepatic fibrosis is found in rare cases of ADPKD with early-onset renal disease. The gene responsible for ARPKD has been mapped to chromosome 6. There is no evidence of genetic heterogeneity [53].

Toxic Nephropathies

TOXIC CAUSES OF CHRONIC TUBULOINTERSTITIAL RENAL DISEASES

Metals (environmental or occupational exposure)
  Lead
  Cadmium
Drugs or additives (use, misuse, or abuse)
  Lithium
  Germanium
  Analgesics
  Cyclosporine
  Mesalazine
Fungus and plant toxins (environmental or latrogenic exposure)
  Ochratoxins
  Aristolochic acids

FIGURE 4-43

Chronic exposure to drugs, occupational hazards, or environmental toxins can lead to chronic interstitial renal diseases. This table lists the major toxic causes of chronic interstitial renal diseases.

CAUSES OF LEAD NEPHROPATHY

Environmental
  Eating paint from lead-painted furniture, woodwork, and toys in children
  Lead-contaminated flour
  Home lead-contaminated drinking water from lead pipes
  Drinking of moonshine whiskey
Occupational
  Lead-producing plants: lead smelters, battery plants

FIGURE 4-44

Lead nephropathy associated with environmental and occupational exposure. Epidemiologic observations have established the relationship between lead exposure and renal failure in association with children eating lead paint in their homes, chronic ingestion of lead-contaminated flour, lead-loaded drinking water in homes, and drinking of illegal moonshine whiskey [54,55]. Occupational exposure in lead-producing industries also has been associated with a higher incidence of renal dysfunction.

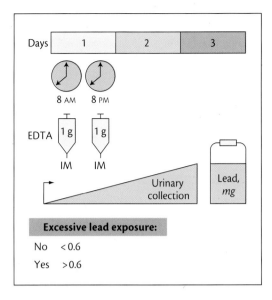

Days | 1 | 2 | 3

8 AM   8 PM

EDTA 1 g   1 g

IM   IM

Urinary collection

Lead, mg

Excessive lead exposure:

No   < 0.6

Yes > 0.6

FIGURE 4-45

Ethylenediamine tetra-acetic acid (EDTA)–lead mobilization test in lead nephropathy. This test consists of a 24-hour urinary lead excretion over 3 consecutive days after administration of 2 g of EDTA by intramuscular route on the first day in divided doses 12 hours apart. Persons without excessive lead exposure excrete less than 0.6 mg of lead during the day after receiving 2 g of EDTA parenterally. In the presence of renal failure, the excretion is delayed; however, the cumulative total remains less than 0.6 mg over 3 days. (*Adapted from* Batuman *et al.* [55].)

LITHIUM NEPHROTOXICITY

Reversible polyuria and polydipsia

Persistent nephrogenic diabetes insipidus

Incomplete distal tubular acidosis

Chronic renal failure (chronic interstitial fibrosis)

FIGURE 4-46

Lithium acts both distally and proximally to antidiuretic hormone–induced generation of cyclic adenosine monophosphatase. Polyuria and polydipsia can occur in up to 40% of patients on lithium therapy and are considered harmless and reversible. However, nephrogenic diabetes insipidus may persist months after lithium has been discontinued [56]. Lithium also induces an impairment of distal urinary acidification. Chronic renal failure secondary to chronic interstitial fibrosis may appear in up to 21% of patients on maintenance lithium therapy for more than 15 years [57]. However, these observations are still a matter of debate [56].

CLINICAL FEATURES OF ANALGESIC NEPHROPATHY

	Cases, %
Daily consumption of analgesic mixtures	100
Women	80
Headache	80
Gastrointestinal disturbances	35–40
Urinary tract infection	30–48
Papillary necrosis (clinical)	20
Papillary calcifications (computed tomography scan)	65

FIGURE 4-47

Classic analgesic nephropathy is a slowly progressive disease resulting from the daily consumption over several years of mixtures containing analgesics usually combined with caffeine, codeine, or both. Caffeine and codeine create psychological dependence. Most cases of analgesic nephropathy occur in women. In 80% of the cases, analgesics were taken for persistent headache. Gastrointestinal complaints are also frequent, as are urinary tract infections. Evidence of clinical papillary necrosis (fever and pain) is present in 20% of cases. Calcifications of papillae (detected by computed tomography scan) are present in 65% of persons who abuse analgesics [58].

EPIDEMIOLOGY OF ANALGESIC NEPHROPATHY AMONG PATIENTS WITH ESRD

	Frequency, %
Australia	20
Belgium	18
Canada	6
Germany	15
South Africa	22
Switzerland	20
United Kingdom	1
United States	5

FIGURE 4-48

Worldwide epidemiology of analgesic nephropathy. The frequency of analgesic nephropathy in patients with end-stage renal diseases (ESRD) varies greatly within and among countries [59,60,61]. The highest prevalence rates of end-stage renal disease from analgesic nephropathy occur in South Africa (22%), Switzerland and Australia (20%), Belgium (18%), and Germany (15%). In Belgium, the prevalence is 36% in the north and 10% in the south. In Great Britain, the rate is 1% nationwide; in Scotland it is 26%. In the United States, the rate is 5% nationwide, 13% in North Carolina, and 3% in Washington, DC. In Canada, the rate is 6% nationwide.

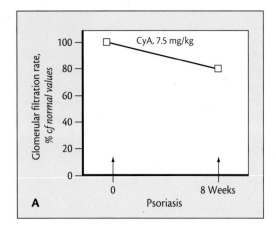

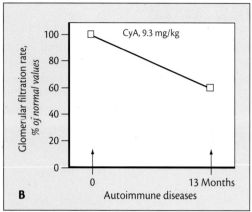

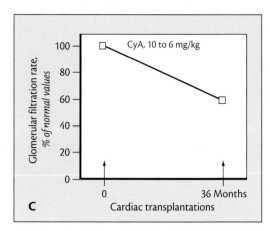

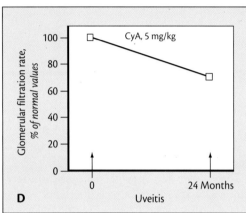

FIGURE 4-49

Cyclosporine (CyA) nephrotoxicity in nonrenal diseases. **A,** Patients treated with cyclosporine (7.5 mg/kg) for psoriasis experienced a median decrease to 84% of the initial values in the glomerular filtration rate after 8 weeks of therapy. **B,** Of patients treated with cyclosporine (9.3 mg/kg) for autoimmune diseases, 21% showed cyclosporine nephropathy on biopsy, with a decrease to 60% of the initial values in renal function. **C,** Patients with cardiac transplantation treated with high doses of cyclosporine (10 to 6 mg/kg) developed a reduction to 57% of the initial values in renal function 36 months after transplantation. Patients treated with azathioprine did not show any reduction in renal function. **D,** Patients receiving cyclosporine (5 mg/kg) for uveitis for 2 years showed a decrease in glomerular filtration rate to 65% of the initial values. (Part *A adapted from* Ellis *et al.* [62]; part *B adapted from* Feutren and Mihatsch [63]; part *C adapted from* Myers and Newton [64]; and part *D adapted from* Deray *et al.* [65].)

CLINICAL FEATURES OF BALKAN NEPHROPATHY

Residence in an endemic area
Occupational history of farming
Progressive renal failure
Microproteinuria of tubular type
Unremarkable urinary sediment
Small and shrunken kidneys
Associated urothelial tumors

FIGURE 4-50

Clinical features in Balkan nephropathy. Balkan nephropathy is characterized by progressive renal failure in residents (generally farmers) living in endemic areas for over 10 years. The urinary sediment is unremarkable and no proteinuria is seen, except for a microproteinuria of tubular type. The kidneys are small and shrunken. Urothelial cancers are frequently associated with Balkan nephropathy [66,67].

CLINICAL FEATURES OF CHINESE HERB NEPHROPATHY

Rapidly progressive renal failure
Microproteinuria of tubular type
Unremarkable urinary sediment
Small and shrunken kidneys
Valvular heart diseases (dexfenfluramine-associated therapy), 30%
Associated urothelial cancers

FIGURE 4-51

The clinical features of Chinese herb nephropathy are characterized by rapidly progressive renal failure without both urinary sediment abnormalities and proteinuria except for a microproteinuria of tubular type. The kidneys are small and shrunken. Vascular heart diseases are associated in 30% of cases (probably owing to dexfenfluramine administered with Chinese herbs for weight loss purposes) [68]. Some cases of associated urothelial cancers also are described [69,70].

Metabolic Causes of Tubulointerstitial Disease

CAUSES OF NEPHROCALCINOSIS

Medullary (total)	97.6*
Primary hyperparathyroidism	32.4
Distal renal tubular acidosis	19.5
Medullary sponge kidney	11.3
Idiopathic hypercalciuria	5.9
Dent's disease	4.3
Milk-alkali syndrome	3.2
Oxalosis	3.2
Hypomagnesemia-hypercalciuria	1.6
Sarcoidosis	1.6
Renal papillary necrosis	1.6
Hypervitaminosis D	1.6
Other†	4.0
Undiscovered causes	6.7
Cortical (total)	**2.4**

* The numbers represent the percentage of the total of 375 patients.

† Other causes include Bartter syndrome, idiopathic Fanconi syndrome, hypothyroidism, and severe acute tubular necrosis.

FIGURE 4-52

Nephrocalcinosis represents calcification of the renal parenchyma. It is primarily medullary in most cases except in dystrophic calcification associated with inflammatory, toxic, or ischemic disease. Nephrocalcinosis can be seen in association with chronic or severe hypercalcemia or in a variety of hypercalciuric states. The spectrum of causes of nephrocalcinosis is described by Wrong [71]. It is likely that the case mix is affected to some extent by Wrong's interests in, renal tubular acidosis (RTA) and Dent's disease, but this is by far the largest published series. As in other studies, the most important causes of nephrocalcinosis are primary hyperparathyroidism, distal RTA, and medullary sponge kidney. The primary factor predisposing patients to renal calcification in many of these conditions is hypercalciuria, as occurs in idiopathic hypercalciuria, Dent's disease, milk-alkali syndrome, sarcoidosis, hypervitaminosis D, and often in distal RTA. In distal RTA and milk-alkali syndrome, relative or absolute urinary alkalinity promote precipitation of calcium phosphate crystals in the tubular lumena and hypocitraturia is an important contributing factor in distal RTA. Causes of cortical nephrocalcinosis in this study included acute cortical necrosis, chronic glomerulonephritis, and chronic pyelonephritis. (*Adapted from* Wrong [71].)

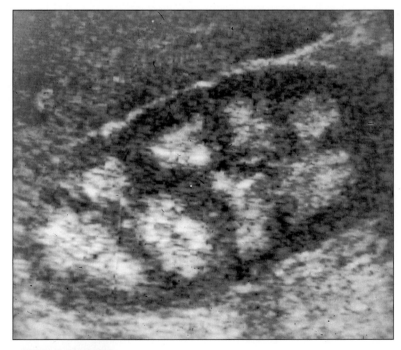

FIGURE 4-53

Nephrocalcinosis. Ultrasound image of right kidney in a patient with primary hyperparathyroidism. Echogenicity of the renal cortex is comparable to that of the adjacent liver. The dense nephrocalcinosis is entirely medullary. (*Courtesy of* R. Botash, MD.)

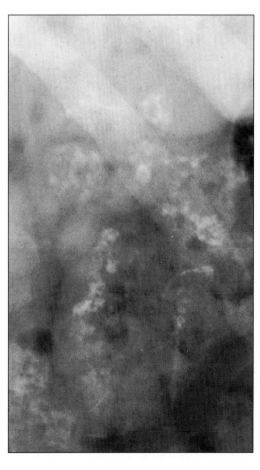

FIGURE 4-54

Noncontrast abdominal radiograph in a 24-year-old man with X-linked nephrolithiasis (Dent's disease). The patient had recurrent calcium nephrolithiasis beginning in childhood and developed end-stage renal disease requiring dialysis at 40 years of age. Extensive medullary calcinosis is evident.

MECHANISMS AND CLINICAL CONSEQUENCES OF HYPEROXALURIA

Type	Mechanism	Clinical consequences
Primary (genetic):		
PH1	Functional deficiency of AGT	Nephrolithiasis
		Nephrocalcinosis and progressive renal failure
		Systemic oxalosis (kidneys, bones, cartilage, teeth, eyes, peripheral nerves, central nervous system, heart, vessels, bone marrow)
PH2	Functional deficiency of DGDH	Nephrolithiasis
Secondary:		
Dietary	Sources: spinach, rhubarb, beets, peanuts, chocolate, and tea	Increased risk of nephrolithiasis
Enteric	Enhanced oxalate absorption because of increased oxalate solubility, bile salt malabsorption, and altered gut flora (eg, inflammatory bowel disease and bowel resection)	Nephrolithiasis Nephrocalcinosis Systemic oxalosis (rarely)
Metabolism from excess of precursors	Ascorbate	Nephrolithiasis
	Ethylene glycol, glycine, glycerol, xylitol, methoxyflurane	Tubular obstruction by crystals leading to acute renal failure
Pyridoxine deficiency	Cofactor for AGT	Nephrolithiasis

FIGURE 4-55

Oxalate is a metabolic end-product of limited solubility in physiologic solution. Thus, the organism is highly dependent on urinary excretion, which involves net secretion. Normal urine is supersaturated with respect to calcium oxalate. Crystallization is prevented by a number of endogenous inhibitors, including citrate. A mild excess of oxalate load, as occurs with excessive dietary intake, contributes to nephrolithiasis. A more severe oxalate overload, as in type 1 primary hyperoxaluria, can lead to organ damage through tissue deposition of calcium oxalate and possibly through the toxic effects of glyoxalate [72].

Two types of primary hyperoxaluria (PH) have been identified, of which type 1 (PH1) is much more common. PH1 results from absolute or functional deficiency of the liver-specific enzyme alanine:glyoxalate aminotransferase (AGT). This deficiency leads to calcium oxalate nephrolithiasis in childhood, with nephrocalcinosis and progressive renal failure. Because the kidney is the main excretory route for oxalate, in the face of excessive oxalate production even mild degrees of renal insufficiency can lead to systemic deposition of oxalate in a wide variety of tissues. It is interesting that the liver itself is spared from calcium oxalate deposition. Clinical consequences include heart block and cardiomyopathy, severe peripheral vascular insufficiency and calcinosis cutis, and bone pain and fractures. Many of these conditions are exacerbated by the effects of end-stage renal disease. In contrast, PH2 is much more rare than is PH1. Patients with PH2 have recurrent nephrolithiasis. Nephrocalcinosis, renal failure, and systemic oxalosis have not been reported in PH2. The metabolic defect in PH2 appears to be a functional deficiency of D-glycerate dehydrogenase (DGDH) [72].

Secondary causes of hyperoxaluria include dietary excess, enteric hyperabsorption, and enhanced endogenous production resulting from either exposure to metabolic precursors of oxalate or pyridoxine deficiency. Normally, dietary sources of oxalate account for only approximately 10% of urinary oxalate. Restriction of dietary oxalate can be effective in some patients with kidney stones who are hyperoxaluric, but even conscientious adherence to dietary restriction is disappointing in many patients who may have mild metabolic hyperoxaluria, an entity that probably exists but is poorly understood. Intestinal absorption of oxalate can be enhanced markedly in patients with bowel disease, particularly inflammatory bowel disease or after extensive bowel resection or jejunoileal bypass. In this setting, several mechanisms have been described including, 1) enhanced oxalate solubility as a consequence of binding of calcium to fatty acids in patients with fat malabsorption; 2) a direct effect of malabsorbed bile salts to enhance absorption of oxalate by intestinal mucosa, and 3) altered gut flora with reduction in the population of oxalate-metabolizing bacteria [72,73]. Because of the important role of the colon in absorbing oxalate, ileostomy abolishes enteric hyperoxaluria [73].

Excessive endogenous production of oxalate occurs in patients ingesting large quantities of ascorbic acid, which may increase the risk of nephrolithiasis. In the setting of acute exposure to large quantities of metabolic precursors, such as ingestion of ethylene glycol or administration of glycine or methoxyflurane, tubular obstruction by calcium oxalate crystals can lead to acute renal failure. Pyridoxine deficiency is associated with increased oxalate excretion clinically in humans and experimentally in animals; it can contribute to mild hyperoxaluria. In all patients with primary hyperoxaluria, a trial of pyridoxine therapy should be given, because some patients will have a beneficial response.

Renal Tubular Disorders

OVERVIEW OF RENAL TUBULAR DISORDERS INHERITED AS MENDELIAN TRAITS

Inherited disorder	Transmission mode	Defective protein
Renal glucosuria	?AR, AD	Sodium-glucose transporter 2
Glucose-galactose malabsorption syndrome	AR	Sodium-glucose transporter 1
Acidic aminoaciduria	AR	Sodium-potassium–dependent glutamate transporter
Cystinuria	AR	Apical cystine-dibasic amino acid transporter
Lysinuric protein intolerance	AR	Basolateral dibasic amino acid transporter
Hartnup disease	?	?
Blue diaper syndrome	AR	Kidney-specific tryptophan transporter
Neutral aminoacidurias: Methioninuria Iminoglycinuria Glycinuria	AR	?
Hereditary hypophosphatemic rickets with hypercalciuria	AR	? Sodium-phosphate cotransporter
X-linked hypophosphatemic rickets	X-linked dominant	Phosphate-regulating with endopeptidase features on the X chromosome
Inherited Fanconi's syndrome isolated disorder	AR and AD	?
Inherited Fanconi's syndrome associated with inborn errors of metabolism	AR	–
Carbonic anhydrase II deficiency	AR	Carbonic anhydrase type II
Distal renal tubular acidosis	AR	?
	AD	Basolateral anion exchanger (AE1)
Bartter-like syndromes:		
Antenatal Bartter variant	AR	NKCC2, ROMK, ClC-K2
Classic Bartter variant	AR	ClC-K2b
Gitelman's syndrome	AR	NCCT
Pseudohypoparathyroidism:		
Type Ia	AD	Guanine nucleotide–binding protein
Type Ib	?	
Low-renin hypertension:		
Glucocorticoid-remediable aldosteronism	AD	Chimeric gene (11β-hydroxylase and aldosterone synthase)
Liddle's syndrome	AD	β and γ subunits of the sodium channel
Apparent mineralocorticoid excess	AR	11-β-hydroxysteroid dehydrogenase
Pseudohypoaldosteronism:		
Type 1	AR and AD	α and β subunits of the sodium channel
Type 2 (Gordon's syndrome)	AD	?
Nephrogenic diabetes insipidus		
X-linked	X-linked recessive	Arginine vasopressin 2 receptor
Autosomal	AR and AD	Aquaporin 2 water channel
Urolithiases		
Cystinuria	AR	Apical cystine–dibasic amino acid transporter
Dent's disease	X-linked	Renal chloride channel (ClC-5)
X-linked recessive nephrolithiasis	X-linked	Renal chloride channel (ClC-5)
X-linked recessive hypophosphatemic rickets	X-linked	Renal chloride channel (ClC-5)
Hereditary renal hypouricemia	AR	? Urate transporter

FIGURE 4-56

Overview of renal tubular disorders. Inherited renal tubular disorders generally are transmitted as autosomal dominant, autosomal recessive, X-linked dominant, or X-linked recessive traits. For many of these disorders, the identification of the disease-susceptibility gene and its associated defective protein product has begun to provide insight into the molecular pathogenesis of the disorder. AD—autosomal dominant; AR—autosomal recessive; ClC-K2—renal chloride channel; NCCT—thiazide-sensitive cotransporter; NKCC2—bumetanide-sensitive cotransporter; ROMK—inwardly rectified.

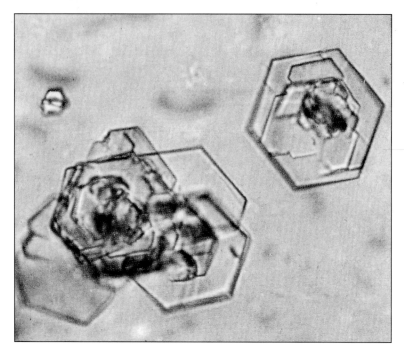

FIGURE 4-57

Urinary cystine crystals. Excessive urinary excretion of cystine (250 to 1000 mg/d of cystine/g of creatinine) coupled with its poor solubility in urine causes cystine precipitation with the formation of characteristic urinary crystals and urinary tract calculi. Stone formation often causes urinary tract obstruction and the associated problems of renal colic, infection, and even renal failure. The treatment objective is to reduce urinary cystine concentration or to increase its solubility. High fluid intake (to keep the urinary cystine concentration below the solubility threshold of 250 mg/L) and urinary alkalization are the mainstays of therapy. For those patients refractory to conservative management, treatment with sulfhydryl-containing drugs, such as D-penicillamine, mercaptopropionylglycine, and even captopril can be efficacious [74,75].

INHERITED RENAL TUBULAR ACIDOSES

Disorder	Transmission mode
Isolated proximal RTA	Autosomal recessive
Carbonic anhydrase II deficiency	Autosomal recessive
Isolated distal RTA	Autosomal dominant
Distal RTA with sensorineural deafness	Autosomal recessive

FIGURE 4-58

Renal tubular acidosis (RTA) is characterized by hyperchloremic metabolic acidosis caused by abnormalities in renal acidification, *eg*, decreased tubular reabsorption of bicarbonate or reduced urinary excretion of ammonium (NH_4^+). RTA can result from a number of disease processes involving either inherited or acquired defects. In addition, RTA may develop from an isolated defect in tubular transport; may involve multiple tubular transport abnormalities, *eg*, Fanconi's syndrome; or may be associated with a systemic disease process. Isolated proximal RTA (type II) is rare, and most cases of proximal RTA occur in the context of Fanconi's syndrome. Inherited forms of classic distal RTA (type I) are transmitted as both autosomal dominant and autosomal recessive traits. Inherited disorders in which RTA is the major clinical manifestation are summarized.

CLINICAL FEATURES DISTINGUISHING BARTTER-LIKE SYNDROMES

Feature	Classic Bartter's syndrome	Gitelman's syndrome	Antenatal Bartter's syndrome
Age at presentation	Infancy, early childhood	Childhood, adolescence	In utero, infancy
Prematurity, polyhydramnios	+/-	-	++
Delayed growth	++	-	+++
Delayed cognitive development	+/-	-	+
Polyuria, polydipsia	++	+	+++
Tetany	Rare	++	-
Serum magnesium	Low in 20%	Low in about 100%	Low-normal to normal
Urinary calcium excretion	Normal to high	Low	Very high
Nephrocalcinosis	+/-	-	++
Urine prostaglandin excretion	High	Normal	Very high
Clinical response to indomethacin	+/-	-	Often life-saving

FIGURE 4-59

Familial hypokalemic, hypochloremic metabolic alkalosis (Bartter's syndrome), is not a single disorder but rather a set of closely related disorders. These Bartter-like syndromes share many of the same physiologic derangements but differ with regard to the age of onset, presenting symptoms, magnitude of urinary potassium and prostaglandin excretion, and extent of urinary calcium excretion. At least three clinical phenotypes have been distinguished: classic Bartter's syndrome, the antenatal hypercalciuric variant (also called *hyperprostaglandin E syndrome*), and hypocalciuric-hypomagnesemic Gitelman's syndrome [76]. (*Adapted from* Guay-Woodford [76].)

INHERITED CAUSES OF UROLITHIASES

Disorder	Stone characteristics	Treatment
Cystinuria	Cystine	High fluid intake, urinary alkalization Sulfhydryl-containing drugs
Dent's disease	Calcium-containing	High fluid intake, urinary alkalization
X-linked recessive nephrolithiasis	Calcium-containing	High fluid intake, urinary alkalization
X-linked recessive hypophos-phatemic rickets	Calcium-containing	High fluid intake, urinary alkalization
Hereditary renal hypouricemia	Uric acid, calcium oxalate	High fluid intake, urinary alkalization Allopurinol
Hypoxanthine-guanine phospho-ribosyltransferase deficiency	Uric acid	High fluid intake, urinary alkalization Allopurinol
Xanthinuria	Xanthine	High fluid intake, dietary purine restriction
Primary hyperoxaluria	Calcium oxalate	High fluid intake, dietary oxalate restriction Magnesium oxide, inorganic phosphates

FIGURE 4-60

Urolithiases are a common urinary tract abnormality, afflicting 12% of men and 5% of women in North America and Europe [77]. Renal stone formation is most commonly associated with hypercalciuria. Perhaps in as many as 45% of these patients, there seems to be a familial predisposition. In comparison, a group of relatively rare disorders exists, each of which is transmitted as a mendelian trait and causes a variety of different crystal nephropathies. The most common of these disorders is cystinuria, which involves defective cystine and dibasic amino acid transport in the proximal tubule. Cystinuria is the leading single gene cause of inheritable urolithiasis in both children and adults [78,79]. Three mendelian disorders (Dent's disease, X-linked recessive nephrolithiasis, and X-linked recessive hypophosphatemic rickets) cause hypercalciuric urolithiasis. These disorders involve a functional loss of the renal chloride channel ClC-5 [80]. The common molecular basis for these three inherited kidney stone diseases has led to speculation that ClC-5 also may be involved in other renal tubular disorders associated with kidney stones. Hereditary renal hypouricemia is an inborn error of renal tubular transport that appears to involve urate reabsorption in the proximal tubule [81].

In addition to renal transport deficiencies, defects in metabolic enzymes also can cause urolithiases. Inherited defects in the purine salvage enzymes hypoxanthine-guanine phosphoribosyltransferase (HPRT) and adenine phosphoribosyltransferase (APRT) or in the catabolic enzyme xanthine dehydrogenase (XDH) all can lead to stone formation [82]. Finally, defective enzymes in the oxalate metabolic pathway result in hyperoxaluria, oxalate stone formation, and consequent loss of renal function [83].

References

1. Eknoyan G: Chronic tubulointerstitial nephropathies. In *Diseases of the Kidney*, edn 6. Edited by Schrier RW, Gottschalk CW. Boston: Little Brown; 1997:1983–2015.

2. Eknoyan G, Qunibi WY, Grissom RT, *et al.*: Renal papillary necrosis: an update. *Medicine* 1982, 61:55–73.

3. Pappas PG: Laboratory in the diagnosis and management of urinary tract infections. *Med Clin North Am* 1991, 75:313–325.

4. Kunin CM, VanArsdale White L, Tong HH: A reassessment of the importance of "low-count" bacteriuria in young women with acute urinary symptoms. *Ann Intern Med* 1993, 119:454–460.

5. Meyrier A, Guibert J: Diagnosis and drug treatment of acute pyelonephritis. *Drugs* 1992, 44:356–367.

6. Meyrier A: Diagnosis and management of renal infections. *Curr Opin Nephrol Hypertens* 1996, 5:151–157.

7. Talner LB, Davidson AJ, Lebowitz RL, *et al.*: Acute pyelonephritis: Can we agree on terminology? *Radiology* 1994, 192:297–306.

8. Roberts JA: Etiology and pathophysiology of pyelonephritis. *Am J Kidney Dis* 1991, 17:1–9.

9. Roshani H, Dabhoiwala NF, Verbeek FJ, Lamers WH: Functional anatomy of the human ureterovesical junction. *Anat Rec* 1996, 245:645–651.

10. Noordzij JW, Dabhoiwala NF: A view on the anatomy of the ureterovesical junction. *Scand J Urol Nephrol* 1993, 27:371–380.

11. Thomson AS, Dabhoiwala NF, Verbeek FJ, Lamers WH: The functional anatomy of the ureterovesical junction. *Br J Urol* 1994, 73:284–291.

12. Politano VA: Vesico-ureteral reflux. In *Urologic Surgery*, edn 2. Edited by Glenn JF. New York: Harper and Row Publishers, 1975:272–293.

13. Lebowitz RL, Olbing H, Parkkulainen K, *et al.*: International system of radiographic grading of vesicoureteral reflux. *Pediatr Radiol* 1985, 15:105.

14. Smellie JM, Edwards D, Hunter N, *et al.*: Vesico-ureteric reflux and renal scarring. *Kidney Int* 1975, 8:s65–s72.

15. Goldraich NP, Goldraich IH, Anselmi OE, Ramos OL: Reflux nephropathy: the clinical picture in South Brazilian children. *Control Nephrol* 1984, 39:52–67.

16. Weiss R, Tamminen-Mobius T, Koskimies O, *et al.*: Characteristics at entry of children with severe primary vesicoureteral reflux recruited for a multicenter international therapeutic trial comparing medical and surgical management. *J Urol* 1992, 148:1644–1649.

17. Astley R, Clark RC, Corkery JJ, *et al.*: Prospective trial of operative vs. non-operative treatment of severe vesicoureteric reflux: two years' observation in 96 children. *Br Med J* 1983, 287:171–174.

18. Olbing H, Claesson I, Ebel K-D, *et al.*: Renal scars and parenchymal thinning in children with vesicoureteral reflux: a 5-year report of the International Reflux Study in Children (European branch). *J Urol* 1992, 148:1653–1656.

19. Taylor CM, White RHR: Prospective trial of operative vs. non-operative treatment of severe vesicoureteric reflux in children: five years' observation. *Br Med J* 1987, 295:237–241.

20. Jodal U, Koskimies O, Hanson E, *et al.*: Infection pattern in children with vesicoureteral reflux randomly allocated to operation or long-term antibacterial prophylaxis. *J Urol* 1992, 148:1650–1652.

21. Goonasekera CDA, Shah V, Wade A, *et al.*: 15-year follow-up of renin and blood pressure in reflux nephropathy. *Lancet* 1996, 347:640–643.

22. Whitherow RO, Whitaker RH: The predictive accuracy of antegrade pressure flow studies in equivocal upper tract obstruction. *Br J Urol* 1981, 53:496.

23. Koff SA, Thrall JN, Keyes JW: Diuretic radionuclide urography. A noninvasive method for evaluating nephroureteral dilatation. *J Urol* 1979, 122:451.

24. Whitfield HN: Furosemide intravenous urography in the diagnosis of pelviureteric junction obstruction. *Br J Urol* 1979, 51:445.

25. Shokeir AA, Nijman RJM, El-Azab M, Provoost AP: Partial ureteral obstruction: effect of intravenous normal saline and furosemide on the resistive index. *J Urol* 1997, 157:1074–1077.

26. Gilkeson GS, Allen NB: Retroperitoneal fibrosis: a true connective tissue disease. *Rheum Dis North Am* 1996, 22:23–38.

27. Kottra JJ, Dunnick NR: Retroperitoneal fibrosis. *Radiol Clin North Am* 1996, 34:1259–1275.

28. Massachusetts General Hospital: Case records–case 27–1996: *N Engl J Med* 1996, 335:650–655.

29. Fick GM, Gabow PA: Hereditary and acquired cystic disease of the kidney. *Kidney Int* 1994, 46:951–964.

30. Welling LW, Grantham JJ: Cystic and developmental diseases of the kidney. In *The Kidney*. Edited by Brenner M. Philadelphia:WB Saunders Company; 1996:1828–1863.

31. Pirson Y, Chauveau D, Grünfeld JP: Autosomal dominant polycystic kidney disease. In *Oxford Textbook of Clinical Nephrology*. Edited by Davison AM, Cameron JS, Grünfeld JP, et al. Oxford:Oxford University Press; 1998:2393–2415.

32. Parfrey PS, Barrett BJ: Hypertension in autosomal dominant polycystic kidney disease. *Curr Opin Nephrol Hypertens* 1995, 4:460–464.

33. Gabow PA: Autosomal dominant polycystic kidney disease. *N Engl J Med* 1993, 329:332–342.

34. Torres WE, Wilson DM, Hattery RR, Segura JW: Renal stone disease in autosomal dominant polycystic kidney disease. *Am J Kidney Dis* 1993, 22:513–519.

35. Choukroun G, Itakura Y, Albouze G, et al.: Factors influencing progression of renal failure in autosomal dominant polycystic kidney disease. *J Am Soc Nephrol* 1995, 6:1634–1642.

36. Schievink WI, Torres VE, Wiebers DO, Huston J III: Intracranial arterial dolichoectasia in autosomal dominant polycystic kidney disease. *J Am Soc Nephrol* 1997, 8:1298–1303.

37. Torra R, Nicolau C, Badenas C, et al.: Ultrasonographic study of pancreatic cysts in autosomal dominant polycystic kidney disease. *Clin Nephrol* 1997, 47:19–22.

38. Schievink WI, Huston J III, Torres VA, Marsh WR: Intracranial cysts in autosomal dominant polycystic kidney disease. *J Neurosurg* 1995, 83:1004–1007.

39. Gabow PA: Autosomal dominant polycystic kidney disease—more than a renal disease. *Am J Kidney Dis* 1990, 16:403–413.

40. Schievink WI, Torres VE: Spinal meningeal diverticula in autosomal dominant polycystic kidney disease. *Lancet* 1997, 349:1223–1224.

41. Chauveau D, Pirson Y, Le Moine A, et al.: Extrarenal manifestations in autosomal dominant polycystic kidney disease. *Adv Nephrol* 1997, 26:265–289.

42. Torres VE: Polycystic liver disease. In *Polycystic Kidney Disease*. Edited by Watson ML, Torres VE. Oxford: Oxford University Press; 1996:500–529.

43. Pirson Y, Chauveau D: Intracranial aneurysms in autosomal dominant polycystic kidney disease. In *Polycystic Kidney Disease*. Edited by Watson ML, Torres VE. Oxford: Oxford University Press; 1996:530–547.

44. Ravine D, Gibson RN, Donlan J, Sheffield LJ: An ultrasound renal cyst prevalence survey: Specificity data for inherited renal cystic diseases. *Am J Kidney Dis* 1993, 22:803–807.

45. Ravine D, Gibson RN, Walker RG, et al.: Evaluation of ultrasonographic diagnostic criteria for autosomal dominant polycystic kidney disease 1. *Lancet* 1994, 343:824–827.

46. Pirson Y, Christophe JL, Goffin E: Outcome of renal replacement therapy in autosomal dominant polycystic kidney diseases. *Nephrol Dial Transplant* 1996, 11 (suppl. 6):24–28.

47. Culleton B, Parfrey PS: Management of end-stage renal failure and problems of transplantation in autosomal dominant polycystic kidney disease. In *Polycystic Kidney Disease*. Edited by Watson ML, Torres VE. Oxford:Oxford University Press; 1996:450–461.

48. Torres VE: Tuberous sclerosis complex. In *Polycystic Kidney Disease*. Edited by Watson ML, Torres VE. Oxford: Oxford University Press; 1996:283–308.

49. Huson SM, Rosser EM: The Phakomatoses. In *Principles and Practice of Medical Genetics*. Edited by Rimoin DL, Connor JM, Pyeritz RE. New York:Churchill Livingstone; 1997: 2269–2302.

50. Michels V: Von Hippel-Lindau disease. In *Polycystic Kidney Disease*. Edited by Watson ML, Torres VE. Oxford: Oxford University Press; 1996:309–330.

51. Neumann HPH, Zbar B: Renal cysts, renal cancer and von Hippel-Lindau disease. *Kidney Int* 1997, 51:16–26.

52. Gagnadoux MF, Broyer M: Polycystic kidney disease in children. In *Oxford Textbook of Clinical Nephrology*. Edited by Davison AM, Cameron JS, Grünfeld JP, et al. Oxford:Oxford University Press; 1998:2385–2393.

53. Zerres K, Mücher G, Bachner L, et al.: Mapping of the gene for autosomal recessive polycystic kidney disease (ARPKD) to chromosome 6p21-cen. *Nature Genet* 1994, 7:429–432.

54. Nuyts GD, Daelemans RA, Jorens PG, et al.: Does lead play a role in the development of chronic renal disease? *Nephrol Dial Transplant* 1991, 6:307–315.

55. Batuman V, Maesaka JK, Haddad B, et al.: The role of lead in gout nephropathy. *N Engl J Med* 1981, 304:520–523.

56. Walker RG: Lithium nephrotoxicity. *Kidney Int* 1993, 44(suppl 42):S93–S98.

57. Bendz H, Aurell M, Balldin J, et al.: Kidney damage in long-term lithium patients: a cross-sectional study of patients with 15 years or more on lithium. *Nephrol Dial Transplant* 1994, 9:1250–1254.

58. Elseviers MM, Bosteels V, Cambier P, et al.: Diagnostic criteria of analgesic nephropathy in patients with end-stage renal failure: results of the Belgian study. *Nephrol Dial Transplant* 1992, 7:479–486.

59. Drukker W, Schwarz A, Vanherweghem JL: Analgesic nephropathy: an underestimated cause of end-stage renal disease. *Int J Artif Organs* 1986, 9:216–243.

60. Klag MJ, Whelton PK, Perneger TV: Analgesics and chronic renal disease. *Curr Opinion Nephrol Hypertens* 1996, 5:236–241.

61. Vanherweghem JL, Even-Adin D: Epidemiology of analgesic nephropathy in Belgium. *Clin Nephrol* 1982, 17:129–133.

62. Ellis CN, Fradin MS, Messana JM, et al.: Cyclosporine for plaque-type psoriasis. *N Engl J Med* 1991, 324:277–284.

63. Feutren G, Mihatsch MJ: Risk factors for cyclosporine-induced nephropathy in patients with autoimmune diseases. *N Engl J Med* 1992, 326: 1654–1660.

64. Myers BD, Newton L: Cyclosporin induced chronic nephropathy: an obliterative renal injury. *J Am Soc Nephrol* 1991, 2:S45–S52.

65. Deray G, Benhmida M, Le Hoang P, et al. Renal function and blood pressure in patients receiving long-term, low-dose cyclosporine therapy for idiopathic autoimmune uveitis. *Ann Intern Med* 1992, 117:578–583.

66. Godin M, Fillastre JP, Simon P, et al.: L'ochratoxine est-elle néphrotoxique chez l'homme ? In *Actualités Néphrologiques*. Edited by Brentano JL, Bach JF, Kreis H, Grunfeld JP. Paris: Flammarion–Medecine Sciences; 1996:225–250.

67. Stefanovic V, Polenakovic MH: Balkan nephropathy: kidney disease beyond the Balkans? *Am J Nephrol* 1991, 11:1–11.

68. Vanherweghem JL: Association of valvular heart disease with Chinese herbs nephropathy. *Lancet* 1997, 350:1858.

69. Cosijns JP, Jadoul M, Squifflet JP: Urothelial malignancy in nephropathy due to Chinese herbs. *Lancet* 1994, 344:118.

70. Vanherweghem JL, Tielemans C, Simon J, Depierreux M: Chinese herbs nephropathy and renal pelvic carcinoma. *Nephrol Dial Transplant* 1995, 10:270–273.

71. Wrong OM: Nephrocalcinosis. In *The Oxford Textbook of Clinical Nephrology*. Edited by Davison AM, *et al*. Oxford: Oxford University Press; 1997:1378–1396.

72. Danpure CJ, Purdue PE: Primay hyperoxaluria. In *The Metabolic and Molecular Bases of Inherited Disease*, edn 6. Edited by Scriver CR, *et al*. New York: McGraw-Hill; 1995:2385–2424.

73. Coe FL, Parks JH, Asplin JR: The pathogenesis and treatment of kidney stones. *N Engl J Med* 1992, 327:1141–1152.

74. Stephens AD: Cystinuria and its treatment: 25 years' experience at St. Bartholomew's Hospital. *J Inherited Metab Dis* 1989, 12:197–209.

75. Perazella M, Buller G: Successful treatment of cystinuria with captopril. *Am J Kidney Dis* 1993, 21:504–507.

76. Guay-Woodford L: Bartter syndrome: unraveling the pathophysiologic enigma. *Am J Med* 1998, 105:151–161.

77. Coe F, Parks J, Asplin J: The pathogenesis and treatment of kidney stones. *N Engl J Med* 1992, 327:1141–1152.

78. Segal S, Thier S: Cystinuria. In *The Metabolic and Molecular Bases of Inherited Diseases*. Edited by Scriver CH, Beaudet AL, Sly WS, Valle D. York: McGraw-Hill; 1995:3581–3602.

79. Polinsky MS, Kaiser BA, Baluarte HJ: Urolithiasis in childhood. *Pediatr Clin North Am* 1987, 34:683–710.

80. Lloyd S, Pearce S, Fisher S, *et al.*: A common molecular basis for three inherited kidney stone diseases. *Nature* 1996, 379:445–449.

81. Grieff M: New insights into X-linked hypophosphatemia. *Curr Opin Nephrol Hypertens* 1997, 6:15–19.

82. Cameron J, Moro F, Simmonds H: Gout, uric acid and purine metabolism in paediatric nephrology. *Pediatr Nephrol* 1993, 7:105–118.

83. Danpure C, Purdue P: Primary Hyperoxaluria. In *The Metabolic and Molecular Bases of Inherited Diseases*. Edited by Scriver CH, Beaudet AL, Sly WS, Valle D. New York: McGraw-Hill; 1995:2385–2424.

Hypertension and the Kidney

Christopher S. Wilcox

John H. Bauer, Lance D. Dworkin, L. Lee Hamm,
Theodore A. Kotchen, L. Gabriel Navar, Charles R. Nolan,
Marc A. Pohl, Garry P. Reams, Douglas C. Shemin,
Stephen T. Textor, Myron H. Weinberger

CHAPTER

5

The Kidney in Blood Pressure Regulation

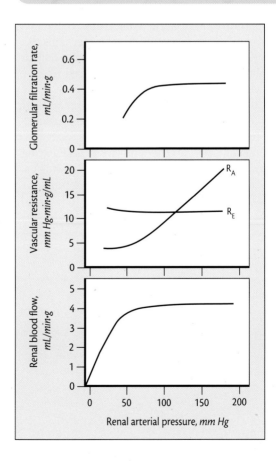

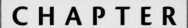

FIGURE 5-1

Renal autoregulatory mechanism. Because the glomerular filtration rate (GFR) is so responsive to changes in the glomerular forces, highly efficient mechanisms have been developed to maintain a stable intrarenal hemodynamic environment [1]. These powerful mechanisms adjust vascular smooth muscle tone in response to various extrinsic disturbances. During changes in arterial pressure, renal blood flow and the GFR are autoregulated with high efficiency as a consequence of adjustments in the vascular resistance of the preglomerular arterioles. Although efferent resistance also can be regulated by other mechanisms, it does not participate significantly over most of the autoregulatory range. The GFR, filtered sodium load, and the intrarenal pressures are maintained stable in the face of various extrarenal disturbances by the autoregulatory mechanism.

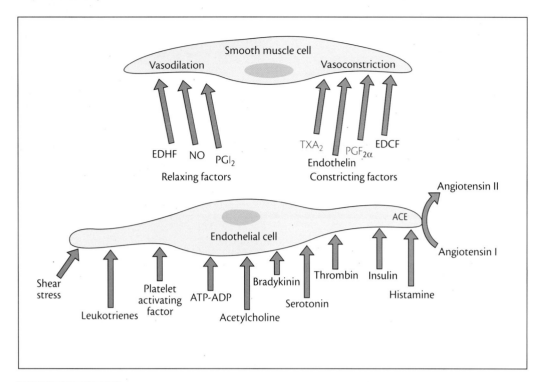

paracrine agents that alter vascular smooth muscle tone and influence tubular transport function. (Examples are shown.) Angiotensin-converting enzyme (ACE) is present on endothelial cells and converts angiotensin I to angiotensin II. Nitric oxide is formed by nitric oxide synthase, which cleaves nitric oxide from L-arginine. Nitric oxide diffuses from the endothelial cells to activate soluble guanylate cyclase and increases cyclic GMP (cGMP) levels in vascular smooth muscle cells, thus causing vasodilation. Agents that can stimulate nitric oxide are shown. The relative amounts of the various factors released by endothelial cells depend on the physiologic circumstances and pathophysiologic status. Thus, endothelial cells can exert vasodilator or vasoconstrictor effects. At least one major influence participating in the normal regulation of vascular tone is nitric oxide. EDCF—endothelial-derived constrictor factor; EDHF—endothelial-derived hyperpolarizing factor; PGF$_{2\alpha}$—prostaglandin F$_{2\alpha}$; PGI$_2$—prostaglandin I$_2$; TXA$_2$—thromboxane A$_2$. (*Adapted from* Navar *et al.* [1].)

FIGURE 5-2

Endothelial-derived factors. In addition to serving as a diffusion barrier, the endothelial cells lining the vasculature participate actively in the regulation of vascular function. They do so by responding to various circulating hormones and physical stimuli and releasing

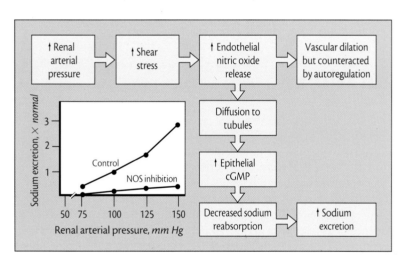

FIGURE 5-3

Nitric oxide in mediation of pressure natriuresis. Several recent studies have demonstrated that nitric oxide also directly affects tubular sodium transport and may be an important mediator of the changes induced by arterial pressure in sodium excretion, as described in Figure 1-5 [9,24]. Increases in arteriolar shear stress caused by increases in arterial pressure stimulate production of nitric oxide. Nitric oxide may exert direct effects to inhibit tubule sodium reabsorptive mechanisms and may elicit vasodilatory actions. Nitric oxide increases intracellular cyclic GMP (cGMP) in tubular cells, which leads to a reduced reabsorption rate through cGMP-sensitive sodium entry pathways [24,25]. When formation of nitric oxide is blocked by agents that prevent nitric oxide synthase activity, sodium excretion is reduced and the pressure natriuresis relationship is markedly suppressed. Thus, nitric oxide may exert a critical role in the regulation of arterial pressure by influencing vascular tone throughout the cardiovascular system and by serving as a mediator of the changes induced by the arterial pressure in tubular sodium reabsorption. (*Adapted from* Vari and Navar [3].)

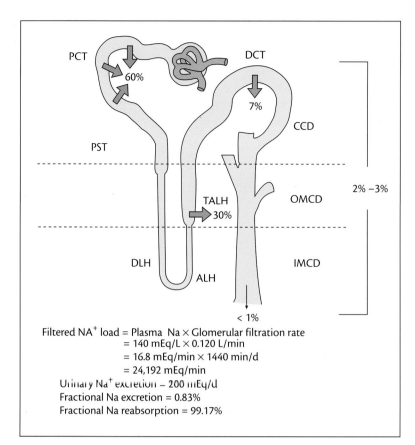

FIGURE 5-4

Tubular transport processes. Sodium excretion is the difference between the very high filtered load and net tubular reabsorption rate such that under normal conditions less than 1% of the filtered sodium load is excreted. The percentage of reabsorption of the filtered load occurring in each nephron segment is shown. The end result is that normally less than 1% of the filtered load is excreted; however, the exact excretion rate can be changed by many mechanisms. Despite the lesser absolute sodium reabsorption in the distal nephron segments, the latter segments are critical for final regulation of sodium excretion. Therefore, any factor that changes the delicate balance existing between the hemodynamically determined filtered load and the tubular reabsorption rate can lead to marked alterations in sodium excretion. ALH—thin ascending limb of the loop of Henle; CCD—cortical collecting duct; DCT—distal convoluted tubule; DLH—thin descending limb of the loop of Henle; IMCD—inner medullary collecting duct; OMCD—outer medullary collecting duct; PCT—proximal convoluted tubule; PST—proximal straight tubule; TALH—thick ascending limb of the loop of Henle.

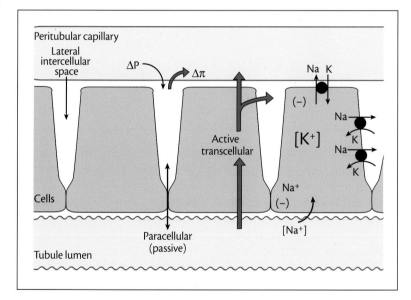

FIGURE 5-5

Proximal tubule reabsorptive mechanisms. The proximal tubule is responsible for reabsorption of 60% to 70% of the filtered load of sodium. Reabsorption is accomplished by a combination of both active and passive transport mechanisms that reabsorb sodium and other solutes from the lumen into the lateral spaces and interstitial compartment. The major driving force for this reabsorption is the basolateral sodium-potassium ATPase (Na^+-K^+ ATPase) that transports Na^+ out of the proximal tubule cells in exchange for K^+. As in most cells, this maintains a low intracellular Na^+ concentration and a high intracellular K^+ concentration. The low intracellular Na^+ concentration, along with the negative intracellular electrical potential, creates the electrochemical gradient that drives most of the apical transport mechanisms. In the late proximal tubule, a lumen to interstitial chloride concentration gradient drives additional net solute transport. The net solute transport establishes a small osmotic imbalance that drives transtubular water flow through both transcellular and paracellular pathways. In the tubule, water and solutes are reabsorbed isotonically (water and solute in equivalent proportions). The reabsorbed solutes and water are then further reabsorbed from the lateral and interstitial spaces into the peritubular capillaries by the colloid osmotic pressure, which establishes a predominant reabsorptive force. ΔP—transcapillary hydrostatic pressure gradient; $\Delta \pi$—transcapillary colloid osmotic pressure gradient.

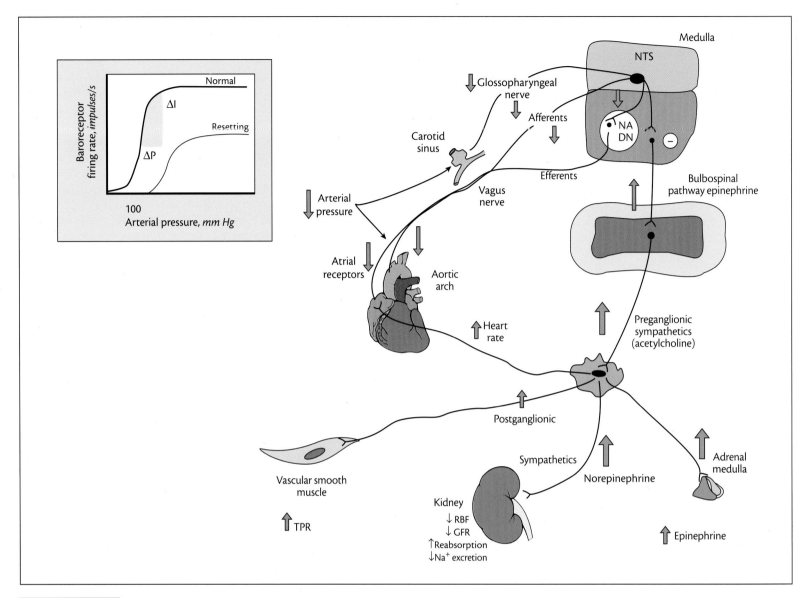

FIGURE 5-6

Neural and sympathetic influences. The neural reflexes serve as the principal mechanisms for the rapid regulation of arterial pressure. The neural reflexes also exert a long-term role by influencing sodium excretion. The pathways and effectors of the arterial baroreflex and atrial pressure-volume reflex are depicted. The *arrows* indicate increased or decreased activity in response to an acute reduction in arterial pressure that is sensed by the baroreceptors in the aortic arch and carotid sinus.

The *insert* depicts the relationship between the arterial blood pressure and baroreflex primary afferent firing rate. At the normal level of mean arterial pressure of approximately 100 mm Hg, the sensitivity ($\Delta I/\Delta P$) is set at the maximum level. After chronic resetting of the baroreceptors, the peak sensitivity and threshold of activation are shifted to a higher level of arterial pressure.

The cardiovascular reflexes involve *high-pressure* arterial receptors in the aortic arch and carotid sinus and *low-pressure* atrial receptors. In response to decreases in arterial pressure or vascular volume, increased sympathetic stimulation participates in short-term control of arterial pressure. This increased stimulation does

so by enhancing cardiac performance and stimulating vascular smooth muscle tone, leading to increased total peripheral resistance and decreased capacitance. The direct effects of the sympathetic nervous system on kidney function lead to decreased sodium excretion caused by decreases in filtered load and increases in tubular reabsorption [2].

The decreases in the glomerular filtration rate (GFR) and filtered sodium load are due to increases in both afferent and efferent arteriolar resistances and to decreases in the filtration coefficient. Sympathetic activation also enhances proximal sodium reabsorption by stimulating the sodium-hydrogen (Na^+-H^+) exchanger mechanism and by increasing the net chloride reabsorption by the thick ascending limb of the loop of Henle. The indirect effects include stimulation of renin secretion and angiotensin II formation, which also stimulates tubular reabsorption. ΔI—change in impulse firing; ΔP—change in pressure; DN—dorsal motor nucleus; NA—nucleus ambiguous; NTS—nucleus tractus solitarii; RBF—renal blood flow; TPR—total peripheral resistance. (*Adapted from* Vari and Navar [3].)

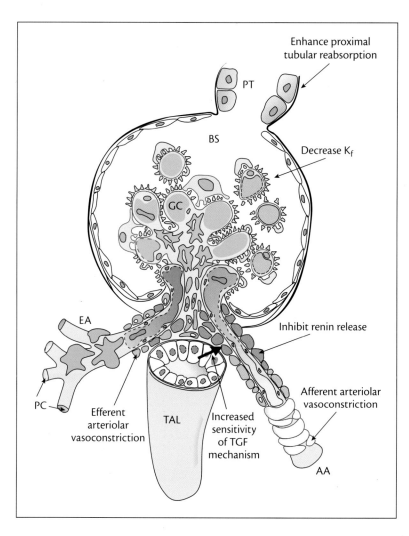

FIGURE 5-7

Angiotensin II actions on renal hemodynamics. Systemic and intrarenal angiotensin II exert powerful vasoconstrictive actions on the kidney to decrease renal blood flow and sodium excretion. At the level of the glomerulus, angiotensin II is a vasoconstrictor of both afferent (AA) and efferent arterioles (EA) and decreases the filtration coefficient K_f. Angiotensin II also directly inhibits renin release by the juxtaglomerular apparatus. Increased intrarenal angiotensin II also is responsible for the increased sensitivity of the tubuloglomerular feedback mechanism that occurs with decreased sodium chloride intake [4–6]. BS—Bowman's space; GC—glomerular capillaries; PC—peritubular capillaries; PT—proximal tubule; TAL—thick ascending limb; TGF—tubuloglomerular feedback mechanism. (*Adapted from* Arendshorst and Navar [4].)

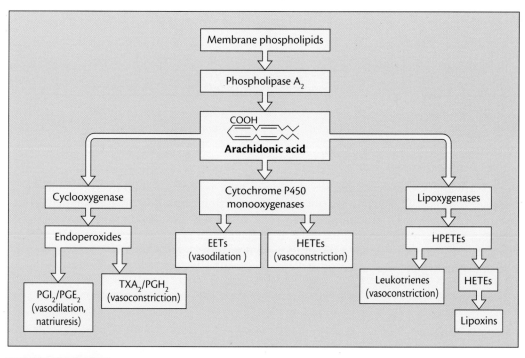

[8,9]. States of volume depletion and hypoperfusion stimulate prostaglandin synthesis [1,4,8].

The vasodilator prostaglandins attenuate the influence of vasoconstrictor substances during activation of the renin-angiotensin system, sympathetic nervous system, or both [10]. These prostaglandins also have transport effects on renal tubules through activation of distinct prostaglandin receptors [11]. In some pathophysiologic conditions, enhanced production of TXA_2 and other vasoconstrictor prostanoids may occur. The vasoconstriction induced by TXA_2 appears to be mediated primarily by calcium influx [4,11].

Leukotrienes are hydroperoxy fatty acid products of 5-hydroperoxyeicosatetraenoic acid (HPETE) that are synthesized by way of the lipoxygenase pathway. Leukotrienes are released in inflammatory and immunologic reactions and have been shown to stimulate renin release. The cytochrome P450 monooxygenases produce several vasoactive agents [1,7,12,13] usually referred to as EETs and hydroxy-eicosatetraenoic acids (HETEs). These substances exert actions on vascular smooth muscle and epithelial tissues [1,12,13].

FIGURE 5-8

Arachidonic acid metabolites. Several eicosanoids (arachidonic acid metabolites) are released locally and exert both vasoconstrictor and vasodilator effects as well as effects on tubular transport [1,7]. Phospholipase A_2 catalyzes formation of arachidonic acid (an unsaturated 20-carbon fatty acid) from membrane phospholipids. The cyclooxygenase pathway and various prostaglandin synthetases are responsible for the formation of endoperoxides (PGH_2), prostaglandins E_2 (PGE_2) and I_2 (PGI_2), and thromboxane (TXA_2)

Renal Parenchymal Disease and Hypertension

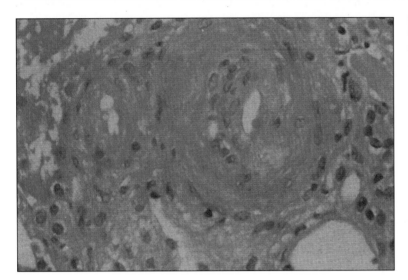

FIGURE 5-9 (*see* Color Plate)
Micrograph of an onion skin lesion from a patient with malignant hypertension.

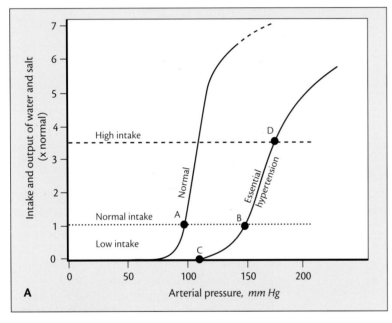

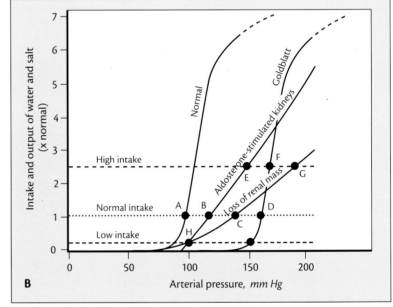

FIGURE 5-10

The relationship between renal artery perfusion pressure and sodium excretion (which defines "pressure natriuresis"). This relationship has been the subject of extensive research. **A,** Essential hypertension is characterized by higher renal perfusion pressures required to achieve daily sodium balance. **B,** Distortion of this relationship routinely occurs in patients with parenchymal renal disease, illustrated here as "loss of renal mass." Similar effects are observed in conditions with disturbed hormonal effects on sodium excretion (aldosterone-stimulated kidneys) or reduced renal blood flow as a result of an arterial stenosis ("Goldblatt" kidneys). In all of these instances, higher arterial pressures are required to maintain sodium balance.

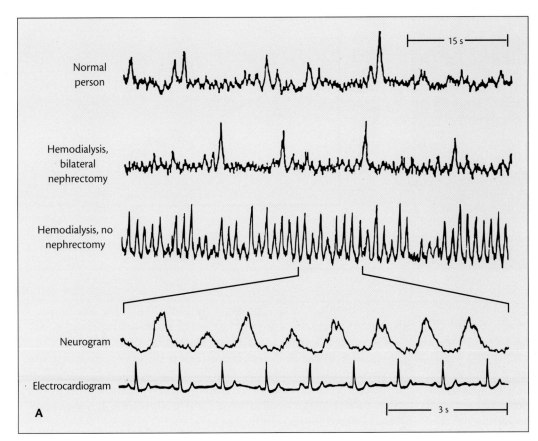

A

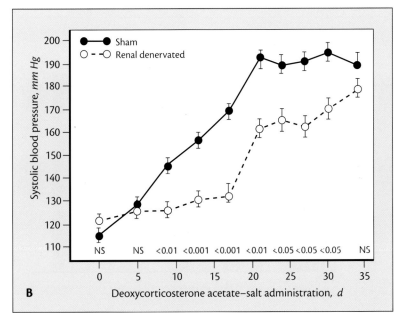

B

FIGURE 5-11

FIGURE 5-11

Sympathetic neural activation in chronic renal disease. Adrenergic activity is disturbed in chronic renal failure and may participate in the development of hypertension. **A,** Microneurographic studies in patients undergoing hemodialysis demonstrate enhanced neural traffic that relates closely to peripheral vascular tone [14]. Studies in patients in whom native kidneys are removed by nephrectomy demonstrate normal levels of neural traffic, suggesting that afferent stimuli from the kidney modulate central adrenergic outflow. **B,** Delayed-onset hypertension in denervated rats. This shows evidence from experimental studies in denervated animals subjected to deoxycorticosterone–salt hypertension. The role of the renal nerves in modifying the development of hypertension is supported by studies of renal denervation that show a delayed onset of hypertension, although no alteration in the final level of blood pressure was achieved. NS—not significant. (*Part A adapted from* Converse *et al.* [14]; *part B adapted from* Katholi *et al.* [15].)

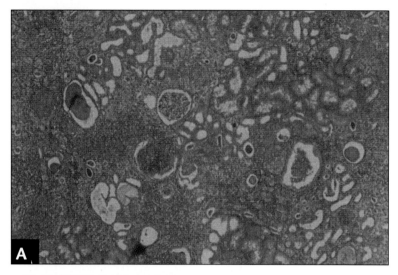

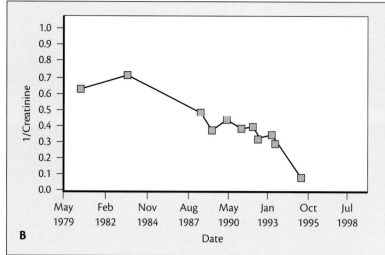

FIGURE 5-12 (see Color Plate)

Hypertension accelerates the rate of progressive renal failure in patients with parenchymal renal disease. **A,** Photomicrograph of malignant phase hypertension. Regardless of the cause of renal disease, untreated hypertension leads to more rapid loss of remaining nephrons and decline in glomerular filtration rates. A striking example of pressure-related injury may be observed in patients with malignant phase hypertension. This image is an open biopsy specimen obtained from a patient with papilledema, an expanding aortic aneurysm, and

blood pressure level at approximately 240/130 mm Hg. The biopsy specimen shows the following features of malignant nephrosclerosis: these patients develop vascular and glomerular injury, which can progress to irreversible renal failure. Before the introduction of antihypertensive drug therapy, patients with malignant phase hypertension routinely proceeded to uremia. Effective antihypertensive therapy can slow or reverse this trend in some but not all patients. **B,** Progressive renal failure in malignant hypertension over 8 years.

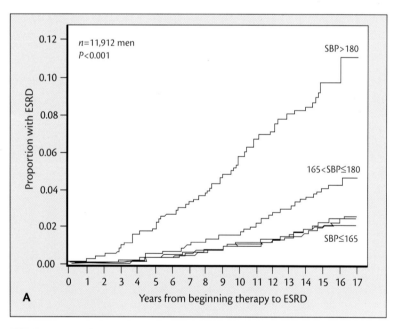

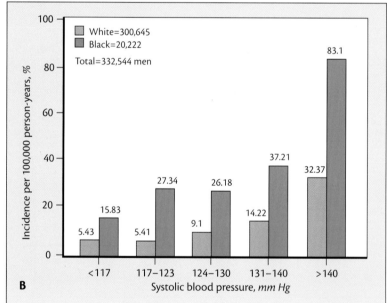

FIGURE 5-13

Blood pressure levels and rates of end-stage renal disease (ESRD). **A,** Line graph showing Kaplan-Meier estimates of ESRD rates; 15-year follow-up. **B,** Age-adjusted 16-year incidence of all-cause ESRD in men in the Multiple Risk Factor Intervention Trial (MRFIT). Large-scale epidemiologic studies indicate a progressive increase in the risk for developing ESRD as a function of systolic blood pressure levels. Follow-up of nearly 12,000 male veterans in the United States established that systolic blood pressure above 165 mm Hg at the initial visit was predictive of progressively higher risk of ESRD over a 15-year

follow-up period [16]. Similarly, follow-up studies after 16 years of more than 300,000 men in MRFIT demonstrated a progressive increase in the risk for ESRD, most pronounced in blacks [17]. These data suggest that blood pressure levels predict future renal disease. However, it remains uncertain whether benign essential hypertension itself induces a primary renal lesion (hypertensive renal disease *nephrosclerosis*) or acts as a catalyst in patients with other primary renal disease, otherwise not detected at initial screening. SBP—systolic blood pressure. (*Part A adapted from* Perry *et al.* [16].)

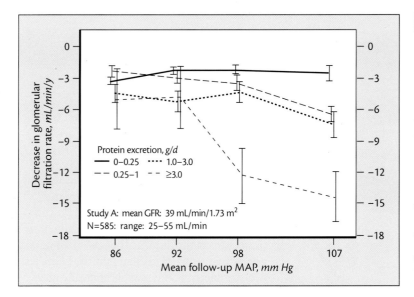

FIGURE 5-14

Blood pressure, proteinuria, and the rate of renal disease progression: results from the Modification of Diet in Renal Disease (MDRD) trial. Shown are rates of decrease of glomerular filtration rate (GFR) for patients enrolled in the MDRD trial, depending on level of achieved treated blood pressure during the trial [18]. A component of this trial included strict versus conventional blood pressure control. The term *strict* was defined as target mean arterial pressure (MAP) of under 92 mm Hg. The term *conventional* was defined as MAP of under 107 mm Hg. The rate of decline in GFR increased at higher levels of achieved MAP in patients with significant proteinuria (>3.0 g/d). No such relationship was evident over the duration of this trial (mean, 2.2 years) for patients with less severe proteinuria. These data emphasize the importance of blood pressure in determining disease progression in patients with proteinuric nondiabetic renal disease. No distinction was made in this study regarding the relative benefits of specific antihypertensive agents. (*From* Peterson *et al.* [18].)

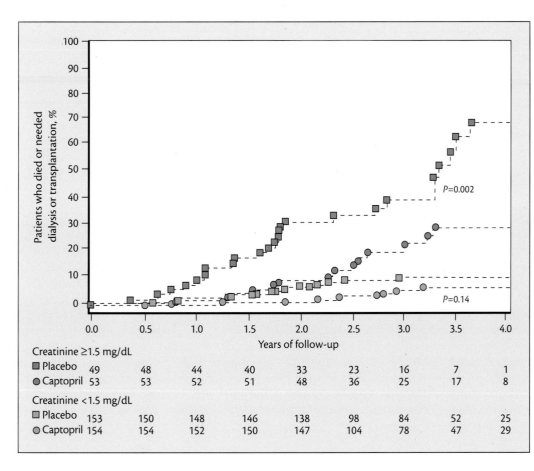

Creatinine ≥1.5 mg/dL

■ Placebo	49	48	44	40	33	23	16	7	1
● Captopril	53	53	52	51	48	36	25	17	8

Creatinine <1.5 mg/dL

■ Placebo	153	150	148	146	138	98	84	52	25
● Captopril	154	154	152	150	147	104	78	47	29

FIGURE 5-15

Angiotensin-converting enzyme (ACE) inhibitors and chronic renal disease. Progression of type I diabetic nephropathy to renal failure was reduced in the ACE inhibitor arm of a trial comparing conventional antihypertensive therapy with a regimen containing the ACE inhibitor captopril. All patients in this trial had significant proteinuria (>500 mg/d). The most striking effect of the ACE inhibitor regimen was seen in patients with higher serum creatinine levels (>1.5 mg/dL) as shown in the top two lines. It should be noted that calcium channel blocking drugs were excluded from this trial and the ACE inhibitor arm had somewhat lower arterial pressures during treatment. These data offer support to the concept that ACE inhibition lowers intraglomerular pressures, reduces proteinuria, and delays the progression of diabetic nephropathy by more mechanisms than can be explained by pressure reduction alone. (*Data from* Lewis *et al.* [19].)

Renovascular Hypertension and Ischemic Nephropathy

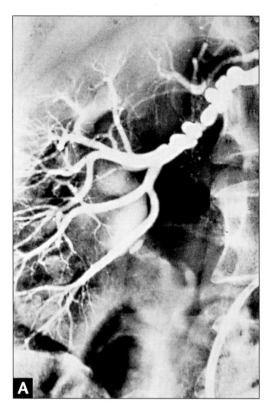

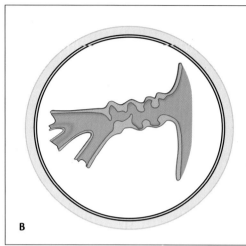

FIGURE 5-16

Arteriogram and schematic diagram of medial fibroplasia. **A,** Right renal arteriogram demonstrating weblike stenosis with interposed segments of dilatation (large beads) typical of medial fibroplasia ("string of beads" lesion). **B,** Schematic diagram of medial fibroplasia.

The lesion of medial fibroplasia characteristically affects the distal half of the main renal artery, frequently extending into the branches, is often bilateral, and angiographically gives the appearance of multiple aneurysms ("string of beads"). Histologically, this beaded lesion is characterized by areas of proliferation of fibroblasts of the media surrounded by fibrous connective tissue (stenosis) alternating with areas of medial thinning (aneurysms). Inspection of the renal angiogram in *part A* indicates that the width of areas of aneurysmal dilatation is wider than the nonaffected proximal renal artery, an angiographic clue to medial fibroplasia. (*Part A from* Pohl [20]; with permission.)

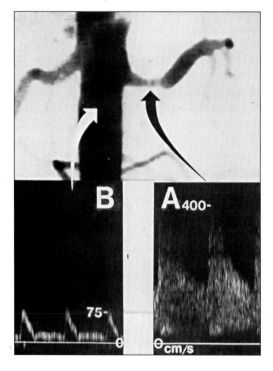

FIGURE 5-17

Renal duplex ultrasound for diagnosis of renal artery stenosis. Duplex ultrasound scanning of the renal arteries is a noninvasive screening test for the detection of renal artery stenosis. It combines direct visualization of the renal arteries (B-mode imaging) with measurement of various hemodynamic factors in the main renal arteries and within the kidney (Doppler), thus providing both an anatomic and functional assessment. Unlike other noninvasive screening tests (*eg*, captopril renography), duplex ultrasonography does not require patients to discontinue any antihypertensive medications before the test. The study should be performed while the patient is fasting. The *white arrow* indicates the aorta and the *black arrow* the left renal artery, which is stenotic. Doppler scans (*bottom*) measure the corresponding peak systolic velocities in the aorta and in the renal artery. The peak systolic velocity in the left renal artery was 400 cm/s, and the peak systolic velocity in the aorta was 75 cm/s. Therefore, the renal-aortic ratio was 5.3, consistent with a 60% to 99% left renal artery stenosis. (*From* Hoffman *et al.* [21]; with permission.)

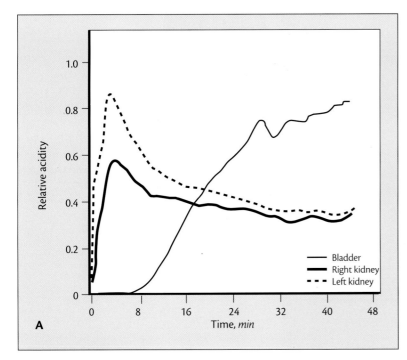

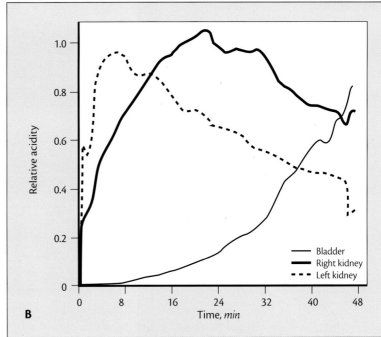

FIGURE 5-18

Captopril renography. **A,** TcDPTA time-activity curves during baseline. **B,** TcDPTA time-activity curves after captopril administration. These curves represent a captopril renogram in a patient with unilateral left renal artery stenosis. This diagnostic test has been used to screen for renal artery stenosis and to predict renovascular hypertension. Captopril renography appears to be highly sensitive and specific for detecting physiologically significant renal artery stenosis. Scintigrams and time-activity curves should both be analyzed to assess renal perfusion, function, and size. If the renogram following captopril administration is abnormal (*part B,* demonstrating delayed time to maximal activity and retention of the radionuclide in the right kidney), another renogram may be obtained without captopril for comparison. The diagnosis of renal artery stenosis is based on asymmetry of renal size and function and on specific, captopril-induced changes in the renogram, including delayed time to maximal activity ($\geq$11 minutes), significant asymmetry of the peak of each kidney, marked cortical retention of the radionuclide, and marked reduction in the calculated glomerular filtration rate of the kidney ipsilateral to the stenosis. One must interpret the clinical and renographic data with caution, as protocols are complex and diagnostic criteria are not well standardized. Nevertheless, captopril renography appears to be an improvement over the captopril provocation test, with many reports indicating sensitivity and specificity from 80% to 95% in predicting an improvement in blood pressure following intervention. (*Adapted from* Nally *et al.* [22].)

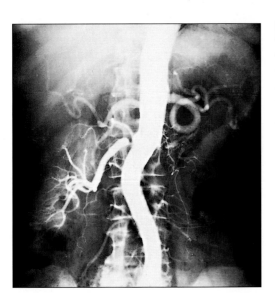

FIGURE 5-19

Aortogram in a 62-year-old white woman demonstrating subtotal occlusion of the left main renal artery supplying an atrophic left kidney and high-grade ostial stenosis of the proximal right renal artery from atherosclerosis. This patient presented in 1977 with a recent appearance of hypertension and a blood pressure of 170/115 mm Hg. Three years previously, when diagnosed with polycythemia vera, an IVP was normal. She was followed closely between 1974 and 1977 by her physician and was always normotensive until the hypertension suddenly appeared. A repeat rapid sequence IVP demonstrated a reduction in the size of the left kidney from 14 cm in height (1974) to 11.5 cm in height (1977). The serum creatinine was 2.6 mg/dL. The renal arteriogram shown here indicates high-grade bilateral renal artery stenosis with the left kidney measuring 11.5 cm in height, and the right kidney measuring 14.5 cm in height. Renal vein renins were obtained and lateralized strongly to the smaller left kidney. The blood pressure was well controlled with inderal and chlorthalidone. Right aortorenal reimplantation was undertaken solely to preserve renal function. Postoperatively the serum creatinine fell to 1.5 mg/dL and remained at this level for the next 13 years. Blood pressure continued to require antihypertensive medication, but was controlled to normal levels with inderal and chlorthalidone.

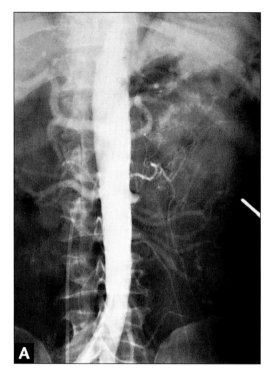
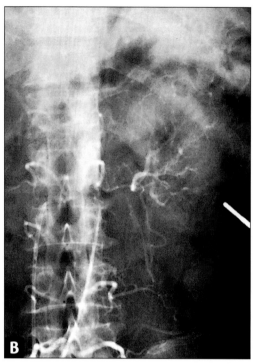

FIGURE 5-20

This abdominal aortogram reveals complete occlusion of the left main renal artery (*part A*) with filling of the distal renal artery branches from collateral supply on delayed films (*part B*). The observation of collateral circulation when the main renal artery is totally occluded proximally suggests viable renal parenchyma. (*From* Novick and Pohl [23]; with permission.)

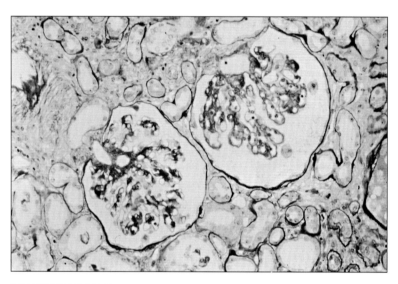

FIGURE 5-21

Renal biopsy of a solitary left kidney in a 67-year-old woman who had been anuric and on chronic dialysis for 9 months. The biopsy shows hypoperfused retracted glomeruli consistent with ischemia. There is no evidence of active glomerular proliferation or glomerular sclerosis. Note intact tubular basement membranes and negligible interstitial scarring. Left renal revascularization resulted in recovery of renal function and discontinuance of dialysis with improvement in scrum creatinine to 2.0 mg/dL. (*From* Novick [24]; with permission.)

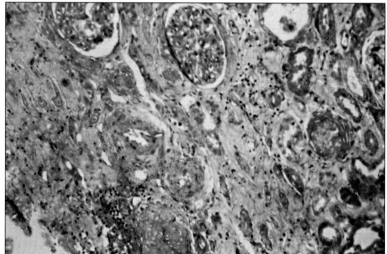

FIGURE 5-22

Pathologic specimen of kidney beyond a main renal artery occlusion in a patient with severe bilateral renal artery stenosis and a serum creatinine of 4.5 mg/dL. The biopsy demonstrates glomerular sclerosis, tubular atrophy, and interstitial fibrosis. The magnitude of glomerular and interstitial scarring predict irreversible loss of kidney viability. (*From* Pohl [20]; with permission.)

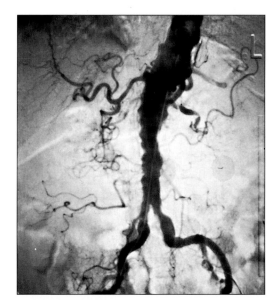

FIGURE 5-23

Severe atherosclerosis involving the abdominal aorta, renal, and iliac arteries. This abdominal aortogram demonstrates a ragged aorta, total occlusion of the right main renal artery, and subtotal occlusion of the proximal left main renal artery. Such patients are at high risk for atheroembolic renal disease following aortography, selective renal arteriography, percutaneous transluminal renal angioplasty, renal artery stenting, or surgical renal revascularization.

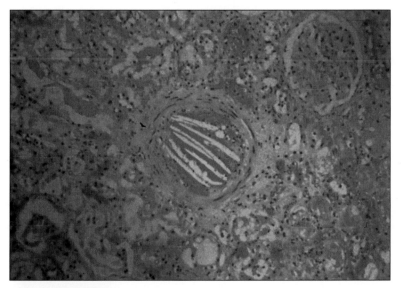

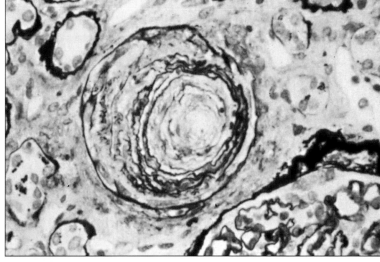

FIGURE 5-24

Pathologic specimen of kidney demonstrating atheroembolic renal disease (AERD). Microemboli of atheromatous material are readily identified by the characteristic appearance of cholesterol crystal inclusions that appear in a biconvex needle-shaped form. In routine paraffin-embedded histologic sections, the cholesterol is not seen because the methods used in preparing sections dissolve the crystals; the characteristic biconvex clefts in the glomeruli (or blood vessels) persist, allowing easy identification. Several patterns of renal failure in patients with AERD are recognized: 1) insult (eg, abdominal aortogram) leads to end-stage renal disease (ESRD) over weeks to months; 2) insult leads to chronic stable renal insufficiency; 3) multiple insults (repeated angiographic procedures) lead to a step-wise rise in serum creatinine eventuating in end-stage renal failure; and 4) insult leading to ESRD over several weeks to months with recovery of some renal function allowing for discontinuance of dialysis.

FIGURE 5-25

Renal biopsy demonstrating severe arteriolar nephrosclerosis. Arteriolar nephrosclerosis is intimately associated with hypertension. The histology of the kidney in arteriolar nephrosclerosis shows considerable variation in intensity and extent of the arteriolar lesions. Thickening of the vessel wall, edema of the smooth muscle cells, hypertrophy of the smooth muscle cells, and hyaline degeneration of the vessel wall may be apparent depending on the severity of the nephrosclerosis. In addition to the vascular lesions of arteriolar nephrosclerosis, there are abnormalities of glomeruli, tubules, and interstitial areas that are believed to be secondary to the ischemia that results from arteriolar insufficiency. Arteriolar nephrosclerosis is observed in patients with longstanding hypertension; the more severe the hypertension, the more severe the arteriolar nephrosclerosis. Arteriolar nephrosclerosis may also be seen in elderly normotensive individuals and is frequently observed in elderly patients with generalized atherosclerosis or essential hypertension.

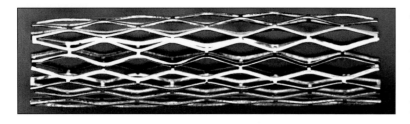

FIGURE 5-26

Palmaz stent, expanded. Because percutaneous transluminal renal angioplasty (PTRA) has suboptimal long-term benefits for athero-sclerotic ostial renal artery stenosis, endovascular stenting has gained wide acceptance. Renal artery stenting may be performed at the time of the diagnostic angiogram, or at some time thereafter, depending on the physician's preference and the risk to the patient of repeated angiographic procedures. From a technical standpoint, indications for renal artery stenting include 1) as a primary procedure for ostial atherosclerotic renal artery disease (ASO-RAD), 2) technical difficulties in conjunction with attempted PTRA, 3) post-PTRA dissection, 4) post-PTRA abrupt occlusion, and 5) restenosis following PTRA. It is unclear what the long-term patency and restenosis rates will be for renal artery stenting for ostial disease. Preliminary observations suggest that the 1-year patency rate for stents is approximately twice that for PTRA.

Adrenal Causes of Hypertension

PHYSIOLOGIC MECHANISMS IN ADRENAL HYPERTENSION

Disorder	Cause	Pathophysiology	Pressure mechanism
Primary aldosteronism	Autonomous hypersecretion of aldosterone (hypermineralocorticoidism)	Increased renal sodium and water reabsorption, increased urinary excretion of potassium and hydrogen ions	Extracellular fluid volume expansion, hypokalemia (?), alkalosis
Cushing's syndrome	Hypersecretion of cortisol (hyperglucocorticoidism)	Increased activation of mineralocorticoid receptor (?), increased angiotensinogen (renin substrate) concentration	Extracellular fluid volume expansion (?), increased angiotensin II (vasoconstriction and increased peripheral resistance)
Pheochromocytoma	Hypersecretion of catecholamines	Vasoconstriction, increased heart rate	Increased peripheral resistance, increased cardiac output

FIGURE 5-27

The causes and pathophysiologies of the three major forms of adrenal hypertension and the proposed mechanisms by which blood pressure elevation results.

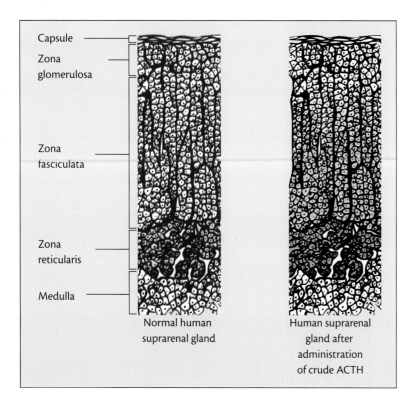

Capsule

Zona glomerulosa

Zona fasciculata

Zona reticularis

Medulla

Normal human suprarenal gland

Human suprarenal gland after administration of crude ACTH

FIGURE 5-28

Histology of the adrenal. A cross section of the normal adrenal before (*left*) and after (*right*) stimulation with adrenocorticotropic hormone (ACTH) [25]. The adrenal is organized into the outer adrenal cortex and the inner adrenal medulla. The outer adrenal cortex is composed of the zona glomerulosa, zona fasciculata, and zona reticularis. The zona glomerulosa is responsible for production of aldosterone and other mineralocorticoids and is chiefly under the control of angiotensin II. The zona fasciculata and zona reticularis are influenced primarily by ACTH and produce glucocorticoids and some androgens. The adrenal medulla produces catecholamines and is the major source of epinephrine (in addition to the organ of Zuckerkandl located at the aortic bifurcation).

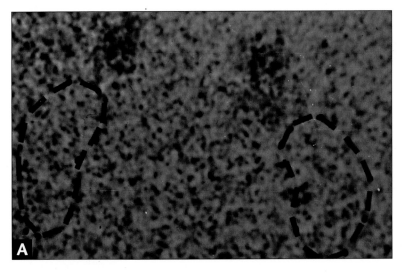
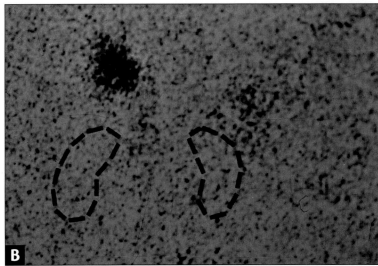

FIGURE 5-29

Normal and abnormal adrenal isotopic scans. **A,** Normal scan. Increased bilateral uptake of I^{131}-labeled iodo-cholesterol of normal adrenal tissue is shown above the indicated renal outlines.

B, Intense increase in isotopic uptake by the left adrenal (as viewed from the posterior aspect) containing an adenoma.

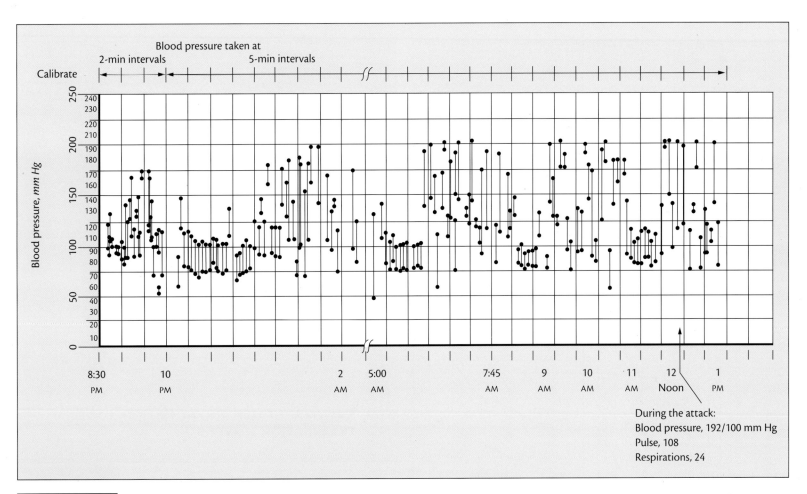

FIGURE 5-30

Paroxysmal blood pressure pattern in pheochromocytoma. Note the extreme variability of blood pressure in this patient with pheochromocytoma during ambulatory blood pressure monitoring [26]. Whereas most levels were within the normal range, episodic increases to levels of 200/140 mm Hg were observed. Such paroxysms can be spontaneous or associated with activity of many sorts. (*Adapted from* Manger and Gifford [26].)

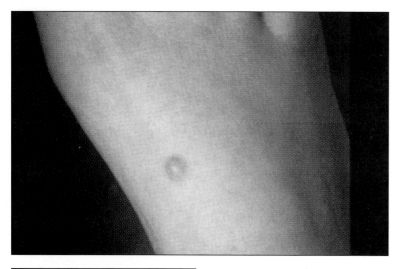

FIGURE 5-31 (*see* Color Plate)

Neurofibroma associated with pheochromocytoma. Neurofibromas are sometimes found in patients with pheochromocytoma. These lesions are soft, fluctuant, and nontender and can appear anywhere on the surface of the skin. These lesions can be seen in profile in Figure 5-32.

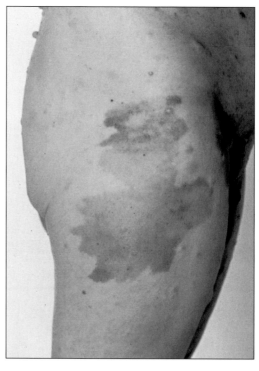

FIGURE 5-32

Café au lait lesions in a patient with pheochromocytoma. These light-brown-colored (coffee-with-cream-colored) lesions, sometimes seen in patients with pheochromocytoma, usually are larger than 3 cm in the largest dimension. In this particular patient, neurofibromas also are present and can be seen in profile.

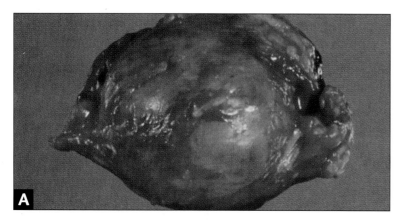

FIGURE 5-33 (*see* Color Plates)

A and B, Pathologic appearance of pheochromocytoma before (*part A*) and after (*part B*) sectioning. This 3.5-cm-diameter tumor had gross areas of hemorrhage noted by the dark areas visible in the photographs.

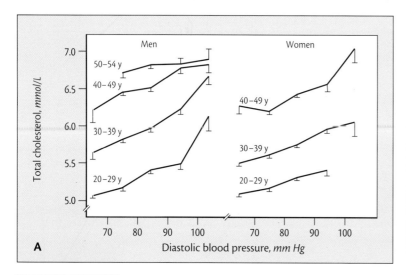

FIGURE 5-34

Hyperlipidemia and hypertension. **A,** Epidemiologic studies document an association between serum cholesterol and blood pressure in men and women. **B,** Based on data from the National Health and Nutrition Examination Survey II, persons with hypertension have a high prevalence of hyperlipidemia and vice versa [27]. (*Part A adapted from* Bonna and Thelle [28].)

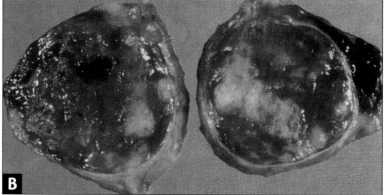

B. NATIONAL HEALTH AND NUTRITION EXAMINATION SURVEY II

1. Persons with blood pressure >140/90 mm Hg or taking medication for hypertension: 40% have cholesterol >240 mg/dL
2. Persons with blood cholesterol >240 mg/dL: 46% have blood pressure >140/90 mm Hg

Insulin Resistance and Hypertension

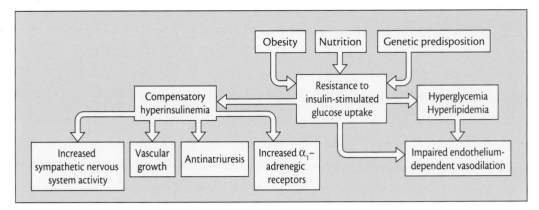

FIGURE 5-35

Hypertension associated with insulin resistance. It is unclear whether hyperinsulinemia associated with insulin resistance causes hypertension, although a number of potential mechanisms have been proposed.

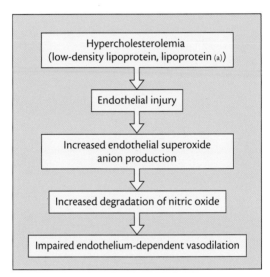

FIGURE 5-36

Metabolic consequences of insulin resistance. These consequences also may affect peripheral vascular resistance. Hypercholesterolemia may result in vascular endothelial injury and, hence, impaired vasodilation.

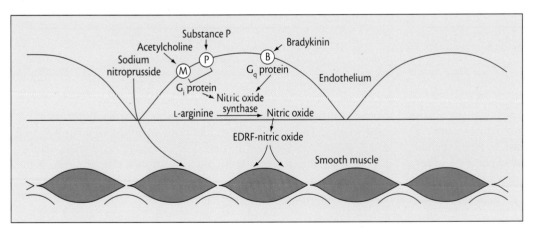

FIGURE 5-37

Impaired endothelium-dependent vascular relaxation and insulin resistance. Insulin resistance is associated with impaired endothelium-dependent vascular relaxation, which is a defect that may be corrected by insulin-sensitizing agents. One approach to evaluating vascular endothelial function is to measure vascular relaxation in response to acetylcholine. EDRF—endothelium-derived relaxing factor.

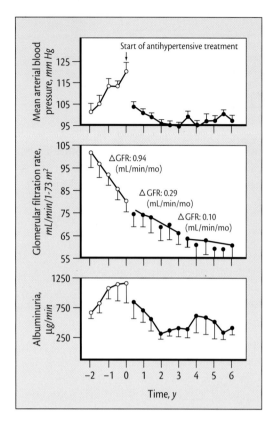

FIGURE 5-38

Course of diabetic nephropathy during effective antihypertensive treatment in patients with overt diabetic nephropathy. Effective antihypertensive therapy with regimens that include diuretics also decreases the rate of progression of renal failure (both the glomerular filtration rate and albumin excretion) in patients with diabetic nephropathy. (*Adapted from* Parving *et al.* [29].)

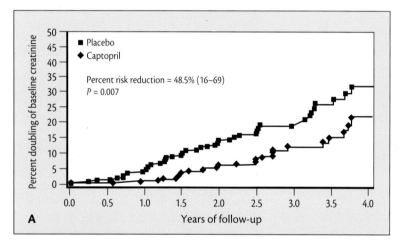

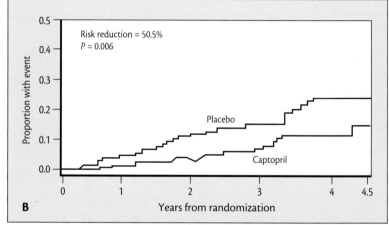

FIGURE 5-39

Cumulative incidence of events in patients with diabetic nephropathy in captopril and placebo groups. **A,** Time to doubling of serum creatinine. **B,** Time to end-stage renal disease or death. In type I diabetic patients with nephropathy and either normal blood pressure or hypertension, treatment with angiotensin-converting enzyme inhibitors decreases proteinuria and retards the rate of progression of renal insufficiency. The cumulative incidence of doubling of serum creatinine concentrations over time and development of end-stage renal disease are less in patients treated with captopril than in those treated with placebo. (*Adapted from* Lewis *et al.* [30].)

The Role of Hypertension in Progression of Chronic Renal Disease

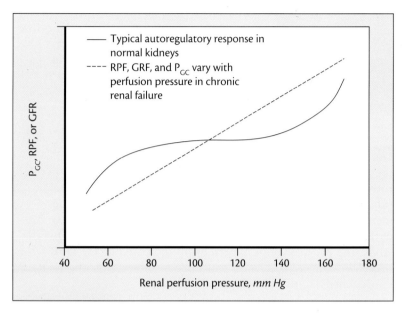

FIGURE 5-40

Imaginary autoregulation curves in normal and diseased kidneys. Plotted on the y-axis are renal plasma flow (RPF), glomerular filtration rate (GFR), and glomerular capillary hydraulic pressure (P_{GC}) with undefined units. Ordinarily, RPF, GFR, and P_{GC} remain relatively constant over a wide range of perfusion pressures within the physiologic range, from approximately 80 to 140 mm Hg. Because autoregulatory ability is impaired in the kidneys of persons with chronic renal disease, these patients who develop systemic hypertension also are likely to have glomerular hypertension.

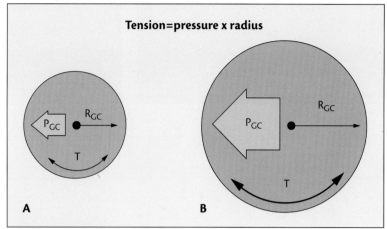

FIGURE 5-41

The wall tension hypothesis. **A,** Normal. **B,** Chronic renal failure. After a partial loss of kidney function, compensatory adaptations within surviving nephrons include renal vasodilation. Vasodilation leads to an increase in glomerular capillary pressure and compensatory renal growth associated with an increase in the radius of the glomerular capillaries. According to the LaPlace equation, wall tension in a blood vessel is equal to the product of the transmural pressure and the radius of the vessel. In a surviving glomerular capillary of a damaged kidney, therefore, wall tension increases not only because of the increase in glomerular pressure but also because of an increase in capillary radius. Elevations in wall tension contribute to progressive renal disease by damaging the endothelial and epithelial cells lining the glomerular capillaries. By reducing wall tension, maneuvers that decrease either glomerular pressure or glomerular capillary radius are predicted to be beneficial. P_{GC}—glomerular capillary hydraulic pressure; R_{GC}—glomerular capillary radius; T—tension. (*Adapted from* Dworkin and Benstein [31].)

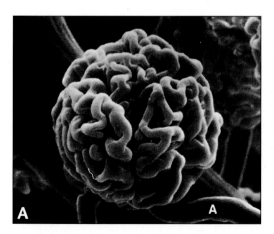 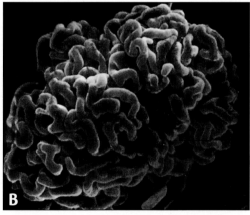

FIGURE 5-42

Scanning electron micrographs of vascular casts of glomeruli from normal or uninephrectomized rats. **A,** A glomerulus from a rat having had a sham operation, showing a uniform capillary pattern. (Parts *B–D* display casts from uninephrectomized rats.) **B,** A uniform pattern with most capillaries being approximately the same size.

(*Continued on next page*)

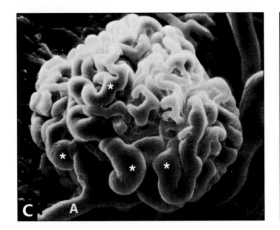
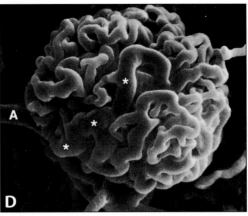

FIGURE 5-42 (continued)

C and D, Nonuniform patterns in which individual capillary loops (indicated by *asterisks*) are markedly dilated. In dilated capillary loops, wall tension is elevated and capillary wall damage is most likely to occur. The segmental nature of the capillary dilation may explain why glomerular sclerosis that eventually develops in remnant kidneys is also focal in early stages of the disease process. (Magnification of parts A through D, × 320.) (*From* Nagata *et al.* [32]; with permission.)

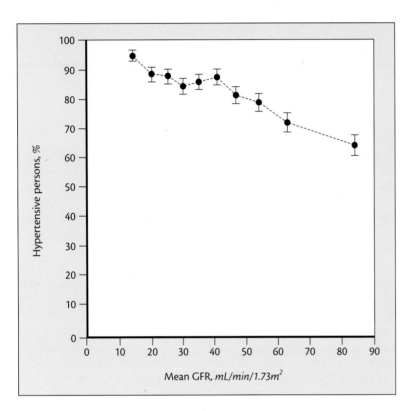

FIGURE 5-43

Hypertension prevalence corresponds with decreased glomerular filtration rate (GFR). Hypertension is common in glomerular, tubular, vascular, and interstitial renal disease and becomes increasingly prevalent as renal function declines. In almost 200 patients screened for the Modification of Diet in Renal Disease study, the prevalence of hypertension increased as the GFR decreased and hypertension was almost universal as the GFR approached 10 mL/min [33].

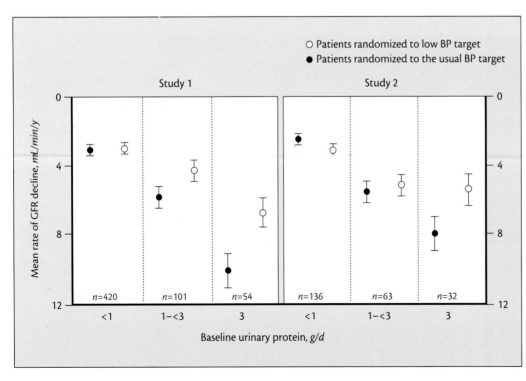

FIGURE 5-44

Two patient groups in the study of diet in renal disease. The Modification of Diet in Renal Disease (MDRD) study involved two patient groups. The group in which patients had moderate renal dysfunction (glomerular filtration rate [GFR] between 25 and 55 mL/min) was called Study 1. The other group, which included patients who had more severe renal dysfunction (with a GFR between 13 and 24 mL/min) was called Study 2. The effects of the lower blood pressure (BP) target on patients with proteinuria in Studies 1 and 2 are shown. The y-axis divides patients in Studies 1 and 2 into three groups, depending on urinary protein excretion. The x-axis represents the rate of GFR decline. In the subset of patients in the MDRD trial in both Studies 1 and 2 who had massive proteinuria (protein over 3 g/24 h), the lower blood pressure had an especially salutary effect: the decline in GFR was much slower [34].

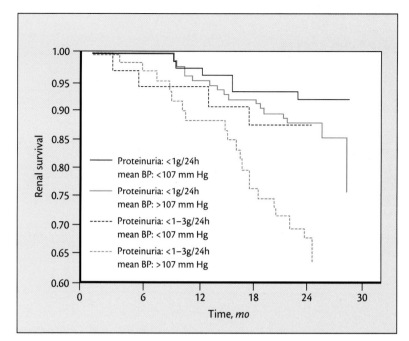

FIGURE 5-45

Proteinuria as a marker for progressive renal disease. Nephrotic proteinuria may be a more important and independent marker for progression of renal disease than is hypertension. That is, patients in whom massive proteinuria and hypertension coexist have the worst renal prognosis. In a study of over 400 patients with renal insufficiency followed over 2 years, Locatelli *et al.* [35] found that patients who had both a mean blood pressure (BP) higher than 107 mm Hg and protein excretion of 1 to 3 g/24 h had the lowest rates of renal survival.

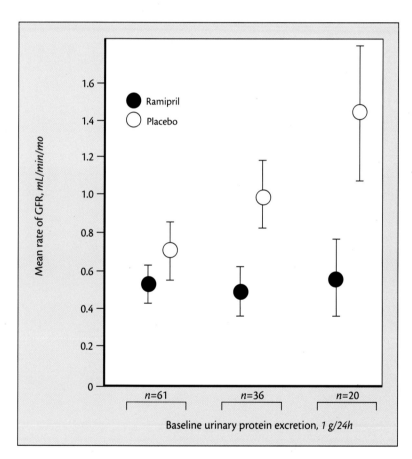

FIGURE 5-46

Study of patients with renal disease not associated with diabetes who were randomly assigned to ramipril or placebo. Blood pressure and proteinuria decreased more significantly in the patients treated with ramipril. This group had significantly lower rates of decline in glomerular filtration rate (GFR) over time. This effect was increasingly striking as the baseline level of proteinuria increased and was most pronounced in patients with a urinary protein excretion of over 7 g per 24 hours.

Pharmacologic Treatment of Hypertension

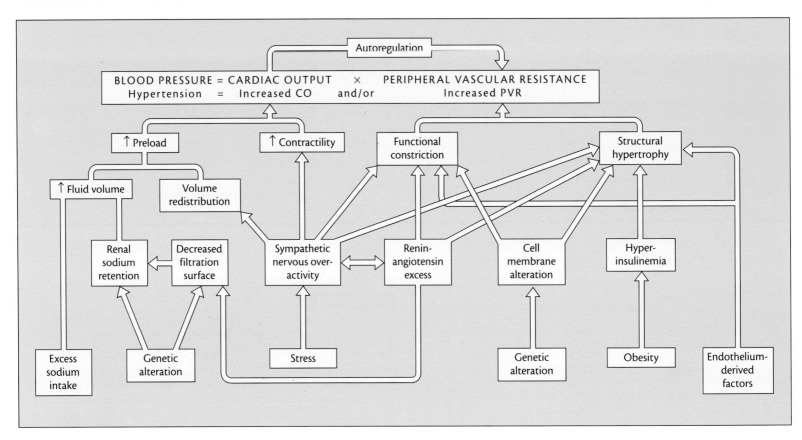

FIGURE 5-47

Pathogenesis of hypertension. Mean arterial pressure (MAP) is the product of cardiac output (CO) and peripheral vascular resistance (PVR). There are a large number of control mechanisms involved in every type of hypertension. (*Adapted from* Kaplan [36].)

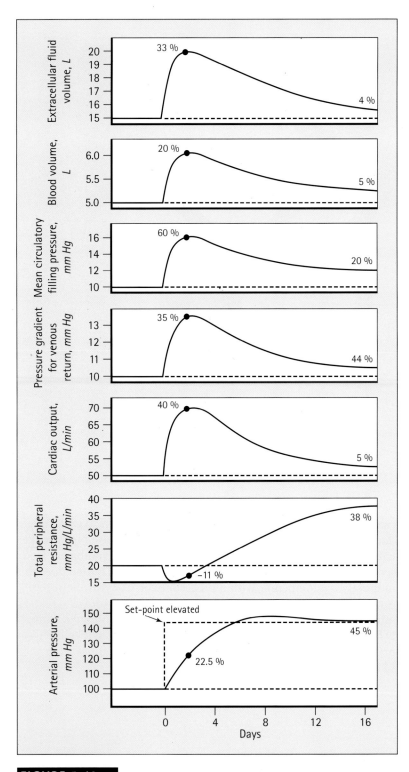

FIGURE 5-48

Cardiac output. An increase in cardiac output has been suggested as a mechanism for hypertension, particularly in its early borderline phase [37,38]. Sodium and water retention have been theorized to be the initiating events. Sequential changes following salt loading are depicted [37]. The resultant high cardiac output perfuses the peripheral tissues in excess of their metabolic requirements, resulting in a normal autoregulatory (vasoconstrictor) pressure. The early phase of high cardiac output and normal peripheral vascular resistance gradually changes to the characteristic feature of the sustained hypertensive state: normal cardiac output and high peripheral vascular resistance. Shown here are segmental changes in the important cardiovascular hemodynamic variables in the first few weeks following the onset of short-term salt-loading hypertension. Note especially that the arterial pressure increases ahead of the increase in total peripheral resistance. (*Adapted from* Guyton *et al.* [37].)

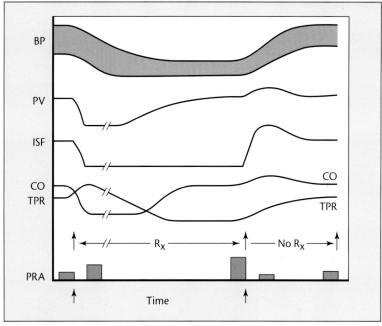

FIGURE 5-49

Hemodynamic response to diuretics. Diuretics reduce mean arterial pressure by their initial natriuretic effect [39]. Acutely, this is achieved by a reduction in cardiac output mediated by a reduction in plasma and extracellular fluid volumes [40]. Initially, peripheral vascular resistance is increased, mediated in part by stimulation of the renin-angiotensin system. During sustained diuretic therapy, cardiac output returns to pretreatment levels, probably reflecting restoration of plasma volume. Chronic blood pressure control now correlates with a reduction in peripheral vascular resistance. BP—blood pressure; CO—cardiac output; ISF—interstitial fluid; PRA—plasma renin activity; PV—plasma volume; Rx—treatment; TPR—total peripheral resistance. (*Adapted from* Tarazi [40].)

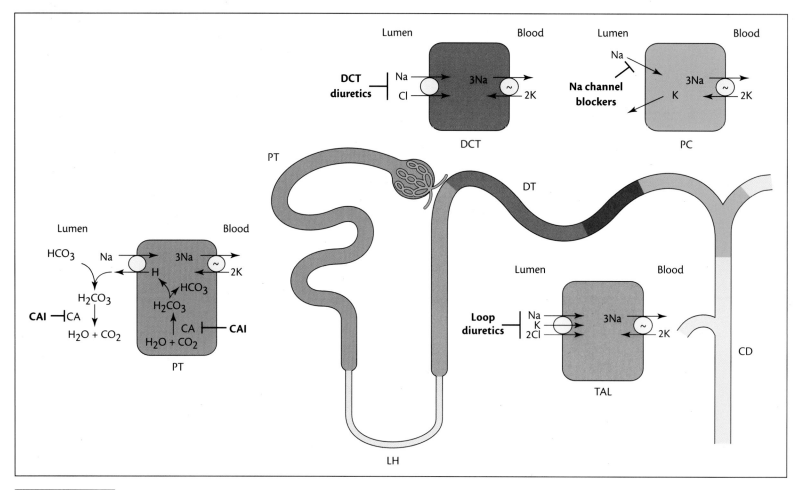

FIGURE 5-50

The major sites and mechanisms of action of diuretic drugs [41]. The diuretic/natriuretic action of benzothiadiazide-type diuretics is predicated on their gaining access to the luminal side of the distal convoluted tubule and inhibiting Na+Cl- cotransport by competing for the chloride site.

The diuretic/natriuretic action of loop diuretics is predicated on their gaining access to the luminal side of the thick ascending limb of the loop of Henle and inhibiting Na+K+2Cl- electroneutral cotransport by competing for the chloride site.

The diuretic/natriuretic action of potassium-sparing diuretics is predicated on their gaining access to the luminal side of the prin-

cipal cells located in the late distal tubule and cortical collecting duct and blocking luminal sodium channels. Because Na+ uptake is blocked, the lumen negative voltage is reduced, inhibiting K+ secretion. The potassium-sparing diuretic spironolactone does this indirectly by competing with aldosterone for its cytosolic receptor. CA—carbonic anhydrase; CAI—carbonic anhydrase inhibitor; CD—collecting duct; DCT—distal convoluted tubule; DT—distal tubule; LH—loop of Henle; PC—principal cell; PT—proximal tubule; TAL—thick ascending limb. (*Adapted from* Ellison [41].)

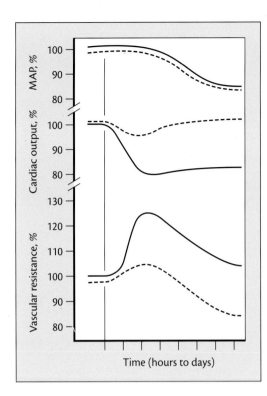

FIGURE 5-51

Hemodynamic changes associated with β-adrenergic blockade. Time course of hemodynamic changes after treatment with a β-adrenergic blocker devoid of partial agonist activity (PAA) (*solid line*) as compared with hemodynamic changes after administration of a β-adrenergic blocker with sufficient PAA to replace basal sympathetic tone (*eg*, pindolol) (*broken line*). MAP—mean arterial pressure. (*Adapted from* Man in't Veld and Schalekamp [42].)

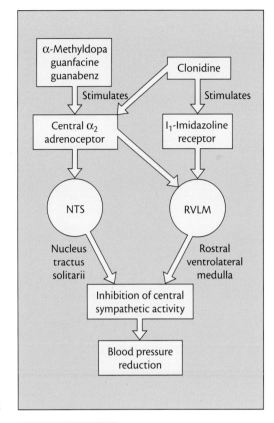

FIGURE 5-52

Physiologic effect of central α₂-adrenergic agonists. Central α₂-adrenergic agonists cross the blood-brain barrier and stimulate α₂-adrenergic receptors in the vasomotor center of the brain stem [39,43]. Stimulation of these receptors decreases sympathetic tone, brain turnover of norepinephrine, and central sympathetic outflow and activity of the preganglionic sympathetic nerves. The net effect is a reduction in norepinephrine release. The central α₂-adrenergic agonist clonidine also binds to imidazole receptors in the brain; activation of these receptors inhibits central sympathetic outflow. Central α₂-adrenergic agonists may also stimulate the peripheral α₂-adrenergic receptors that mediate vasoconstriction; this effect predominates at high plasma drug concentrations and may precipitate an increase in blood pressure. The usual physiologic effect is a decrease in peripheral resistance and slowing of the heart rate; however, output is either unchanged or mildly decreased. Preservation of cardiovascular reflexes prevents postural hypotension.

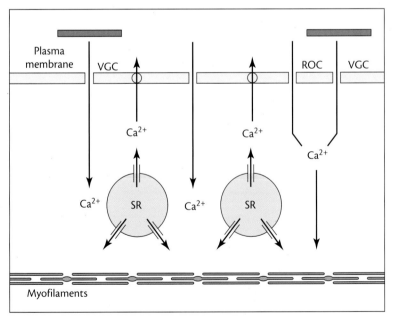

FIGURE 5-53

Calcium antagonists. The calcium antagonists share a common antihypertensive mechanism of action: inhibition of calcium ion movement into smooth muscle cells of resistance arterioles through L-type (long-lasting) voltage-operated channels [39,43]. The ability of these drugs to bind to voltage-operated channels, causing closure of the gate and subsequent inhibition of calcium flux from the extracellular to the intracellular space, inhibits the essential role of calcium as an intracellular messenger, uncoupling excitation to contraction. Calcium ions may also enter cells through receptor-operated channels. The opening of these channels is induced by binding neurohumoral mediators to specific receptors on the cell membrane. Calcium antagonists inhibit the calcium influx triggered by the stimulation of either α-adrenergic or angiotensin II receptors in a dose-dependent manner, inhibiting the influence of α-adrenergic agonist and angiotensin II on vascular smooth muscle tone. The net physiologic effect is a decrease in vascular resistance.

Although all the calcium antagonists share a basic mechanism of action, they are a highly heterogeneous group of compounds that differ markedly in their chemical structure, pharmacologic effects on tissue specificity, pharmacologic behavior side effect profile, and clinical indications [39,43,44]. Thus, calcium antagonists have been subdivided into several distinct classes: phenylalkamines, dihydropyridines, and benzothiazepines. ROC—receptor-operated channel; SR—sarcoplasmic reticulum; VGC—voltage-gated channels.

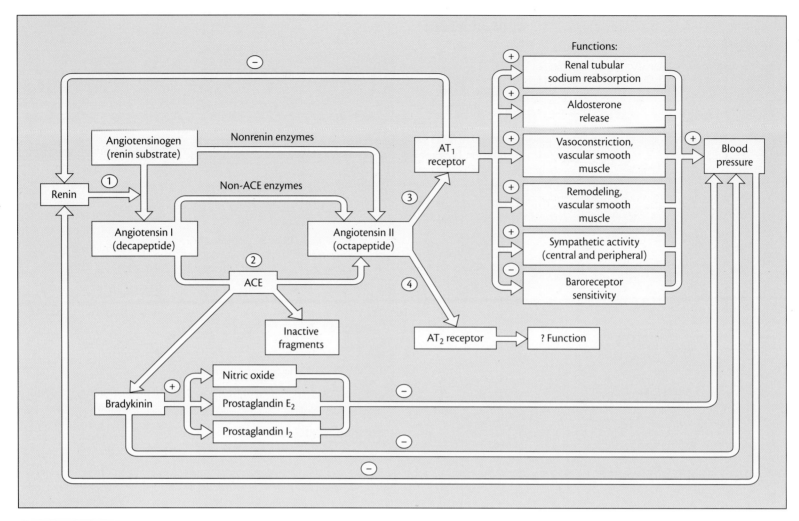

FIGURE 5-54

Mechanisms for decrease in peripheral vascular resistance. Angiotensin-converting enzyme (ACE) inhibitors and angiotensin II type I receptor antagonists lower blood pressure by decreasing peripheral vascular resistance; there is usually little change in heart rate or cardiac output [39,43,45]. Mechanisms proposed for the observed decrease in peripheral resistance are shown [45]. Sites of pharmacologic blockade in the renin angiotensin system include 1) renin inhibitors, 2) ACE inhibitors, 3) angiotensin II type I receptor antagonists, and 4) angiotensin II type II receptor antagonists.

JNC VI CLASSIFICATION OF HYPERTENSION

Category*	Systolic (mm Hg)		Diastolic (mm Hg)
Optimal†	<120	and	<80
Normal	<130	and	<85
High normal	130–139	or	85–89
Hypertension‡			
Stage 1	140/159	or	90/99
Stage 2	160/179	or	100/109
Stage 3	≥-180	or	≥110

*Not taking antihypertensive drugs and not acutely ill. When systolic and diastolic blood pressures fall into different categories, the higher category should be selected to classify the individual's blood pressure status. For example, 160/92 mm Hg should be classified as stage 2 hypertension, and 174/120 mm Hg should be classified as stage 3 hypertension. Isolated systolic hypertension is defined as systolic blood pressure of 140 mm Hg or greater and diastolic blood pressure of less than 90 mm Hg and staged appropriately (eg, 170/82 mm Hg is defined as stage 2 isolated hypertension). In addition to classifying stages of hypertension on the basis of average blood pressure levels, clinicians should specify presence of target organ disease and additional risk factors. This specifically is important for risk classification.

†Optimal blood pressure with respect to cardiovascular risk is below 120/80 mm Hg. Unusually low readings should be evaluated for clinical significance.

‡Based on the average of two or more readings taken at each of two or more visits after an initial screening.

FIGURE 5-55

Prevention and treatment of high blood pressure. The aim of antihypertensive therapy is risk reduction. Because the relationship between blood pressure and cardiovascular risk is continuous, the goal of treatment might be the maximum tolerated reduction in blood pressure. There is controversy concerning what constitutes hypertension and how far systolic or diastolic blood pressure should be lowered, however. The Sixth Report of the Joint National Committee on Detection, Evaluation, and Treatment of High Blood Pressure (JNC VI) [46] provides a new classification of hypertension and recommends that risk stratification be used to determine if lifestyle modification or drug therapy with adjunctive lifestyle modification be initiated according to the patient's blood pressure classification. Major risk factors include smoking, dyslipidemia, diabetes mellitus, an age of 60 or older, male sex or postmenopausal state for women, and a family history of cardiovascular disease in women younger than 65 and in men younger than 55. Target organ damage includes heart disease (left ventricular hypertrophy, angina pectoris, prior myocardial infarction, heart failure), stroke or transient ischemic attack, and nephropathy. Prevention and management of hypertension-related morbidity and mortality may best be accomplished by achieving a systolic blood pressure below 140 mm Hg and a diastolic blood pressure below 90 mm Hg; lower if tolerable. Recently, more aggressive blood pressure control has been advocated in patients with renal disease and hypertension, particularly in those patients with a urinary protein excretion of greater than 1 g/d. Blood pressure control in the range of 125/80 mm Hg (mean arterial pressure of 108 mm Hg) has been shown to slow the progression of renal disease [47,48]. This targeted blood pressure control may therefore be advisable in the majority of patients with hypertension. Regardless, each patient should be treated according to their cerebrovascular, cardiovascular, or renal risks; their specific pathophysiology or target organ damage; and their concurrent disease states. A uniform blood pressure goal (target) probably does not exist for all hypertensive patients, and lower may not always be better. JNC—Joint National Committee.

JNC VI DECISION ANALYSIS FOR TREATMENT

Blood pressure stages (mm Hg)	Risk group A (no risk factors, no TOD/CCD)*	Risk group B (at least 1 risk factor, not including diabetes; no TOD/ CCD)	Risk Group C (TOD/CCD and/or diabetes, with or without other risk factors)†
High normal (130–139/85–89)	Lifestyle modification	Lifestyle modification	Drug therapy‡
Stage 1 (140–159/90–99)	Lifestyle modification (up to 12 months)	Lifestyle modification (up to 6 months)	Drug therapy
Stages 2 and 3 (>160/≥100)	Drug therapy	Drug therapy	Drug therapy

Lifestyle modification should be adjunctive therapy for all patients recommended for pharmacologic therapy.

*TOD/CCD indicates target organ disease/clinical cardiovascular disease.

†For patients with multiple risk factors, clinicians should consider drugs as initial therapy plus lifestyle modifications.

‡For those with heart failure, renal insufficiency, or diabetes.

FIGURE 5-56

Decision analysis for treatment based on the Sixth Report of the Joint National Committee on Detection, Evaluation, and Treatment of High Blood Pressure (JNC VI) [46].

Hypertensive Crises

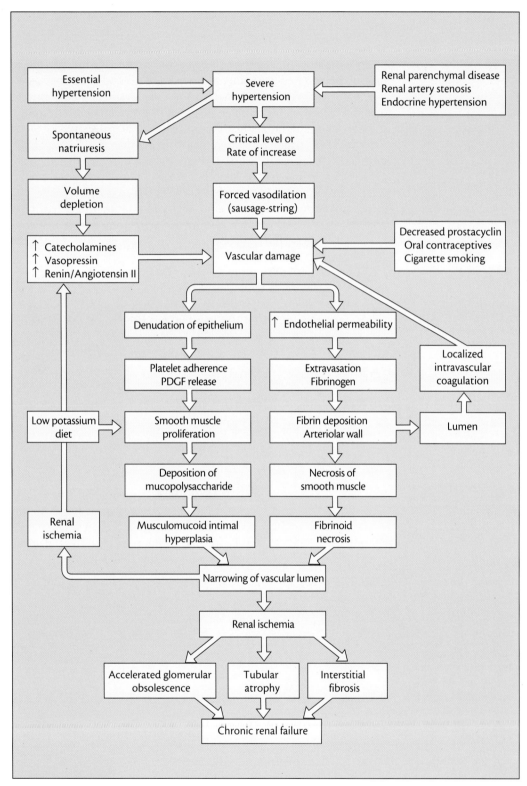

in thickening and remodeling of arteriolar walls that may be an adaptive mechanism to prevent vascular damage from the mechanical stress of hypertension. However, when the blood pressure increases suddenly or increases to a critical level, these adaptive mechanisms may be overwhelmed, resulting in vascular damage. As a result of the mechanical stress of increased transmural pressure, focal segments of the arteriolar vasculature become dilated, producing a *sausage-string* pattern. Endothelial permeability increases in the dilated segments, leading to extravasation of fibrinogen, fibrin deposition in the media, and necrosis of smooth muscle cells (fibrinoid necrosis). Platelet adherence to damaged endothelium with release of platelet-derived growth factor induces migration of smooth muscle cells to the intima where they proliferate (neointimal proliferation) and produce mucopolysaccharide. These cells also produce collagen, resulting in proliferative endarteritis, musculomucoid hyperplasia, and eventually, fibrotic obliteration of the vessel lumen. Occlusion of arterioles leads to accelerated glomerular obsolescence and end-stage renal disease. Other factors may synergize with hypertension to damage the arterial vasculature. Renal ischemia leads to activation of the renin-angiotensin system that can cause further elevation of blood pressure and progressive vascular damage. Spontaneous natriuresis early in the course of malignant hypertension leads to volume depletion with activation of the renin-angiotensin system or catecholamines that further elevates blood pressure. It also is possible that angiotensin II may be directly vasculotoxic. Activation of the clotting cascade within the lumen of damaged vessels may lead to fibrin deposition with localized intravascular coagulation. Thus, microangiopathic hemolytic anemia is a common finding in malignant hypertension. Cigarette smoking and oral contraceptive use may contribute to development of malignant hypertension by decreasing prostacyclin production in the vessel wall and thereby inhibiting repair of hypertension-induced vascular injury. Low dietary intake of potassium may help promote vascular smooth muscle proliferation and therefore predisposes to the development of malignant hypertension in blacks with severe essential hypertension. PDGF—platelet-derived growth factor.

FIGURE 5-57

Pathophysiology of malignant hypertension. The vicious cycle of malignant hypertension is best demonstrated in the kidneys. This cycle also applies equally well to the vascular beds of the retina, pancreas, gastrointestinal tract, and brain [49]. In this scheme, severe hypertension is central. Hypertension may be either essential or secondary to any one of a variety of causes. Because not all patients develop malignant hypertension despite equally severe hypertension, the interaction between the level of blood pressure and the adaptive capacity of the vasculature may be important. In this regard, chronic hypertension results

COMMON CAUSES OF MALIGNANT HYPERTENSION

Primary (essential) malignant hypertension*
Secondary malignant hypertension
  Primary renal disease
    Chronic glomerulonephritis*
    Chronic pyelonephritis*
    Analgesic nephropathy*
    IgA nephropathy*
    Acute glomerulonephritis
    Radiation nephritis
  Renovascular hypertension*
  Oral contraceptives
  Atheroembolic renal disease (cholesterol embolism)
  Scleroderma renal crisis
  Antiphospholipid antibody syndromes
  Chronic lead poisoning
  Endocrine hypertension
    Aldosterone-producing adenoma (Conn's syndrome)
    Cushing's syndrome
    Congenital adrenal hyperplasia
    Pheochromocytoma

*Most common causes of malignant hypertension.

FIGURE 5-58

Common causes of malignant hypertension. Malignant hypertension is not a single disease entity but, rather, a syndrome in which the hypertension can be either primary (essential) or secondary to any one of a number of different causes [50]. Among black patients, the underlying cause is almost always essential hypertension that has entered a malignant phase. The most common secondary causes of malignant hypertension are primary renal parenchymal disorders. Chronic glomerulonephritis is thought to be the cause of malignant hypertension in up to 20% of cases. Unless a history of an acute nephritic episode or long-standing hematuria or proteinuria is available, the underlying glomerulonephritis may only become apparent when a renal biopsy is performed. Recently, immunoglobulin A (IgA) nephropathy has been reported as an increasingly frequent cause of malignant hypertension. In one series of 66 patients with IgA nephropathy, 10% developed malignant hypertension [51]. Chronic atrophic pyelonephritis in children, often a result of underlying vesicoureteral reflux, is the most common cause of malignant hypertension [52]. In Australia, malignant hypertension complicates up to 7% of cases of analgesic nephropathy [53]. Transient malignant hypertension responsive to volume expansion has been reported in analgesic nephropathy. It has been suggested that interstitial disease with salt-wasting is important in the pathogenesis by causing profound volume depletion with activation of the renin-angiotensin axis. Malignant hypertension is both an early and late complication of radiation nephritis that can occur up to 11 years after radiotherapy. Renovascular hypertension from either fibromuscular dysplasia or atherosclerosis is a well-recognized cause of malignant hypertension. In a series of 123 patients with malignant hypertension, renovascular hypertension was found in 43% of whites and 7% of blacks [54]. Among women of childbearing age, oral contraceptives can cause malignant hypertension [55]. In the absence of underlying renal disease, with discontinuation of the drug, long-term prognosis is excellent. Severe hypertension that may become malignant is a common complication of atheroembolic renal disease. In patients presenting with malignant hypertension in the weeks to months after an arteriographic procedure, a careful history and physical should be performed to look for evidence of atheroembolism. Scleroderma renal crisis is the most life-threatening complication of progressive systemic sclerosis. Scleroderma renal crisis is characterized by hypertension that may enter the malignant phase. Even in the absence of hypertensive neuroretinopathy suggesting malignant hypertension, the renal lesion in scleroderma renal crisis is virtually indistinguishable from primary malignant nephrosclerosis [56]. Patients with antiphospholipid antibody syndrome, either primary or secondary to systemic lupus erythematosus, can develop malignant hypertension with renal insufficiency as a result of thrombotic microangiopathy [57]. The endocrine causes of hypertension only rarely lead to malignant hypertension. Pheochromocytoma can cause hypertensive crises owing to hypertensive encephalopathy or acute hypertensive heart failure in the absence of hypertensive neuroretinopathy (malignant hypertension).

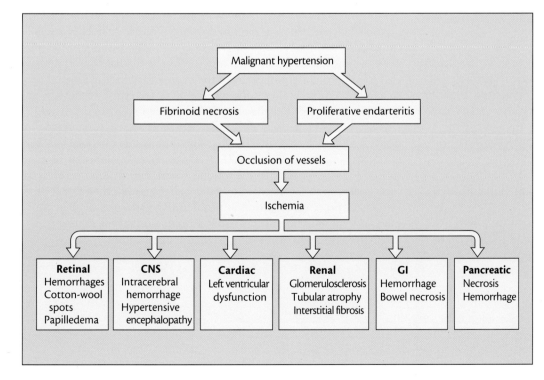

FIGURE 5-59

Distribution of vascular lesions in malignant hypertension. Malignant hypertension is essentially a systemic vasculopathy induced by severe hypertension. Fibrinoid necrosis and proliferative endarteritis occur throughout the body in numerous vascular beds, leading to ischemic changes. In the retina, striate hemorrhages and cotton-wool spots develop. The finding of hypertensive neuroretinopathy is the clinical *sine qua non* of malignant hypertension. Vascular lesions in the gastrointestinal (GI) tract can lead to hemorrhage or bowel necrosis. Hemorrhagic pancreatitis also can occur. Cerebrovascular lesions can lead to cerebral infarction or intracerebral hemorrhage. Hypertensive encephalopathy also can develop as a result of failure of autoregulation with cerebral overperfusion and edema. Vascular lesions also can develop in the myocardium; however, acute hypertensive heart failure is largely the result of acute diastolic dysfunction induced by the marked increase in afterload that accompanies malignant hypertension. CNS—central nervous system.

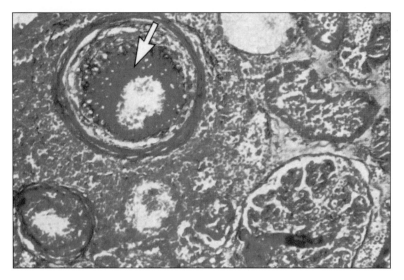

FIGURE 5-60 (*see* Color Plate)

Micrograph of fibrinoid necrosis in malignant hypertension. Fibrinoid necrosis of the afferent arterioles and interlobular arteries has traditionally been regarded as the hallmark of malignant hypertension. The characteristic finding is the deposition in the arteriolar wall of a granular material that is a bright-pink color on hematoxylin and eosin staining. On Masson trichrome staining, as illustrated, the granular fibrinoid material is bright red (*arrow*). The fibrinoid material usually is found in the media of the vessel; however, deposition in the intima also may occur. Whole or fragmented erythrocytes may be extravasated into the arteriolar wall. These hemorrhages account for the petechial hemorrhages that give rise to the peculiar flea-bitten appearance of the capsular surface of the kidney in malignant hypertension. Fibrinoid necrosis is thought to result from the mechanical stress placed on the vessel wall by severe hypertension. Forced vasodilation occurs when there is failure of autoregulation of renal blood flow, which leads to endothelial injury with seepage of plasma proteins into the vessel wall. Contact of plasma constituents with smooth muscle cells activates the coagulation cascade, and fibrin is deposited in the wall. Fibrin deposits then cause necrosis of smooth muscle cells (*fibrinoid necrosis*). (Masson trichrome stain, original magnification × 100.)

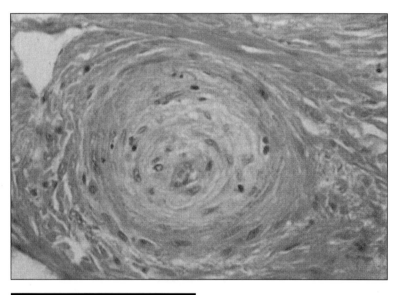

FIGURE 5-61 (*see* Color Plate)

Micrograph of proliferative endarteritis in malignant hypertension (*musculomucoid intimal hyperplasia*). In malignant nephrosclerosis, the interlobular (cortical radial) arteries reveal characteristic lesions. These lesions are variously referred to as proliferative endarteritis, endarteritis fibrosa, musculomucoid intimal hyperplasia, or the onion skin lesion. The typical finding is marked thickening of the intima that obstructs the vessel lumen. In severely affected vessels the luminal diameter may be reduced to the caliber of a single erythrocyte. Occasionally, complete obliteration of the lumen by a superimposed fibrin thrombus occurs.

Traditionally, three patterns of intimal thickening have been described [58]: 1) The onionskin pattern consists of pale layers of elongated concentrically arranged myointimal cells along with delicate connective tissue fibrils that give rise to a lamellar appearance. The media often appears as an attenuated layer stretched around the expanded intima. 2) In the mucinous pattern, intimal cells are sparse. Seen is an abundance of lucent, faintly basophilic-staining amorphous material. 3) In fibrous intimal thickening, seen are few cells with an abundance of hyaline deposits, reduplicated bands of elastica, and coarse layers of collagen. The renal histology in blacks with malignant hypertension demonstrates a characteristic finding in the larger arterioles and interlobular arteries known as *musculomucoid intimal hyperplasia*, with an abundance of cells and a small amount of myxoid material (that is light blue in color on hematoxylin and eosin staining) between the cells [59,60]. These various intimal findings may represent progression over time from an initially cellular lesion to fibrosis of the intima. Electron microscopy demonstrates that in each type of intimal thickening the most abundant cellular element is a modified smooth muscle cell. This cell is called a *myointimal cell*. Proliferative endarteritis is thought to occur as a result of phenotypic modulation of medial smooth muscle cells that dedifferentiate from the normal contractile phenotype to acquire a more embryologic proliferative-secretory phenotype. It has been proposed that the endothelial injury in malignant hypertension results in attachment of platelets with release of platelet-derived growth factor (PDGF) that may induce the phenotypic change in smooth muscle cells. PDGF stimulates chemotaxis of medial smooth muscles to the intima, where they proliferate and secrete mucopolysaccharide and later collagen and other extracellular matrix proteins, resulting in proliferative endarteritis, musculomucoid hyperplasia, and ultimately fibrous intimal thickening. (Hematoxylin and eosin stain, original magnification × 100.)

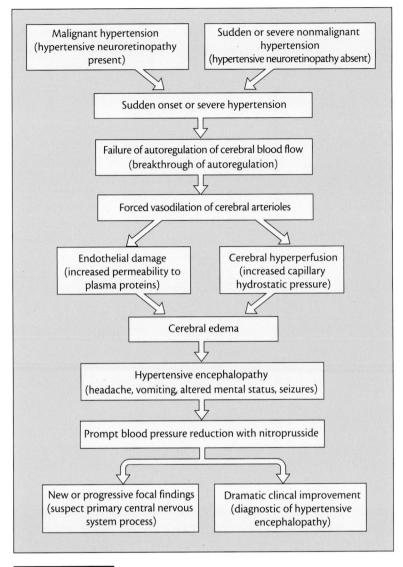

FIGURE 5-62

Pathogenesis and treatment of hypertensive encephalopathy. *Hypertensive encephalopathy* is a hypertensive crisis in which acute cerebral dysfunction is attributed to sudden or severe elevation of blood pressure [61–63]. Hypertensive encephalopathy is one of the most serious complications of malignant hypertension. However, malignant hypertension (hypertensive neuroretinopathy) need not be present for hypertensive encephalopathy to develop. Hypertensive encephalopathy also can occur in the setting of severe or sudden hypertension of any cause, especially if an acute elevation of blood pressure occurs in a previously normotensive person, *eg*, from

postinfectious glomerulonephritis, catecholamine excess states, or eclampsia. Under normal circumstances, autoregulation of the cerebral microcirculation occurs, and therefore, cerebral blood flow remains constant over a wide range of perfusion pressures. However, in the setting of sudden severe hypertension, autoregulatory vasoconstriction fails and there is forced vasodilation of cerebral arterioles with endothelial damage, extravasation of plasma proteins, and cerebral hyperperfusion with the development of cerebral edema. This breakthrough of cerebral autoregulation underlies the development of hypertensive encephalopathy. In patients with chronic hypertension, structural changes occur in the cerebral arterioles that lead to a shift in the autoregulation curve such that much higher blood pressures can be tolerated without breakthrough. This phenomenon may explain the clinical observation that hypertensive encephalopathy occurs at much lower blood pressure in previously normotensive persons than it does in those with chronic hypertension. Clinical features of hypertensive encephalopathy include severe headache, blurred vision or occipital blindness, nausea, vomiting, and altered mental status. Focal neurologic findings can sometimes occur. If aggressive blood pressure reduction is not initiated, stupor, convulsions, and death can occur within hours. The *sine qua non* of hypertensive encephalopathy is the prompt and dramatic clinical improvement in response to antihypertensive drug therapy. When a diagnosis of hypertensive encephalopathy seems likely, antihypertensive therapy should be initiated promptly without waiting for the results of time-consuming radiographic examinations. The goal of therapy, especially in previously normotensive patients, should be reduction of blood pressure to normal or near-normal levels as quickly as possible. Theoretically, cerebral blood flow could be jeopardized by rapid reduction of blood pressure in patients with chronic hypertension in whom the lower limit of cerebral blood flow autoregulation is shifted to a higher blood pressure. However, clinical experience has shown that prompt blood pressure reduction with the avoidance of frank hypotension is beneficial in patients with hypertensive encephalopathy [61]. Of the conditions in the differential diagnosis of hypertension with acute cerebral dysfunction, only cerebral infarction might be adversely affected by the abrupt reduction of blood pressure. Pharmacologic agents that have rapid onset and short duration of action such as sodium nitroprusside should be used so that the blood pressure can be titrated carefully, with close monitoring of the patient's neurologic status. A prompt improvement in mental status with blood pressure reduction confirms the diagnosis of hypertensive encephalopathy. Conversely, when blood pressure reduction is associated with new or progressive focal neurologic deficits, the presence of a primary central nervous system event, such as cerebral infarction, should be considered.

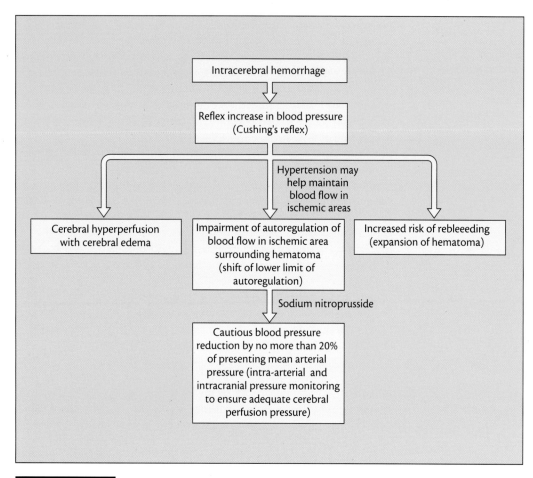

FIGURE 5-63

Hypertensive crises due to intracerebral hemorrhage. Chronic hypertension is the major risk factor for intracerebral hemorrhage. The most common sites of hemorrhage are the small-diameter penetrating cerebral end-arteries in the basal ganglia, pons, thalamus, cerebellum, and deep hemispheric white matter. Lacunar infarcts arise from the same vessels and are similarly distributed. Intracerebral hemorrhage characteristically begins abruptly with headache and vomiting followed by steadily increasing focal neurologic deficits and alteration of consciousness [64]. More than 90% of hemorrhages rupture through brain parenchyma into the ventricles, producing bloody cerebrospinal fluid. Patients presenting with intracerebral hemorrhage are invariably hypertensive. In contrast to cerebral infarction, the hypertension does not tend to decrease spontaneously during the first week. The patient's condition worsens steadily over a period of minutes to days until either the neurologic deficit stabilizes or the patient dies. When death occurs, most often it is due to herniation caused by the expanding hematoma and surrounding edema. Treatment of hypertension in the setting of intracerebral hemorrhage is controversial. An increase in intracranial pressure accompanied by a reflex increase in systemic blood pressure almost always occurs. Because cerebral perfusion pressure is a function of the difference between arterial pressure and intracranial pressure, reduction of blood pressure could compromise cerebral perfusion. Moreover, as in cerebral infarction, autoregulation is impaired in the area of marginal ischemia surrounding the hemorrhage. In contrast, cerebral vasogenic edema may be exacerbated by hypertension. Moreover, hypertension may increase the risk of rebleeding with expansion of the hematoma. Thus, in deciding to treat hypertension in the setting of intracerebral hemorrhage, a precarious balance must be struck between beneficial reduction in cerebral edema on the one hand, and deleterious reduction of cerebral blood flow on the other. Studies have shown that the lower limit of autoregulation after intracerebral hemorrhage is approximately 80% of the initial blood pressure; therefore, a 20% decrease in mean arterial pressure should be considered the maximal goal of blood pressure reduction during the acute stage [45]. Antihypertensive therapy should be undertaken only in conjunction with intracranial and intra-arterial pressure monitoring to allow for assessment of cerebral perfusion pressure. The short duration of action of nitroprusside makes its use preferable over other agents with a longer duration of action and the risk of sustained overshoot hypotension, despite the theoretic concern that nitroprusside treatment could lead to an increase in intracranial pressure by way of dilation of cerebral veins and arteries.

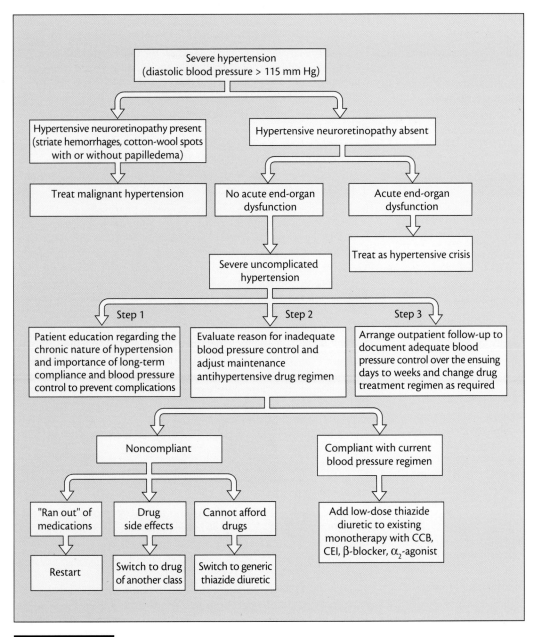

exhibits severe hypertension (diastolic blood pressure >115 mm Hg) in the absence of hypertensive neuroretinopathy or acute end-organ damage that would signify a true crisis. This entity, known as *severe uncomplicated hypertension*, is very commonly seen in the emergency department or other acute-care settings. Of patients with severe uncomplicated hypertension, 60% are entirely asymptomatic and present for prescription refills or routine blood pressure checks, or are found to have elevated pressure during routine physical examinations. The other 40% of patients initially exhibit nonspecific findings such as headache, dizziness, or weakness in the absence of evidence of acute end-organ dysfunction. In the past, this entity was referred to as *urgent hypertension*, reflecting the erroneous notion that acute reduction of blood pressure, over a few hours before discharge from the acute-care facility, was essential to minimize the risk of short-term complications from severe hypertension. Commonly employed treatment regimens included oral clonidine loading or sublingual nifedipine. However, in recent years the practice of acute blood pressure reduction in severe uncomplicated hypertension has been questioned [65,66]. In the Veterans Administration Cooperative Study of patients with severe hypertension, there were 70 placebo-treated patients who had an average diastolic blood pressure of 121 mm Hg at entry. Among these untreated patients, 27 experienced morbid events at a mean of 11 ± 8 months of follow-up. However, the earliest morbid event occurred only after 2 months [67]. These data suggest that in patients with *severe uncomplicated hypertension* in which severe hypertension is not accompanied by evidence of malignant hypertension or acute end-organ dysfunction, eventual complications from stroke, myocardial infarction, or congestive heart failure tend to occur over months to years, rather than hours to days.

FIGURE 5-64

Severe uncomplicated hypertension. The benefits of acute reduction in blood pressure in the setting of true hypertensive crises are obvious. Fortunately, true hypertensive crises are relatively rare events that almost never affect hypertensive patients. Another type of presentation that is much more common than are true hypertensive crises is that of the patient who initially

References

1. Navar LG, Inscho EW, Majid DSA, *et al.*: Paracrine regulation of the renal microcirculation. *Physiol Rev* 1996, 76:425–536.

2. DiBona GF, Kopp UC: Neural control of renal function. *Physiol Rev* 1997, 77:75–197.

3. Vari RC, Navar LG: Normal regulation of arterial pressure. In *Principles and Practice of Nephrology*, edn 2. Edited by Jacobson HR, Striker GE, Klahr GE. St. Louis: Mosby-Yearbook; 1995:354–361.

4. Arendshorst WJ, Navar LG: Renal circulation and glomerular hemodynamics. In *Diseases of the Kidney*, edn 6. Edited by Schrier RW, Gottschalk CW. Boston: Little-Brown; 1997:59–106.

5. Mitchell KD, Braam B: Navar LG: Hypertensinogenic mechanisms mediated by renal actions of renin-angiotensin system. *Hypertension* 1992, 19(suppl I):I-18–I-27.

6. Mitchell KD, Navar LG: Intrarenal actions of angiotensin II in the pathogenesis of experimental hypertension. In *Hypertension: Pathophysiology, Diagnosis, and Management*, edn 2. Edited by Laragh JH, Brenner BM. New York: Raven Press; 1995:1437–1450.

7. Capdevila JH, Falck JR, Estabrook RW: Cytochrome P450 and the arachidonate cascade. *FASEB J* 1992, 6:731–736.

8. Smith WL: Prostanoid biosynthesis and mechanisms of action. *Am J Physiol (Renal Fluid Electrolyte Physiol 32)* 1992, 263:F181–F191.

9. Frazier LW, Yorio T: Eicosanoids: their function in renal epithelia ion transport. *Proceedings of the Society for Experimental Biology and Medicine* 1992, 201:229–243.

10. Jamison RL, Canaan-Kuhl S, Pratt R: The natriuretic peptides and their receptors. *Am J Kidney Dis* 1992, 20:519–530.

11. Breyer MD, Jacobson HR, Breyer RM: Functional and molecular aspects of renal prostaglandin receptors. *J Am Soc Nephrol* 1996, 7:8–17.

12. McGiff JC: Cytochrome P-450 metabolism of arachidonic acid. *Ann Rev Pharmacol Toxicol* 1991, 31:339–369.

13. Imig JD, Zou A-P, Stec DE, *et al.*: Formation and actions of 20-hydroxyeicosatetraenoic acid in rat renal arterioles. *Am J Physiol (Regulat Integrative Comp Physiol 39)* 1996, 270:R217–R227.

14. Converse RL, Jacobsen TN, Toto RD, *et al.*: Sympathetic overactivity in patients with chronic renal failure. *N Engl J Med* 1992, 327:1912–1918.

15. Katholi RE, Nafilan AJ, Oparil S: Importance of renal sympathetic tone in the development of DOCA-salt hypertension in the rat. *Hypertension* 1980, 2:266–273.

16. Perry HM, Miller JP, Fornoff JR, *et al.*: Early predictors of 15-year end-stage renal disease in hypertensive patients. *Hypertension* 1995, 25(part 1):587–594.

17. Klag MJ, Whelton PK, Randall BL, *et al.*: End-stage renal disease in African-American and White men. *JAMA* 1997, 277:1293–1298.

18. Peterson JC, Adler S, Burkart JM, *et al.*: Blood pressure control, proteinuria and the progression of renal disease. *Ann Intern Med* 1995, 123:754–762.

19. Lewis EJ, Hunsicker LG, Bain RP, Rohde RD: The effect of angiotensin-converting-enzyme inhibition on diabetic nephropathy. *N Engl J Med* 1993, 329:1456–1462.

20. Pohl MA: Renal artery stenosis, renal vascular hypertension and ischemic nephropathy. In *Diseases of the Kidney*, edn 6. Edited by Schrier RW, Gottschalk CW. Boston: Little, Brown & Co; 1997: 1367–1427.

21. Hoffmann U, Edwards JM, Carter S, *et al.*: Role of duplex scanning for the detection of atherosclerotic renal artery disease. *Kidney Int* 1991, 39:1232–1239.

22. Nally JV, Olin JW, Lammert MD: Advances in noninvasive screening for renovascular hypertension disease. *Cleve Clin J Med* 1994, 61:328–336.

23. Novick AC, Pohl MA: Atherosclerotic renal artery occlusion extending into branches: successful revascularization in situ with a branched saphenous vein graft. *J Urol* 1979, 122:240–242.

24. Novick AC: Patient selection for intervention to preserve renal function in ischemic renal disease. In *Renovascular Disease*. Edited by Novick AC, Scoble J, Hamilton G. London: WB Saunders; 1996:323–335.

25. Netter FH: Endocrine system and selected metabolic diseases. In *Ciba Collection of Medical Illustrations*, vol. 4; 1981:Section III, Plates 5, 26.

26. Manger WM, Gifford RW Jr: *Pheochromocytoma*. New York: Springer-Verlag; 1977:97.

27. National High Blood Pressure Education Program and National Cholesterol Education Program: Working Group Report on Management of Patients with Hypertension and High Blood Cholesterol. National Institutes of Health Publication No. 90-2361. National Institutes of Health, 1990.

28. Bonna KH, Thelle DJ: Association between blood pressure and serum lipids in a population: the Tromso study. *Circulation* 1991, 83:1305–1324.

29. Parving H-H, Andersen AR, Smidt UM, *et al.*: Effect of antihypertensive treatment on kidney function in diabetic nephropathy. *Br Med J* 1987, 294:1443–1447.

30. Lewis EJ, Hunsicker LG, Bain RP, *et al.*: The effect of angiotensin-converting-enzyme inhibition on diabetic nephropathy. *N Engl J Med* 1993, 329:1456–1462.

31. Dworkin LD, Benstein JA: Antihypertensive agents, glomerular hemo-dynamics and glomerular injury. In *Calcium Antagonists and the Kidney*. Edited by Epstein M, Loutzenhiser R. Philadelphia, Hanley & Belfus; 1990:155–176.

32. Nagata M, Scharer K, Kriz W: Glomerular damage after uninephrec-tomy in young rats. I. Hypertrophy and distortion of the capillary architecture. *Kidney Int* 1992, 42:136–147.

33. Klahr S, Levey AS, Beck GJ, *et al.*: The effects of dietary protein restriction and blood-pressure control on the progression of chronic renal disease. Modification of Diet in Renal Disease Study Group. *N Engl J Med* 1994, 330:877–884.

34. Peterson JC, Adler S, Burkart JM, *et al.* for the Modification of Diet in Renal Disease Study Group. *Ann Intern Med* 1995, 123:754–762.

35. Locatelli F, Marcelli D, Comelli M, *et al.* for the Northern Italian Cooperative Study Group: proteinuria and blood pressure as causal components of progression to end-stage renal failure. *Nephrol Dial Transplant* 1996, 11:461–467.

36. Kaplan NM: *Clinical Hypertension*, edn 6. Baltimore: Williams & Wilkins; 1994:50.

37. Guyton AC, Coleman TG, Yang DB, *et al.*: Salt balance and long-term blood pressure control. *Annu Rev Med* 1980, 31:15–27.

38. Julius S, Krause L, Schork NJ: Hyperkinetic borderline hypertension in Tecumseh, Michigan. *J Hypertens* 1991, 9:77–84.

39. Bauer JH, Reams GP: Mechanisms of action, pharmacology, and use of antihypertensive drugs. In *The Principles and Practice of Nephrology*. Edited by Jacobson HR, Striker GE, Klahr S. St. Louis: Mosby; 1995:399–415.

40. Tarazi RC: Diuretic drugs: mechanisms of antihypertensive action. In *Hypertension: Mechanisms and Management. The 26th Hahnemann Symposium*. Edited by Oneti G, Kim KE, Moer JH. New York: Grune and Stratton; 1973:255.

41. Ellison DH: The physiologic basis of diuretic synergism: its role in treating diuretic resistance. *Ann Intern Med* 1991, 114:886–894.

42. Man in't Veld AJ, Schalekamp MADH: How intrinsic sympathomimetic activity modulates the haemodynamic responses to β-adrenoceptor antagonists: a clue to the nature of their antihypertensive mechanism. *Br J Clin Pharmacol* 1982, 13:2455–2575.

43. Bauer JH, Reams GP: Antihypertensive drugs. In *The Kidney*, edn 5. Edited by Brenner BM. Philadelphia: W.B. Saunders Co.; 1995: 2331–2381.

44. Entel SI, Entel EA, Clozel J-P: T-type Ca^{2+} channels and pharmacological blockade: potential pathophysiological relevance. *Cardiovasc Drugs Ther* 1997, 11:723—739.

45. Bauer JH, Ream GP: The angiotensin II type 1 receptor antagonists. *Arch Intern Med* 1995, 155:1361–1368.

46. JNC VI: The Sixth Report of the Joint National Committee on Detection, Evaluation, and Treatment of High Blood Pressure. *Arch Intern Med* 1993, 153:154–183.

47. Peterson JC, Adler S, Burkart JM, *et al.*: Blood pressure control, proteinuria, and the progression of renal disease. *Ann Intern Med* 1995, 123:754–762.

48. Hebert LA, Kusek JW, Greene T, *et al.*: Effects of blood pressure con-trol on progressive renal disease in blacks and whites. *Hypertension* 1997, 30 (part 1):428–435.

49. Nolan CR, Linas SL: Malignant hypertension and other hypertensive crises. In *Diseases of the Kidney,* edn 6. Edited by Schrier RW, Gottschalk CW. Boston: Little, Brown; 1997:1475–1554.

50. Derow HA, *et al.*: The nature of malignant hypertension. *Ann Intern Med* 1941, 14:1768.

51. Perez-Fontan M, *et al.*: Idiopathic IgA nephropathy presenting as malignant hypertension. *Am J Nephrol* 1986, 6:482.

52. Holland NH, *et al.*: Hypertension in children with chronic pyelonephritis. *Kidney Int* 1975, 8(suppl):S234.

53. Nanra RS, *et al.*: Analgesic nephropathy: etiology, clinical syndrome, and clinicopathologic correlations in Australia. *Kidney Int* 1978, 13:79.

54. Davis BA, *et al.*: Prevalence of renovascular hypertension in patients with grade III or grade IV hypertensive neuroretinopathy. *N Engl J Med* 1979, 301:1273.

55. Lim K, *et al.*: Malignant hypertension in women of childbearing age and its relation to the contraceptive pill. *Br Med J* 1987, 294:1057.

56. Traub YM, *et al.*: Hypertension and renal failure (scleroderma renal crisis) in progressive systemic sclerosis. *Medicine* 1983, 62:335.

57. Cacoub P, *et al.*: Malignant hypertension with antiphospholipid syndrome without overt lupus nephritis. *Clin Exp Rheumatol* 1993, 11:479–485.

58. Sinclair RA, Antonovych TT, Mostofi FL: Renal proliferative arteri-opathies and associated glomerular changes: a light and electron microscopy study. *Hum Pathol* 1976, 7:565.

59. Pitcock JA, *et al.*: Malignant hypertension in blacks: malignant intrarenal arterial disease as observed by light and electron microscopy. *Hum Pathol* 1976, 7:33.

60. Jones DB: Arterial and glomerular lesions associated with severe hypertension. *Lab Invest* 1974, 31:303.

61. Gifford RW Jr, *et al.*: Hypertensive encephalopathy: mechanisms, clinical features, and treatment. *Progr Cardiovasc Dis* 1974, 17:115.

62. Dinsdale HB: Hypertensive encephalopathy. *Neurol Clin* 1983, 1:83.

63. Ziegler DK, *et al.*: Hypertensive encephalopathy. *Arch Neurol* 1965, 12:472.

64. Cuneo RA, *et al.*: The neurologic complications of hypertension. *Med Clin North Am* 1977, 61:565.

65. Fagan TC: Acute reduction of blood pressure in asymptomatic patients with severe hypertension. An idea whose time has come–and gone. *Arch Intern Med* 1989, 149:2169.

66. Ferguson RK, Vlasses PH: Hypertensive emergencies and urgencies. *JAMA* 1986, 255:1607.

67. Veterans Administration Cooperative Study Group on Antihypertensive Agents. Effects of treatment on morbidity in hypertension. Result in patients with diastolic blood pressure averaging 115 through 129 mm Hg. *JAMA* 1967, 202:1028.

Transplantation as Treatment of End-Stage Renal Disease

William M. Bennett

John M. Barry, Laurence Chan, Connie L. Davis,
Angelo M. de Mattos, Marvin R. Garovoy, Robert S. Gaston,
Bertram L. Kasiske, Lauralynn K. Lebeck, Jeremy B. Levy,
Jeanne A. Mowry, Jon S. Odorico, John D. Pirsch, Hans W. Sollinger

CHAPTER

6

Histocompatibility Testing and Organ Sharing

MHC I AND II CHARACTERISTICS

Class I	Class II
Composed of HLA-A, -B, and -C	Composed of HLA-DR, -DQ, and -DP
Ubiquitous distribution	Restricted distribution
Autosomal codominant	Autosomal codominant
Target for immune effector mechanism	Major role in immune response induction
Serologic and molecular detection	Serologic, molecular, and cellular detection
Heterodimer noncovalently linked	Heterodimer noncovalently linked
Heavy chain (α):	α Chain:
Contains variable regions	Nonvariable in HLA-DR
Confers HLA specificity	Contains variable regions in HLA-DQ and -DP
Light chain (β_2-microglobulin):	β Chain:
Invariant	Contains variable regions
	Confers most of HLA-DR specificity

FIGURE 6-1

Human leukocyte antigens (HLAs) are heterodimeric cell-surface glycoproteins. HLAs are divided into two classes, according to their biochemical structure and respective functions. Class I antigens (A, B, and C) have a molecular weight of approximately 56,000 D and consist of two chains: a glycoprotein heavy chain (α) and a light chain (β_2-microglobulin). The α chain is attached to the cell membrane, whereas β_2-microglobulin is associated with the α chain but is not covalently bonded. The HLA class I molecules are found on almost all cells; however, only vestigial amounts remain on mature erythrocytes. Class II antigens (HLA-DR, DQ, and DP) have a molecular weight of approximately 63,000 D and consist of two dissimilar glycoprotein chains, designated α and β, both of which are attached to the membrane. Each chain consists of two extramembranous amino acid domains, and the outer domains of each molecule contain the variable regions corresponding to class II alleles. Although class I antigens are expressed on all nucleated cells of the body, the expression of class II antigens is more restricted. Class II antigens are found on B lymphocytes, activated T lymphocytes, monocyte-macrophages, dendritic cells, early hematopoietic cells, and (of importance in transplantation) endothelial cells.

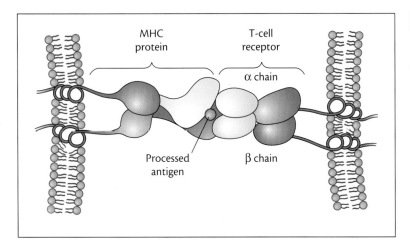

FIGURE 6-2

Biology of the major histocompatibility complex (MHC). The biologic function of MHC antigens is to present antigenic peptides to T lymphocytes. In fact, it is an absolute requirement of T-lymphocyte activation for the T cells to "see" the antigenic peptide bound to an MHC molecule. This *MHC restriction* has been defined on a molecular basis with the elucidation of the crystalline structures of classes I and II MHC molecules.

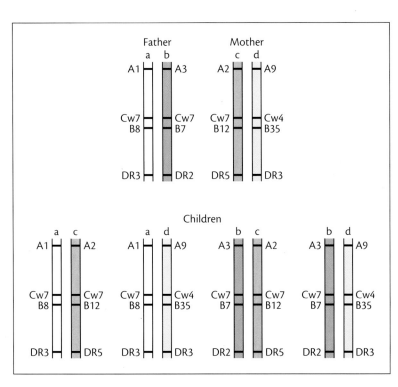

FIGURE 6-3

Genetic principles of the major histocompatibility complex (MHC). The MHC demonstrates a number of genetic principles. Each person has two chromosomes and thus two MHC haplotypes, each inherited from one parent. Because the human leukocyte antigen (HLA) genes are autosomal and codominant, the phenotype represents the combined expression of both haplotypes. Each child receives one chromosome and hence one haplotype from each parent. Because each parent has two different number 6 chromosomes, four different combinations of haplotypes are possible in the offspring. This inheritance pattern is an important factor in finding compatible related donors for transplantation. Thus, an individual has a 25% chance of having an HLA-identical or a completely dissimilar sibling and a 50% chance of having a sibling matched for one haplotype. The genes of the HLA region occasionally (≈ 1%) demonstrate chromosomal crossover. These recombinations are then transmitted as new haplotypes to the offspring.

CROSSMATCH METHODS

Lymphocytotoxicity
  Auto–crossmatch *vs* allo–crossmatch
  T or B cell
  Short/long/wash/AHG methods
  IgG *vs* IgM
Flow cytometry
Enzyme-linked immunosorbent assay

FIGURE 6-4

Crossmatch methods. Early reports correlating a positive crossmatch between recipient serum and donor lymphocytes with hyperacute rejection of transplanted kidneys led to establishing tests of recipient sera as the standard of practice in transplantation. However, controversy remains regarding 1) the level of sensitivity needed for crossmatch testing; 2) the relevance of B-cell crossmatches, a surrogate for class II incompatibilities; 3) the relevance of immunoglobulin class and subclass of donor-reactive antibodies; 4) the significance of historical antibodies, ie, antibodies present previously but not at the time of transplantation; 5) the techniques and type of analyses to be performed for serum screening; and 6) the appropriate frequency and timing of serum screening. Despite a number of variables, when the data from reported studies are considered collectively, several observations can be made. Human leukocyte antigen–donor-specific antibodies present in the recipient at the time of transplantation are a serious risk factor that significantly diminishes graft function and graft survival. Antibodies specific for human leukocyte antigen class II antigens (HLA-DR and -DQ) are as detrimental as are those specific for class I antigens (HLA-A, -B, and -C). The degree of risk resulting from HLA-specific antibodies varies among immunoglobulin classes, with immunoglobulin G antibodies representing the most serious risk. AHG—antiglobulin-augmented lymphocytotoxicity.

Transplant Rejection and Its Treatment

A. VARIETIES OF REJECTION

Types of rejection	Time taken	Cause
Hyperacute	Minutes to hours	Preformed antidonor antibodies and complement
Accelerated	Days	Reactivation of sensitized T cells
Acute	Days to weeks	Primary activation of T cells
Chronic	Months to years	Both immunologic and nonimmunologic factors

B. IMMUNE MECHANISMS OF RENAL ALLOGRAFT REJECTION

Type	Humoral	Cellular
Hyperacute	+++	−
Accelerated	++	+
Acute		
Cellular	+	+++
Vascular	+++	+
Chronic	++	+?

FIGURE 6-5

Varieties of rejection (*part A*) and immune mechanisms (*part B*). On the basis of the pathologic process and the kinetics of the rejection response, rejection of renal allografts can be commonly divided into hyperacute, accelerated, acute, and chronic types.

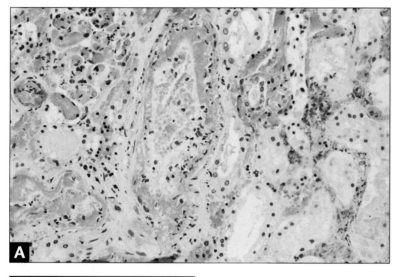

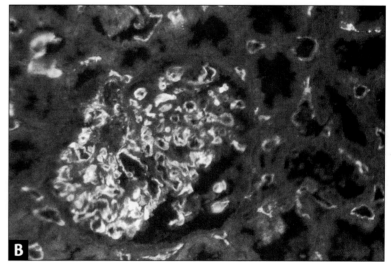

FIGURE 6-6 (*See Color Plate*)

Histologic features of hyperacute rejection. Hyperacute rejection is very rare and is caused by antibody-mediated damage to the graft. The clinical manifestation of hyperacute rejection is a failure of the kidney to perfuse properly on release of the vascular clamps just after vascular anastomosis is completed. The kidney initially becomes firm and then rapidly turns blue, spotted, and flabby. The presence of neutrophils in the glomeruli and peritubular capillaries in the kidney biopsy confirms the diagnosis. **A,** Hematoxylin and eosin stain of biopsy showing interstitial hemorrhage and extensive coagulative necrosis of tubules and glomeruli, with scattered interstitial inflammatory cells and neutrophils. **B,** Immunofluorescence stain of kidney with hyperacute rejection showing positive staining of fibrins.

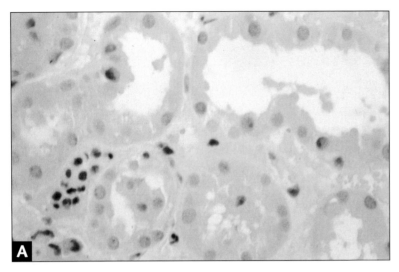

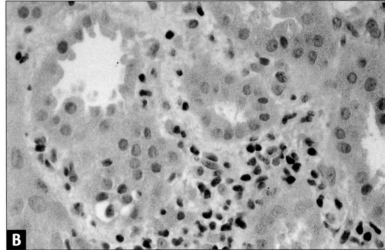

FIGURE 6-7

Histologic features of acute cellular rejection. **A,** Mild tubulitis. **B,** Moderate to severe tubulitis. Acute rejection episodes may occur as early as 5 to 7 days, but are generally seen between 1 and 4 weeks after transplantation. The classic acute rejection episode of the earlier era (*ie*, azathioprine-prednisolone) was accompanied by swelling and tenderness of the kidney and the onset of oliguria with an associated rise in serum creatinine; these symptoms were usually accompanied by a significant fever. However, in patients who have been treated with cyclosporine, the clinical features of an acute rejection are really quite minimal in that there is perhaps some swelling of the kidney, usually no tenderness, and there may be a minimal to moderate degree of fever. Because such an acute rejection may occur at a time when there is a distinct possibility of

acute cyclosporine toxicity, the differentiation between the two entities may be extremely difficult.

The differential diagnosis of acute rejection, acute tubular necrosis, and cyclosporine nephrotoxicity may be difficult, especially in the early posttransplant period when more than one cause of dysfunction can occur together [1]. Knowledge of the natural history of several clinical entities is extremely helpful in limiting the differential diagnosis. Reversible medical and mechanical causes should be excluded first. Percutaneous biopsy of the renal allograft using real-time ultrasound guide is a safe procedure. It provides histologic confirmation of the diagnosis of rejection, aids in the differential diagnosis of graft dysfunction, and allows for assessment of the likelihood of a response to antirejection treatment.

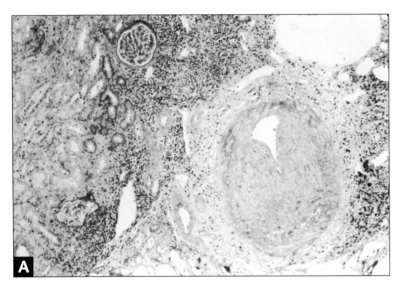

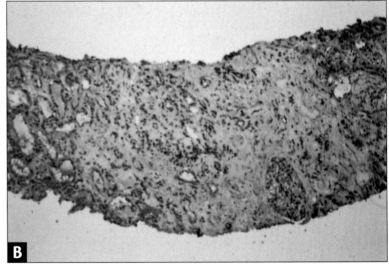

C. CHRONIC ALLOGRAFT REJECTION

Typical clinical presentation
  Gradual increase in creatinine (months)
  Non-nephrotic–range proteinuria
  No recent nephrotoxic events
Key pathologic features
  Interstitial fibrosis
  Arterial fibrosis and intimal thickening

FIGURE 6-8

Features of chronic rejection. **A,** Arterial fibrosis and intimal thickening. **B,** Interstitial fibrosis and tubular atrophy. **C,** Typical presentation and pathologic features. Chronic rejection occurs during a span of months to years. It appears to be unresponsive to current treatment and has emerged as the major problem facing transplantation [2]. Because chronic rejection is thought to be the end result of uncontrolled repetitive acute rejection episodes or a slowly progressive inflammatory process, its onset may be as early as the first few weeks after transplantation or any time thereafter.

(*Continued on next page*)

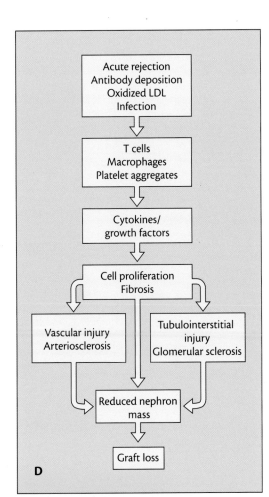

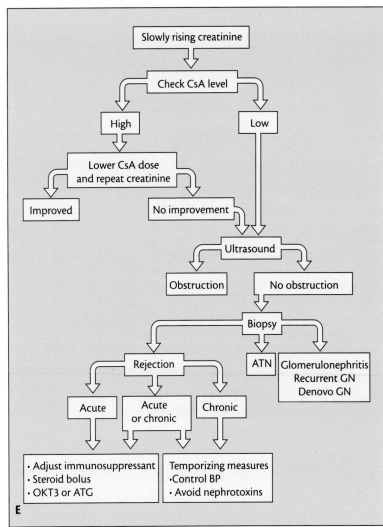

FIGURE 6-8 (*continued*)

D, The likely sequence of events in chronic rejection and potential mediating factors for key steps. Progressive azotemia, proteinuria, and hypertension are the clinical hallmarks of chronic rejection. Immunologic and nonimmunologic mechanisms are thought to play a role in the pathogenesis of this entity. Immunologic mechanisms include antibody-mediated tissue destruction that occurs possibly secondary to antibody-dependent cellular cytotoxicity, leading to obliterative arteritis, growth factors derived from macrophages and platelets leading to fibrotic degeneration, and glomerular hypertension with hyperfiltration injury due to reduced nephron mass leading to progressive glomerular sclerosis. Nonimmunologic causes can also contribute to the decline in renal function. Atheromatous renovascular disease of the transplant kidney may also be responsible for a significant number of cases of progressive graft failure. E, Diagnostic and therapeutic approach to chronic rejection. ATG—antithymocyte globulin; ATN—acute tubular necrosis; BP—blood pressure; CsA—cyclosporine; LDL—low-density lipoprotein.

A. INDUCTION PROTOCOLS

Standard induction
Corticosteroids
Azathioprine or mycophenolate
Cyclosporine or FK506
Antibody induction
OKT3 or antithymocyte gamma globulin

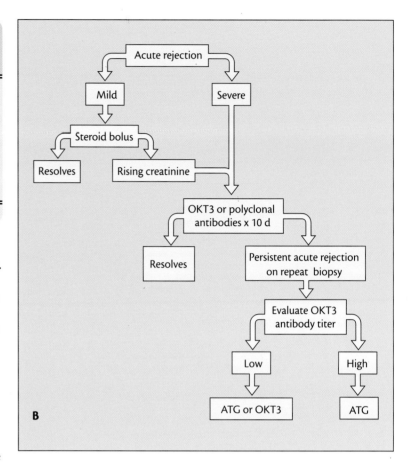

B

FIGURE 6-9

Treatment of acute rejection. **A,** Typical antirejection therapy regimens. **B,** Treatment algorithm. A biopsy should be performed whenever possible. The first-line treatment for acute rejection in most centers is pulse methylprednisolone, 500 to 1000 mg, given intravenously daily for 3 to 5 days. The expected reversal rate for the first episode of acute cellular rejection is 60% to 70% with this regimen [3–5]. Steroid-resistant rejection is defined as a lack of improvement in urine output or the plasma creatinine concentration within 3 to 4 days. In this setting, OKT3 or polyclonal anti–T-cell antibodies should be considered [6]. The use of these potent therapies should be confined to acute rejections with acute components that are potentially reversible, *eg,* mononuclear interstitial cell infiltrate with tubulitis or endovasculitis with acute inflammatory endothelial infiltrate [7,8]. ATG—antithymocyte globulin; ICAM-1—intercellular adhesion molecule-1; LFA-1—leukocyte function-associated antigen-1.

Posttransplant Infections

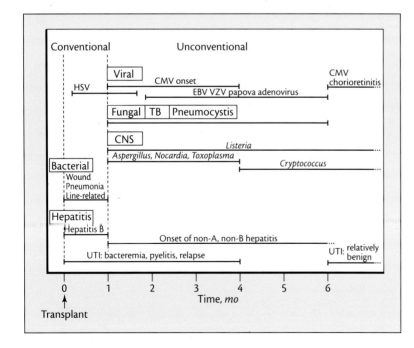

FIGURE 6-10

Timetable for the occurrence of infection in the renal transplant patient. Exceptions to this chronology are frequent. CMV—cytomegalovirus; CNS—central nervous system; EBV—Epstein-Barr virus; HSV—herpes simplex virus; UTI—urinary tract infection; VZV—varicella-zoster virus. (*Adapted from* Rubin *et al.* [9].)

INFECTIOUS DISEASE HISTORY TO BE TAKEN PRIOR TO TRANSPLANTATION

1. Past immunizations
2. Past infections or exposures to infections
   A. Bacterial
      Rheumatic fever, sinusitis, ear infections, urinary tract infections, pyelonephritis, pneumonia, diverticulitis, tuberculosis
   B. Viral
      Measles, mumps, varicella, rubella, hepatitis
3. Chronic or recurrent infections, such as pneumonia, sinusitis, urinary tract infection, or diverticulitis
4. Surgical history, such as splenectomy
5. Transfusion or previous transplant history and dates
6. Past travel history, including military service
7. Past immunosuppressive drug treatment (*eg*, for asthma, renal disease, or rheumatologic disease)
8. Lifestyle
   A. Smoking, drinking, illicit drug use, marijuana smoking
   B. Sexual partners, orientation, unprotected contact and date, safety practices used, sexually transmitted diseases, genital warts
   C. Food, consumption of raw fish or meat, consumption of unpasteurized products such as milk, cheese, fruit juices, or tofu
   D. Avocation—gardening and the use of gloves, cleaning sheds, hiking, camping, water sources, bathing pets, cleaning pet litter and cages, hunting practices
   E. Vocation—jobs that require exposure to possible infectious agents, such as daycare, ministry, small closed offices, garbage collections or dump workers, construction workers, forestry workers, health care, veterinarians, farmers

FIGURE 6-11

Infectious disease history to be taken prior to transplantation.

PRETRANSPLANT VIRAL SEROLOGIES TO CHECK AT THE PRETRANSPLANT VISIT

Viral serology	Treatment, work-up modification, or change in posttransplant treatment
Herpes simplex virus 1, 2	If positive, treat early posttransplant with acyclovir, famciclovir, or ganciclovir
Epstein-Barr virus	If negative, consider posttransplant ganciclovir. Test donor due to risk of posttransplant lymphoma with primary infection
Varicella-zoster virus	Consider vaccination with Oka strain live attenuated virus if negative or treatment with acyclovir following clinical exposure
Cytomegalovirus	If the recipient is positive or donor positive, consider prophylactic or preemptive antiviral treatment
HBsAg	If positive, check HBeAg and HBDNA and biopsy. If HBDNA positive, consider pretransplant antiviral treatment with interferon if biopsy allows. Consult hepatologist regarding other treatment options
Hepatitis C virus	If positive, check HCV RNA status by polymerase chain reaction. If positive biopsy even with normal transaminase values and consider pretransplant treatment with interferon
HIV	Consider safety of transplantation if true positive. More data are required to make an informed decision

FIGURE 6-12

Pretransplant viral serologies to check at the pretransplant visit.

INFECTIONS TRANSMITTED TO TRANSPLANT RECIPIENTS VIA THE DONOR ORGAN

Virus	Bacteria	Fungi	Parasitic
HIV, cytomegalovirus, herpes simplex virus, Epstein-Barr virus, hepatitis B virus, hepatitis C virus, hepatitis D virus (?), hepatitis G virus, adenovirus (?), parvovirus (?), papillomavirus, rabies, Creutzfeldt-Jakob	Aerobe (gram positive), aerobe (gram negative), anaerobes, *Mycobacterium tuberculosis*, atypical mycobacteria	*Candida albicans*, *Histoplasma capsulatum*, *Cryptococcus neoformans*, *Marosporium apiospermum*	Malaria toxoplasmosis, trypanosomiasis, strongyloidiasis

FIGURE 6-13

Infections transmitted to transplant recipients via the donor organ.

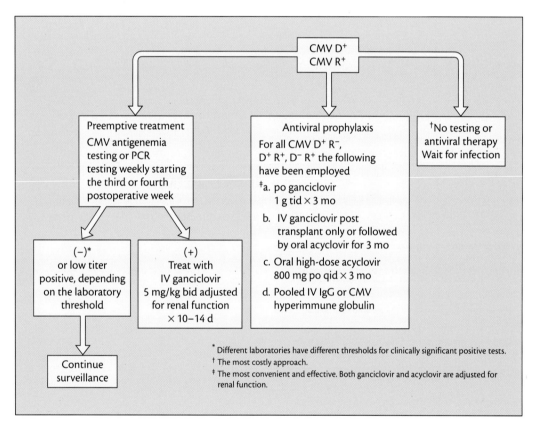

FIGURE 6-14

The "prevention" of cytomegalovirus (CMV) disease. This figure shows the different strategies for the management of CMV-positive transplant recipients or recipients of CMV-positive organs.

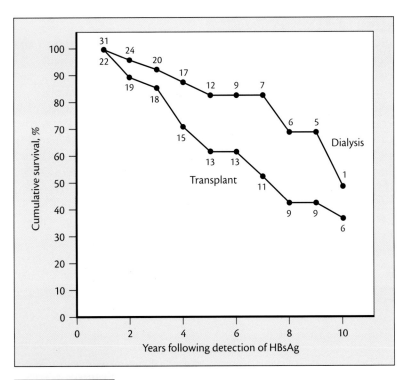

FIGURE 6-15

Survival of hepatitis B virus (HBV)–infected patients with end-stage renal disease treated with either dialysis or transplantation. Patients infected with HBV (hepatitis B surface antigen [HBsAg] positive) on hemodialysis were matched for age with 22 previously transplanted HBsAg-positive patients. This study shows the reason for concern and investigation as to the safety of transplantation in HBV-infected patients. Although there are other studies showing a significantly decreased survival in patients transplanted with HBV infection, most currently show equivalent survival of over 10 years. The cause of death in the HBV-infected group, however, may more often be from infection and liver failure than from cardiac disease.

The safety of transplantation in HBsAg-positive patients has been debated for over 25 years. Increased mortality, if seen, is usually seen beyond 10 years following transplantation and is often secondary to liver failure or sepsis. The acquisition of hepatitis B infections posttransplant, however, does carry a worse prognosis. Virtually all patients with severe chronic active hepatitis, and 50% to 60% of those with mild chronic active hepatitis on liver biopsy prior to transplantation, will progress to cirrhosis. Patients with chronic persistent hepatitis usually do not show histologic progression over 4 to 5 years of follow-up, although mild lesions do not guarantee preservation of hepatic function over longer periods. The complete natural history of hepatitis B following transplantation is not known, as biopsies have been performed largely in those who have abnormal liver function tests; however, one recent study that included analyses of all individuals who were HBsAg positive around the time of transplantation has shown histologic progression in 85.3% of those who were rebiopsied, with the development of hepatocellular carcinoma in eight of 35 patients who developed cirrhosis. A key to management of patients who were HBsAg positive following transplantation is to periodically monitor the liver by ultrasound and to perform a serum α-fetoprotein level to detect hepatocellular carcinoma at the earliest possible stage. The key to minimizing the effects of hepatitis B infections following transplantation, however, is to administer the hepatitis B vaccine as early as possible in the treatment for end-stage renal disease. It is noted that 60% will develop antihepatitis B titers when vaccinated while on dialysis compared with only 40% of those who have already been transplanted. Co-infection with hepatitis C may result in more aggressive liver disease but so far has not led to a marked decrease in patient survival. Because of the high risk of acute renal failure or rejection with the use of interferon posttransplant, treatment of hepatitis B with interferon following renal transplantation is not advised. Lamivudine or other experimental antihepatitis agents may be used pretransplant for patients with hepatitis B infection. (*Adapted from* Harnett *et al.* [10].)

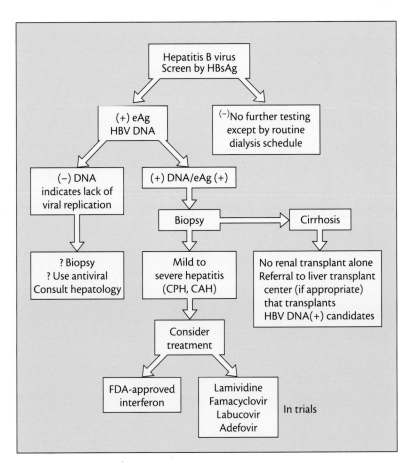

FIGURE 6-16

Hepatitis screening in renal transplant candidates. CAH—chronic active hepatitis; CPH—chronic persistent hepatitis; HBsAg—hepatitis B surface antigen; HBV—hepatitis B virus.

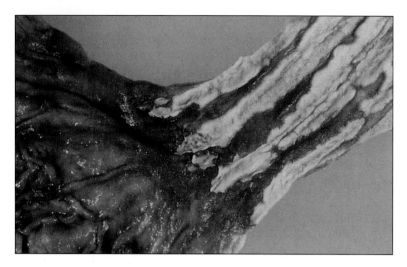

FIGURE 6-17 (*see* Color Plate)

Linear esophageal ulcers caused by herpes simplex virus (HSV) and *Candida*. Infection with HSV-1 and -2 leads to stomatitis and esophagitis posttransplantation without acyclovir prophylaxis. Additionally, paronychia, corneal ulcers, encephalitis, genital lesions, disseminated involvement of the gastrointestinal tract, pancreas, and liver, and interstitial nephritis has been seen. HSV-6 causes exanthem subitum in children, mononucleosis, and hepatitis. There has been some evidence that reactivation infections may be associated with rejection in transplant recipients. Both reactivation and reinfection may occur. HSV-8 is associated with Kaposi's sarcoma. Prevention of these infections has been achieved using prophylactic acyclovir following transplantation. If clinical symptoms occur from HSV, they usually are treated with acyclovir adjusted for renal function.

CAUSES OF HEADACHE IN THE TRANSPLANT RECIPIENT

Medications
  OKT3 (aseptic meningitis)
  ATG
  IVIgG
  Cyclosporine
  Tacrolimus
  Antihypertensives
    Calcium channel blockers
    ACE inhibitors
  Nitrates
  Hydralozine
  Minoxidil
Hypertension
Neck "tension," muscle pulls, ligamental irritation
Sinusitis
Ocular abnormalities
Excessive vomiting
Migraine headaches exacerbated by cyclosporine, tacrolimus, and
  calcium channel blockers
Stroke
Infection of the central nervous system

FIGURE 6-18

Causes of headache in the transplant recipient. ACE—angiotensin-converting enzyme; CNS—central nervous system; ATG—antithymocyte globulin.

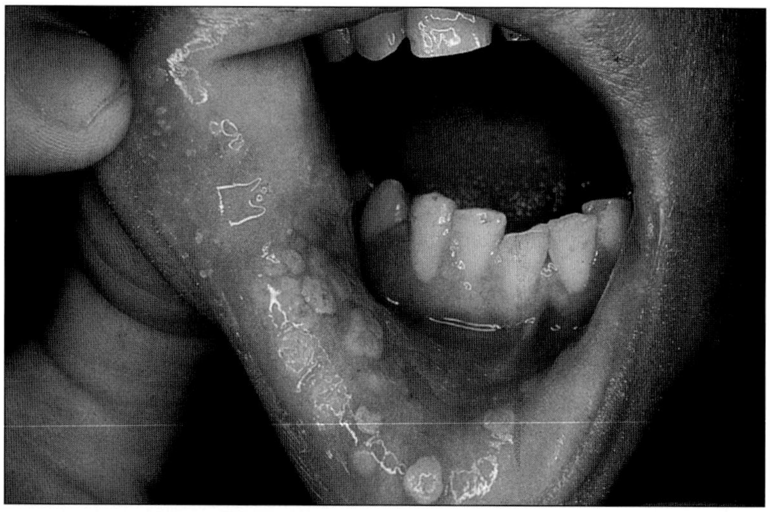

FIGURE 6-19 (*see* Color Plate)

Primary oral herpes simplex. Vesicles and ulceration are visible in the mucosal membrane.

Immunosuppressive Therapy and Protocols _____

AGENTS USED IN RENAL TRANSPLANTATION

Drug	Dosage	Adverse reactions
Cyclosporine Sandimmune (Sandoz Pharmaceuticals, East Hanover, NJ)	Starting dose: 7–10 mg/kg/d in 2 divided doses Maintenance: based on blood levels	Nephrotoxicity, hypertension, gingival overgrowth, hirsutism, hepatotoxicity, neurotoxicity, hypomagnesia, hyperkalemia
Neoral (Sandoz Pharmaceuticals, East Hanover, NJ)	Starting dose: 7–10 mg/kg/d in 2 divided doses Maintenance: based on blood levels IV Csa equals one third of oral Csa; IV cyclosporine is given by continuous infusion over 24 h	Same
Azathioprine Imuran (Glaxo Wellcome, Research Triangle Park, NC) Azathioprine (Roxane Laboratories, Columbus, OH) Azathioprine sodium (injectable) (Bedford Laboratories, Bedford, OH)	Starting and maintenance dose: 1–3 mg/kg/d; IV dose equals half of oral dose Decrease dose by half for 50% decrease in leukocyte count Hold dose for leukocyte count of <3000	Leukopenia, anemia, thrombocytopenia, hepatitis, pancreatitis, alopecia, skin cancer, aplastic anemia (rare)
OKT3 (Ortho Pharmaceutical, Raritan, NJ) Muromonab-cd3	Induction: 2 mg/d (low-dose) 5 mg/d (standard) Rejection treatment: 5 mg/d Hold (delay) dose for weight gain >3% or temperature >39°C Increase dose based on CD3+ cell count and CD3 density (suggested) Discontinue if anti-OKT3 antibody titer >1:1000	Cytokine release syndrome: fever, chills, chest pain, dyspnea, wheezing, noncardiogenic pulmonary edema, nausea, vomiting, diarrhea, headache, aseptic meningitis, seizures, skin rash
Antithymocyte globulin Atgam (Upjohn Co, Kalamazoo, MI)	Starting dose: 15–30 mg/kg/d Decrease (or hold) dose for leukocytes <3000 or platelets <100,000 Starting dose: 500 to 1000-mg infusion for 3–5 d	Leukopenia, thrombocytopenia, fever, chills, skin rash, back pain, headache, nausea, vomiting, diarrhea, horse serum sickness
Prednisone Deltasone (Upjohn Co, Kalamazoo, MI)	Maintenance: taper schedule (variable)	Fat redistribution, increased appetite, weight gain, hyperlipidemia, hypertension, peripheral edema, hyperglycemia, skin atrophy, poor healing, acne, night sweats, insomnia, mood changes, blurred vision, cataracts, glaucoma, osteoporosis
FK-506, tacrolimus Prograf (Fujisawa USA, Inc, Deerfield, IL)	Starting dose: 0.15–0.3 mg/kg/d in 2 divided doses Avoid IV (0.05–0.1 mg/kg/d as a continuous infusion over 24 h) Maintenance: based on blood levels	Nephrotoxicity, hypertension, hepatotoxicity, pancreatitis, diabetes, seizures, headache, insomnia, tremor, paresthesia
Mycophenolate mofetil CellCept (Roche Laboratories, Nutley, NJ)	Starting dose: 2–3 g/d orally in 2 divided doses (IV preparation in clinical trials) Maintenance: based on GI and bone marrow toxicities	Nausea, vomiting, diarrhea, leukopenia, anemia, thrombocytopenia
Daclizumab (Roche Laboratories, Nutley, NJ)	1 mg/kg/d every 2 wk for a total of 5 doses	Reported same as placebo
Simulect (Novartis Pharmaceuticals Inc., East Hanover, NJ)	20 mg/d, given on days 0 and 4 posttransplant	Reported same as placebo

CD3—monomorphic membrane coreceptor present in T lymphocytes; Csa—cyclosporine; GI—gastrointestinal. (*Adapted from* de Mattos *et al*. [11,12].)

FIGURE 6-20

This table summarizes the immunosuppressive agents currently used in human renal transplantation. Dosages and costs are subject to local variation. CD3—monomorphic membrane coreceptor present in T lymphocytes; Csa—cyclosporine; GI—gastrointestinal. (*Adapted from* de Mattos *et al*. [11,12].)

CLINICALLY RELEVANT DRUG INTERACTIONS WITH IMMUNOSUPPRESSIVE DRUGS

Drug	Effect	Mechanism
Cyclosporin A and tacrolimus		
Diltiazem	Increased blood levels	Decreased metabolism (inhibition of cytochrome P-450-IIIA 4)
Nicardipine		
Verapamil		
Erythromycin	Increased blood levels	Decreased metabolism (inhibition of cytochrome P-450-IIIA 4)
Clarithromycin		
Ketoconazole	Increased blood levels	Decreased metabolism (inhibition of cytochrome P-450-IIIA 4)
Fluconazole		
Itraconazole		
Methylprednisolone (high dose only)	Increased blood levels	Unknown
Carbamazepine	Decreased blood levels	Increased metabolism (inhibition of cytochrome P-450-IIIA 4)
Phenobarbital		
Phenytoin		
Rifampin		
Aminoglycosides	Increased renal dysfunction	Additive nephrotoxicity
Amphotericin B		
Cimetidine	Increased serum creatinine	Competition for tubular secretion
Lovastatin	Decreased metabolism	Myositis, increased creatine phosphokinase, rhabdomyolysis
Azathioprine		
Allopurinol	Increased bone marrow toxicity	Inhibiting xantine oxidase
Warfarin	Decreased anticoagulation effect	Increased prothrombin synthesis or activity
ACE inhibitors	Increased bone marrow toxicity	Not established
Mycophenolate mofetil		
Acyclovir-ganciclovir (high doses only)	Increased levels of acyclovir-ganciclovir and mycophenolate mofetil	Competition for tubular secretion
Antacids	Decreased absorption	Binding to mycophenolate mofetil
Cholestyramine	Decreased absorption	Interferes with enterohepatic circulation

FIGURE 6-21

Clinical relevant drug interactions with immunosuppressive agents. Close monitoring of drug levels is required periodically with concomitant use of drugs with potential interaction. Drug level monitoring is clinically available for cyclosporin A and tacrolimus. Monitoring of nonimmunosuppressive drug level is also important when used with potential interacting immunosuppressive agents. ACE—angiotensin-converting enzyme. (*Adapted from* de Mattos *et al.* [11,12].)

Evaluation of Prospective Donors and Recipients

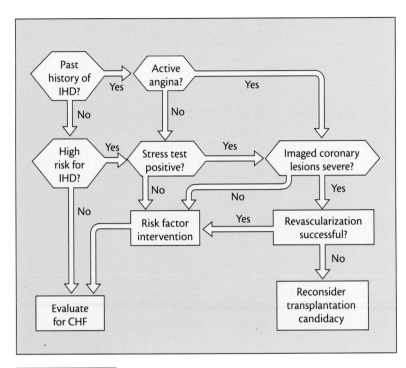

FIGURE 6-22

Ischemic heart disease (IHD). The incidence of IHD is several-fold higher in renal transplantation recipients compared with the general population. Patients with IHD before transplantation are at high risk to develop IHD events after transplantation. Therefore, angiography should be considered in candidates for transplantation who have angina pectoris. Candidates with currently asymptomatic IHD and those at high risk for IHD should undergo a stress test. Patients with severe coronary artery disease on angiography must be considered for a revascularization procedure before transplantation. Aggressive management of risk factors is appropriate for all patients, with or without IHD. (*Adapted from* Kasiske *et al.* [13].)

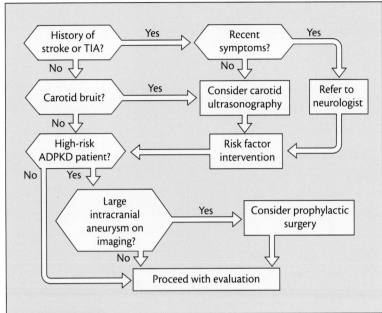

FIGURE 6-23

Cerebral vascular disease (CVD). Patients must not undergo surgery within 6 months of a stroke or transient ischemic attack (TIA). Asymptomatic patients with a carotid bruit should be considered for carotid ultrasonography because patients with severe carotid disease may be candidates for prophylactic surgery. Patients with autosomal dominant polycystic kidney disease (ADPKD) and either a previous episode or a positive family history of a ruptured intracranial aneurysm must be screened with computed tomography or magnetic resonance imaging. Patients found to have an aneurysm over 7 mm in diameter may benefit from prophylactic surgery. (*Adapted from* Kasiske *et al.* [13].)

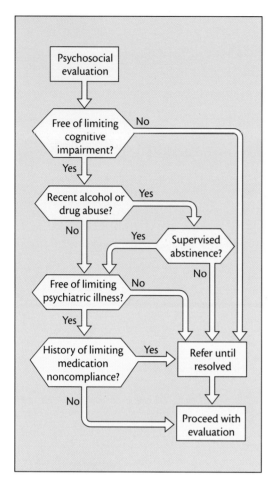

FIGURE 6-24

Psychosocial evaluation. Patients must be free of cognitive impairments and able to give informed consent. Most transplantation centers require patients with a history of alcohol or drug abuse to demonstrate a period of supervised abstinence, generally 6 months or more [12]. Similarly, patients with a past history of medication adherence poor enough to suspect that the immunosuppressive regimen will be compromised may need to delay transplantation until reasonable adherence can be demonstrated [12]. (*Adapted from* Kasiske *et al.* [13].)

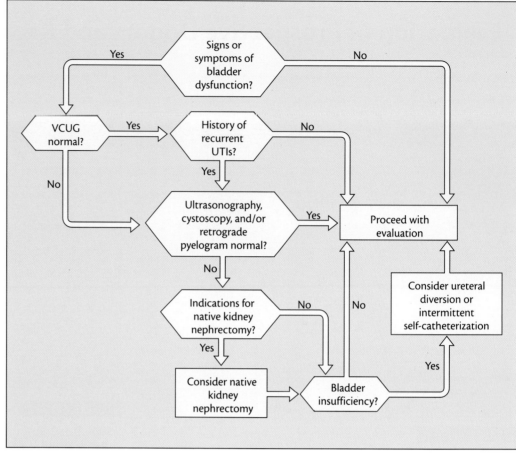

FIGURE 6-25

Urologic evaluation of transplantation recipients. Patients without signs and symptoms of bladder dysfunction generally do not need additional urologic testing. However, patients with bladder dysfunction must be evaluated to ensure that the bladder is functional after transplantation and that potential sources of urinary tract infection (UTI) are eliminated. Such patients can be screened initially with voiding cystourethrography (VCUG). (*Adapted from* Kasiske *et al.* [13].)

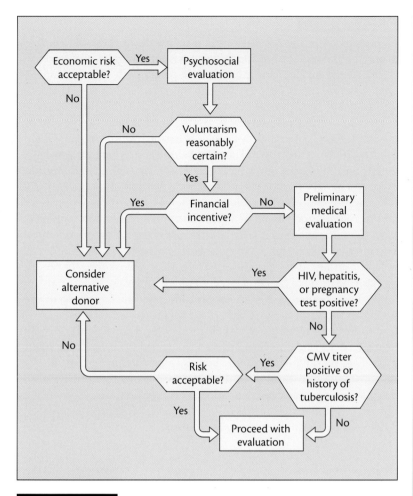

FIGURE 6-26

Preliminary evaluation of a living prospective donor. The prospective donor must be made aware of the possible costs associated with donation, including travel to and from the transplantation center and time away from work. The prospective donor must undergo a psychologic evaluation to ensure the donation is voluntary. A preliminary medical evaluation should assess the risks of transmitting infectious diseases with the kidney, *eg*, infection with HIV and cytomegalovirus (CMV). (*Adapted from* Kasiske *et al.* [14].)

FIGURE 6-27

Risk assessment for living donor. Older age may place the living prospective donor at greater surgical risk and may be associated with reduced graft survival for the recipient. The prospective donor must be informed of both the short-term surgical risks (very low in the absence of cardiovascular disease and other risk factors) and the long-term consequences of having only one kidney. With regard to long-term risks, it should be considered whether there is a familial disease that the living donor may be at risk to acquire and whether having only one kidney would alter the natural history of renal disease progression. These questions are often most pertinent for relatives of patients with diabetes. (*Adapted from* Kasiske *et al.* [14].)

Medical Complications of Renal Transplantation

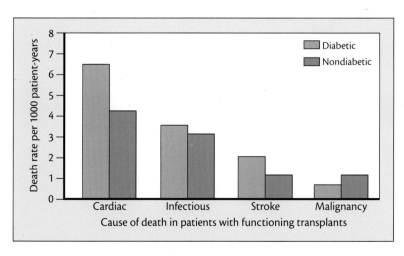

FIGURE 6-28

Causes of death in renal allograft recipients. Cardiovascular diseases are the most common cause of death, largely reflecting the high prevalence of coronary artery disease in this population [15]. The risks are particularly high among recipients who have diabetes, as many as 50% of whom, even if asymptomatic, may have significant coronary disease at the time of transplantation evaluation [16]. Effective management of cardiac disease after transplantation mandates documentation of preexisting disease in patients at greatest risk [17].

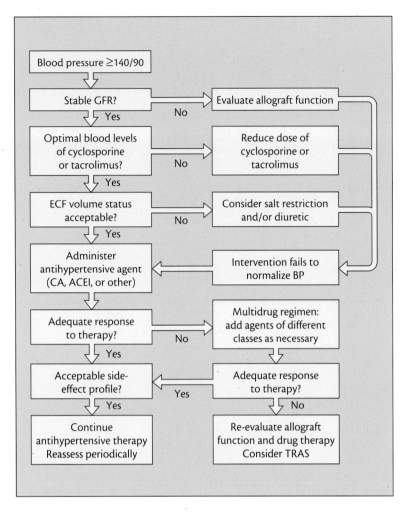

FIGURE 6-29

Hypertension in the renal transplant recipient. In these patients it may be possible to approach diagnosis and therapy in a fairly standardized fashion. In transplant recipients with blood pressure readings consistently over 140/90 mm Hg, intervention is warranted. The initial approach includes assessment of allograft function, extracellular fluid volume (ECF) status, and immunosuppressive dosing. If these variables are stable, it is reasonable to proceed with antihypertensive therapy. Calcium antagonists (CA) are effective agents and may offer the added benefit of attenuating cyclosporine-induced changes in renal hemodynamics. Verapamil, diltiazem, nicardipine, and mibefradil increase blood levels of cyclosporine and tacrolimus and should be used with caution. Common problems with CAs that may limit their use include cost, refractory edema, and gingival hyperplasia. Angiotensin antagonists (ACEIs and receptor antagonists) are also effective; their use requires close monitoring of renal function, serum potassium levels, and hematocrit levels. Diuretics frequently are useful adjuncts to therapy in recipients owing to the salt retention that often accompanies cyclosporine use. Other antihypertensive medications offer no particular benefits or drawbacks and can be employed as needed. The rationale of multidrug therapy is to employ agents that block hypertensive responses via interruption of differing pathogenetic pathways. As antihypertensive drugs are added, this consideration should remain paramount [18,19]. GFR—glomerular filtration rate; TRAS—transplanted renal artery stenosis.

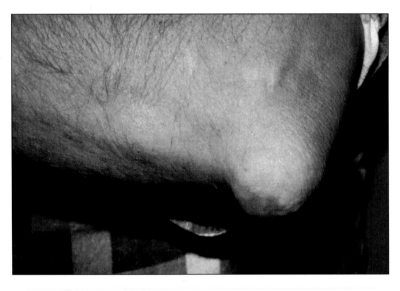

FIGURE 6-30

Photograph of gouty inflammation of joints (tophus). Gout is the clinical manifestation of hyperuricemia. After transplantation, cyclosporine can exacerbate hyperuricemia, and severe gout can be problematic even in the presence of chronic immunosuppression. Management of gouty arthritis usually involves some combination of colchicine and judicious use of short courses of nonsteroidal anti-inflammatory drugs. Concomitant administration of allopurinol and azathioprine can cause profound bone marrow suppression and is avoided by most physicians who treat transplant recipients. Because the metabolism of mycophenolate mofetil (MMF) is not dependent on xanthine oxidase, use of allopurinol in patients treated with MMF is relatively safe [20,21].

Technical Aspects of Renal Transplantation _____

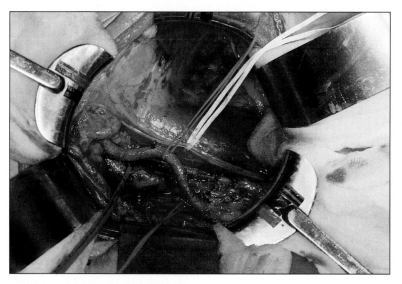

FIGURE 6-31 (*see* Color Plate)

Exposure of the right iliac fossa. The contents of the iliac fossa are exposed by incising the skin, subcutaneous tissues, anterior rectus sheath, external and internal oblique muscles, and the transversalis muscle and fascia. The inferior epigastric artery is divided between ligatures, the spermatic cord is preserved (in women, the round ligament is divided between ligatures), and the rectus muscle and peritoneum are retracted medially. This exposes the genitofemoral nerve (*white umbilical tape*), the external iliac vein (*blue tape*), and the external and internal iliac arteries (*red tapes*).

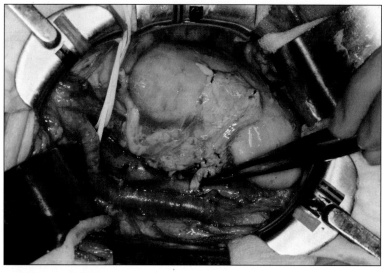

FIGURE 6-32

Determining "best fit." The kidney graft is placed in the wound and the renal vessels stretched to the recipient vessels to determine the best sites for the arterial and venous anastomoses.

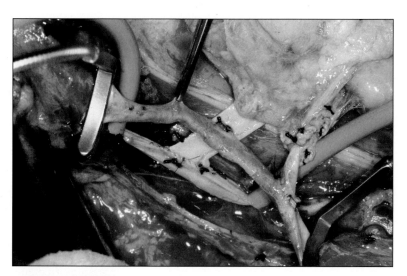

FIGURE 6-33

Completed venous and arterial anastomoses.

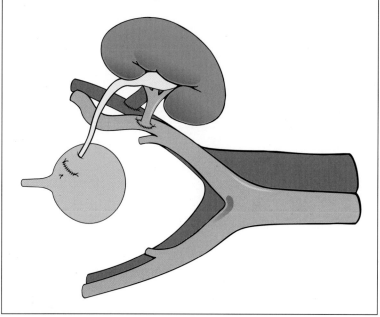

FIGURE 6-34

The completed kidney transplantation.

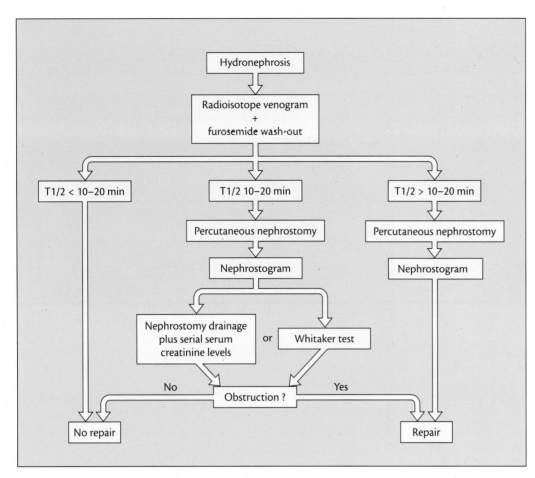

FIGURE 6-35

Algorithm for evaluation of kidney transplantation hydronephrosis [22]. The generally accepted criterion for exclusion of upper urinary tract obstruction is a washing out of half of the radioisotope from the renal pelvis in less than 10 minutes. Obstruction is considered to be present when this value is over 20 minutes. Percutaneous nephrostomy allows anatomic definition of the obstruction and temporary drainage of the hydronephrotic kidney. A generally accepted criterion for the diagnosis of obstruction with the percutaneous pressure-flow Whitaker test is fluid infusion into the pelvis at the rate of 10 mL/min, resulting in a renal pelvic pressure over 20 cm H_2O.

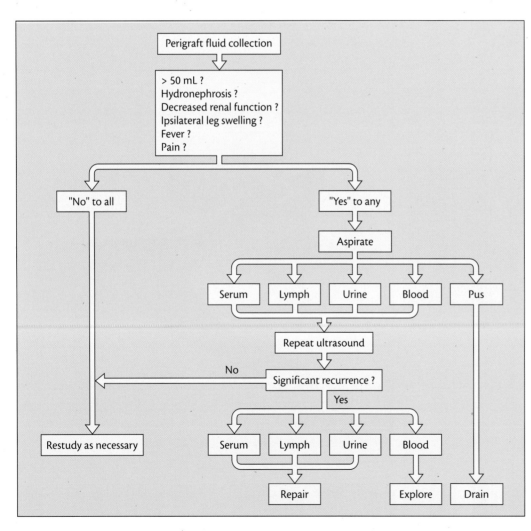

FIGURE 6-36

Algorithm for evaluation and treatment of perigraft fluid collection [22]. Perigraft fluid collection is one of the two most common urologic complications for which invasive therapy is required, the other being hydronephrosis owing to ureteral obstruction. Serum, urine, lymphatic fluid, blood, and pus can be differentiated by creatinine and hematocrit determinations and by microscopic examination of the fluid. Urine has a high creatinine level, serum and lymphatic fluid have low creatinine levels, and blood has a relatively high hematocrit level. Lymphocytes are present in lymphatic fluid, and polymorphonuclear leukocytes with or without organisms are present in pus. Open surgical drainage is usually necessary for fluid collections showing infection. Significant lymphoceles have been successfully treated with percutaneous sclerosis or by marsupialization into the peritoneal cavity by either a laparoscopic or open surgical technique. Persistent urinary extravasation often requires open surgical repair. Significant bleeding requires exploration and control of bleeding.

Kidney-Pancreas Transplantation

EXCLUSION CRITERIA FOR PANCREAS TRANSPLANTATION

Significant cardiac disease

Substance abuse

Psychiatric illness

History of noncompliance

Extreme obesity

Active infection or malignancy

No secondary complications of diabetes

The exclusion criteria for pancreas transplantation include significant cardiac disease, substance abuse, psychiatric illness, and a history of noncompliance. Extreme obesity, active infection, and malignancy are relative contraindications to transplantation. Patients with few or very mild secondary complications of diabetes may be candidates for kidney transplantation alone.

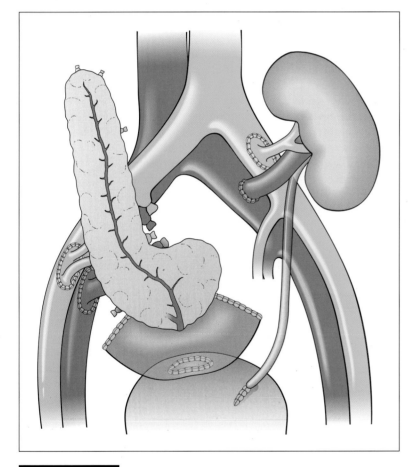

FIGURE 6-38

Simultaneous pancreas-kidney allograft procedure. Most pancreas transplantations performed in the United States are whole organ pancreaticoduodenal allografts from cadaveric donors transplanted simultaneously with the kidney from the same donor [23]. Because the pancreas from a patient with diabetes still subserves digestive function, it is not removed. Therefore, the pancreaticoduodenal allograft is transplanted to an ectopic location, usually the right iliac fossa. Similarly, the kidney allograft is transplanted ectopically to the contralateral iliac fossa. The reconstructed arterial supply to the pancreas is anastomosed to the common or external iliac artery. The portal vein of the allograft is anastomosed to the common iliac vein or distal inferior vena cava. Likewise, on the left side the renal artery and vein are anastomosed to the common iliac artery and vein, respectively. To restore the continuity of the urinary tract, a standard ureteroneocystostomy is constructed to the dome of the bladder.

Because the pancreas has dual endocrine and exocrine functions, it is necessary to perform another anastomosis to handle exocrine secretions. A variety of techniques to manage pancreatic exocrine secretions have been proffered over the years with less than satisfactory results. These include duct occlusion, open drainage into the peritoneal cavity, and creation of a button of duodenum and anastomosing this or the pancreatic duct directly to the bladder. Currently, the most commonly performed technique in the United States is drainage of pancreatic exocrine secretions into the bladder [23]. The bladder drainage (BD) technique involves fashioning a short segment of donor duodenum, which is transplanted along with the pancreas. Then the donor duodenum is anastomosed to the dome of the recipient bladder in a side-to-side manner. In this way exocrine secretions, including enzymes, proenzymes, water, and sodium bicarbonate, are diverted into the urinary tract. This technique is safe, reliable, and well tolerated; however, it is associated with a number of specific urinary tract complications.

As a consequence of implantation into the iliac fossa, the pancreatic allograft is drained into the systemic venous circulation, as depicted. This results in systemic venous, rather than portal venous, insulin release, and peripheral hyperinsulinemia. An alternative approach practiced by some surgeons is portal venous drainage. In this approach the portal vein of the allograft is anastomosed to the superior mesenteric vein of the recipient in an end-to-side fashion. This technique establishes drainage of insulin into the portal venous blood flow, perhaps a more physiologic situation (procedure not shown). The results of the two techniques are largely comparable. Fortunately, patients have suffered no adverse effects of systemic venous drainage and hyperinsulinemia.

Solitary pancreaticoduodenal allografts are implanted into either iliac fossa, at whichever point the iliac vessels permit vascular anastomoses. This procedure is done, usually and preferentially, on the right side. Otherwise, the operative sequence duplicates that of the combined procedure.

IMMUNOSUPPRESSIVE PROTOCOLS

SPK	PAK and PTA
ATGAM (20 mg/kg/d for 10 d)	ATGAM (20 mg/kg/d for 10 d) or
MMF (3 g/d)	OKT3 (5–10 mg/d for 10 d)
Neoral® (8 mg/kg/d)	MMF (2 g/d)
Prednisone (500 mg intraoperatively; 250	FK506 (8 mg/d)
mg on postoperative days 1 and 2; 30	Prednisone (500 mg intraoperatively; 250
mg/d thereafter)	mg on postoperative days 1 and 2; 30
	mg/d thereafter)

FIGURE 6-39

Because the best treatment of rejection is prevention, the most efficacious regimen of immunosuppressive drugs should be used first.

Quadruple-drug immunosuppressive regimens, including the use of antithymocyte globulin (ATGAM) or OKT3 (muromonab, murine antihuman CD3 monoclonal antibody), have been accepted as standard at most pancreas transplant centers. Recent data from the United Network for Organ Sharing and several smaller retrospective comparative trials provide evidence that anti–T-cell antibody induction therapy may lessen the severity and delay the onset of rejection and may improve short-term graft survival in recipients of simultaneous pancreas-kidney (SPK) transplants [23–25]. This is the current practice. The development of newer more specific immunosuppressive agents, however, recently has changed the face of modern immunosuppression in solid organ transplantation and raises the possibility of successful pancreas transplantation without induction therapy. Mycophenolate mofetil (MMF) has recently replaced azathioprine (AZA) as maintenance immunosuppressive therapy in kidney transplantation alone, SPK, and pancreas transplantation alone. MMF is a potent noncompetitive reversible inhibitor of inosine monophosphate dehydrogenase (IMPDH). IMPDH is an essential enzyme in the *de novo* purine synthetic pathway upon which lymphocyte DNA synthesis and proliferation are strictly dependent. Compared with AZA, MMF has no association with pancreatitis and has less association with leukopenia. Moreover, whereas AZA is not useful in treating ongoing rejection, MMF can salvage refractory acute renal allograft rejection in up to half of patients. By virtue of this mechanism of action, MMF provides more effective and specific immunosuppression with less risk compared with AZA.

Similarly, Neoral, a microemulsified formulation of cyclosporine (CsA) has replaced standard CsA therapy with Sandimmune (both drugs from Sandoz Pharmaceuticals, East Hanover, NJ). Because of gastroparesis and autonomic dysfunction, patients with diabetes exhibit unpredictable absorption of CsA. The new formulation of CsA has an increased rate and extent of drug absorption with lower inter- and intra-individual pharmacokinetic variability than does Sandimmune, particularly in patients with diabetes. Improved bioavailability and more reliable pharmacokinetics may translate into fewer rejection episodes and improved graft survival. Experience with tacrolimus (FK506) in pancreas transplantation for induction, maintenance, and rescue therapy has demonstrated that it is safe, well tolerated, and has a low risk of glucose intolerance. Moreover, particularly for solitary pancreas transplants, strikingly improved short-term graft survival results have been reported [26,27]. The mechanism of action of FK506 as a calcineurin inhibitor is similar to that of CsA. FK506 has a better side-effect profile compared with CsA, causing less hirsutism, less hyperlipidemia, but somewhat more neurotoxicity. Unlike CsA, FK506 can rescue patients with refractory rejection and treat ongoing rejection. One caveat when using FK506 in combination with MMF is the risk of overimmunosuppression. Several studies have highlighted the fact that FK506 may increase blood levels of the active metabolite of MMF, mycophenolic acid, in a clinically relevant manner [27]. By reducing the incidence of rejection, these modern immunosuppressants have resulted in improved short- and long-term graft survival. Fewer rejection episodes will likely translate into an overall reduction in the glucocorticoid dosage being given in the perioperative period. This reduction may favorably impact short-term infectious complications and long-term steroid-related adverse side effects.

EFFECTS OF PANCREAS TRANSPLANTATION ALONE ON SECONDARY COMPLICATIONS OF DIABETES

Maintenance of normoglycemia	Beneficial
Neuropathy	Stabilization and improvement
Prevention of recurrent nephropathy	Beneficial
Quality of life	Major
Retinopathy	None
Vascular disease	Minimal

FIGURE 6-40

Multiple studies have been performed on the effects of pancreas transplantation on the secondary complications of diabetes. Unfortunately, most of these studies were performed with small numbers of patients and were not randomized controlled studies. There are four major benefits of pancreas transplantation for the secondary complications of diabetes: 1) normoglycemia has been demonstrated for an extended period of time as long as the pancreas is functioning, 2) nephropathy has been shown to improve, 3) pancreas transplantation appears to prevent recurrent diabetic nephropathy in the transplanted kidney, and 4) improved quality of life. Complete freedom from insulin injections appears to be the major benefit of pancreas transplantation. Unfortunately, pancreas transplantation does not appear to reverse established diabetic nephropathy in patients with their own kidneys, and established retinopathy and vascular disease do not appear to improve.

Transplantation in Children

DISEASES CAUSING END-STAGE RENAL DISEASE

Disease category	Children <18 years, %*	Adults 20–64 years, %†,
Urologic malformations	26	4
Renal dysplasia	17	0.3
Other congenital causes	15	5
Focal segmental glomerulosclerosis	11	2
Other glomerulonephrites and immunologic diseases	14	17
Hypertensive nephropathy	0	22
Diabetic nephropathy	0.1	40
All other causes	17	10

*Data from North American Pediatric Renal Transplant Cooperative Study.
†Data from United States Renal Data Source.

FIGURE 6-41

Different diseases causing end-stage renal disease in children and adults. The leading causes of chronic renal failure in young children are inherited disorders or congenital abnormalities of the urinary tract, especially obstructive uropathy and reflux nephropathy. Focal segmental glomerulosclerosis and other glomerular disorders are seen more often in older children. Almost no children develop end-stage renal disease as a result of diabetic nephropathy and hypertension, the leading causes of end-stage renal disease in adults. (*Adapted from* Harmon [29].)

RISK FACTORS ASSOCIATED WITH GRAFT FAILURE

Cadaveric donor	Relative risk increase	P value
Recipient age (<2 y)	2.03	0.001
Donor age (<6 y)	1.47	0.001
Previous transplantation	1.36	0.004
ATG, ALG, OKT3 early administration (none)	1.36	0.001
More than 5 lifetime transfusions	1.37	0.001
No DR matches	1.23	0.01
Annual cohort (1992 vs 1987)	1.29	0.04
Living related donor		
Recipient age <2 y	1.4	0.08
Black race	1.9	<0.001
More than 5 previous transfusions	1.7	<0.001

FIGURE 6-42

Risk factors associated with graft failure in a proportional hazards model for recipients of donor grafts. ALG—antilymphocytic globulin; ATG—antithrombocytic globulin. (*Adapted from* Warady *et al.* [30].)

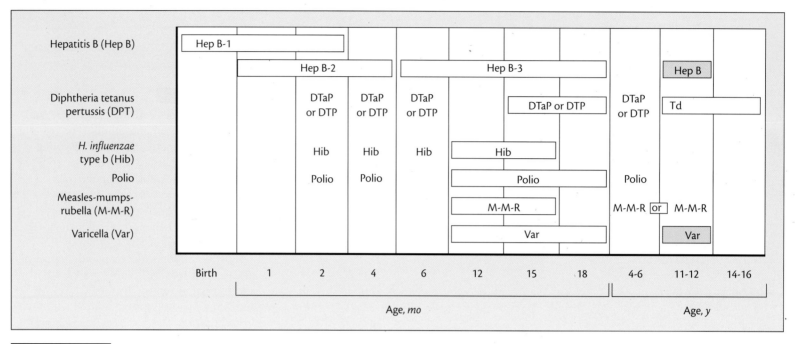

FIGURE 6-43

Infection remains a major cause of morbidity and mortality in pediatric transplantation recipients. Many infections can be successfully prevented by immunization. The recommended US immunization schedule for children (January–December 1997) before transplantation is outlined. Diphtheria-tetanus-pertussis vaccine, *Haemophilus influenza* type b vaccine, inactivated poliovirus vaccine, and hepatitis B immunizations can be given after transplantation but their efficacy may be suboptimal. The live attenuated vaccines, oral polio vaccine (OPV), measles-mumps-rubella (M-M-R) vaccine, and varicella virus vaccine, usually are recommended to be given only after immunosuppressive therapy has been discontinued for 3 months. Influenza A vaccines also should be administered yearly in the fall to pediatric transplantation recipients. The advent of the varicella virus vaccine may decrease the chances of pediatric transplantation recipients developing severe chickenpox and the incidence of zoster [31]. A recent survey by the North American Pediatric Renal Transplant Cooperative Study found that almost 90% of centers recommend the use of influenza vaccine, whereas only 60% of centers recommend pneumococcal vaccine for children with renal disease. Between 5% and 12% of centers recommend live viral vaccines, including OPV, M-M-R vaccine, and varicella virus vaccine, for immunosuppressed patients after renal transplantation.

Vaccines are listed under the routinely recommended ages. *Bars* indicate the range of acceptable ages for vaccination. *Shaded bars* indicate *catch-up vaccination*: at 11 to 12 years of age, hepatitis B vaccine should be administered to children not previously vaccinated, and varicella virus vaccine should be administered to children not previously vaccinated who lack a reliable history of having had chickenpox. This schedule indicates the recommended age for routine administration of currently licensed childhood vaccines. Some combination vaccines are available and may be used whenever administration of all components of the vaccine is indicated. Providers should consult the manufacturers' package inserts for detailed recommendations. Approved by the Advisory Committee on Immunization Practices (ACIP), American Academy of Pediatrics (AAP), and American Academy of Family Physicians (AAFP). (*See* Red Book [31] for more information.) (*Adapted from* Furth *et al.* [32].)

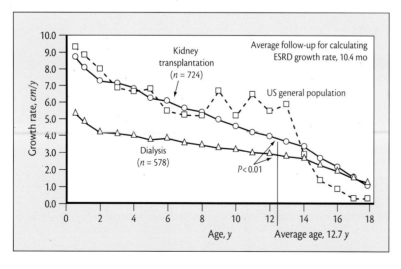

FIGURE 6-44

Chronic renal insufficiency and end-stage renal disease (ESRD) resulting in physical growth and sexual development well below the potential for age and gender [33]. One of the benefits of transplantation in children has been to improve the growth rate; however, this may not occur in all patients [34–36]. Depicted is the overall comparison between adjusted annualized growth rates by age for prevalent pediatric transplantation and dialysis patients (1990 USRDS data) [37] and the US general population (1976–1980 data from the National Center for Health Statistics) [38]. Shown are the results of a linear regression analysis of growth rates for 578 patients on dialysis and 724 transplantation recipients. Growth rates were adjusted to reflect the average characteristics of patients with ESRD at each age with regard to gender, race, ethnicity, baseline height, and duration of ESRD. At almost all ages, growth rates were higher for transplantation recipients compared with patients on dialysis; however, the degree of advantage declined with age. No pubertal growth spurt was seen in either treatment group. Although growth rates in adolescents between 15 and 18 years of age were higher than expected for both the dialysis and transplantation groups, the average height achieved at the end of the study was still lower than expected. (*Adapted from* Turenne *et al.* [39].)

FIGURE 6-45

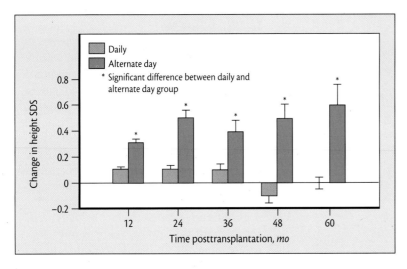

Corticosteroids are an integral part of pediatric renal transplantation immunosuppressive protocols. In addition to hypertension and hyperlipidemia, one of the main adverse effects of daily steroid dosing in children is growth retardation. A review of North American Pediatric Renal Transplant Cooperative Study data, looking at the change in the height standard deviation score (SDS) from 30 days after transplantation to 12 to 60 months after transplantation analyzed the difference between the 1477 children treated continuously on a daily or alternate-day steroid regimen. The mean change in SDS was significantly greater for the alternate-day group at each 12-month interval ($P < 0.05$). Of note is the fact that at 12 months, those children on alternate-day steroids had a mean serum creatinine of 1.06 ± 0.04 mg/dL as compared with 1.28 ± 0.02 mg/dL for those on daily steroids ($P < 0.001$). Alternate-day therapy also was more common in children without a rejection episode in the first 12 months after transplantation, recipients of living donor grafts, white recipients, and children 2 to 12 years of age at the time of transplantation. (*Adapted from* Jabs *et al.* [40].)

DIAGNOSIS OF ACUTE REJECTION

Clinical picture

Fever, weight gain, enlargement and tenderness of graft, hypertension, reduced urinary output, decreased renal function, reduced urinary sodium excretion, and increased proteinuria

Cyclosporine trough blood level

When these levels are higher than expected, cyclosporine nephrotoxicity is suspected; however, this does not rule out rejection—very low levels, in the presence of elevated serum creatinine, suggest acute rejection, perhaps as a result of noncompliance

Radionuclide renal studies

Provide information about blood flow and the excretion index, and aid in excluding extravasation and obstruction

Renal sonography with Doppler ultrasonography

Provides information about kidney size, renal blood flow, corticomedullary differentiation, pyramid shape, and the collecting system; establishes the diagnosis of obstruction, extravasation, and renal artery stenosis

Renal arteriogram

Establishes the diagnosis of major renal vessel stenosis or occlusion

Magnetic resonance imaging

Establishes the diagnosis of obstruction, renal vessel stenosis, or occlusion; aids in evaluating the corticomedullary junction and pyramid shape

Fine-needle aspiration biopsy

Identifies inflammatory cells in the graft, tubular damage, cyclosporine toxicity, and cytomegalovirus infection; aids in differentiating rejection, acute tubular necrosis, cytomegalovirus infection, and cyclosporine nephrotoxicity

Renal biopsy

Remains the gold standard for determining rejection and cyclosporine nephrotoxicity

FIGURE 6-46

When impaired graft function occurs in pediatric renal transplantation recipients, rejection is the most common cause. A number of other conditions exist that also can result in an increase in serum creatinine and blood urea nitrogen, a decrease in urine output, or both, which must be differentiated from rejection. In small children with large allografts, the most sensitive indication of rejection is hypertension. It is important to remember that in small children, a small increase in serum creatinine can reflect a significant decrease in the glomerular filtration rate. Several methods to establish the cause of renal allograft dysfunction are described; however, the diagnostic gold standard is the allograft core biopsy. Biopsy can easily be performed percutaneously in most children and should not be postponed once other variables have been eliminated and rejection is likely. (*Adapted from* Yadin *et al.* [41].)

GRAFT FAILURE FROM RECURRENT DISEASE

Disease	Recurrence rate, %	Clinical severity	Those with recurrence whose graft failed, %
FSGS	25–30	High	40–50
MPGN type I	70	Mild	12–30
MPGN type II	100	Low	10–20
SLE	5–40	Low	5
HSP	55–85	Low to mild	5–20
HUS			
Classic	12–20	Moderate	0–10
Atypical	±25	High	40–50

FIGURE 6-47

Recurrence rates and graft failure from recurrent disease. Some primary renal diseases may recur in the allograft, making the underlying disease an important consideration when evaluating a child for renal transplantation. Focal segmental glomerular sclerosis and atypical hemolytic uremic syndrome recur in roughly 25% of cases. These diseases are severe clinically and lead to the highest percentage of graft failures, *ie*, 40% to 50%. In contrast, membranoproliferative glomerulonephritis type II recurs in all cases; however, it is not very severe clinically and leads to graft failure in only 10% to 20% of patients. FSGS—focal segmental glomerulosclerosis; HSP—Henoch-Schönlein purpura; HUS—hemolytic-uremic syndrome; MPGN—membranoproliferative glomerulonephritis; SLE—systemic lupus erythematosus. (*Adapted from* Fine and Ettenger [42].)

Recurrent Disease in the Transplanted Kidney

DIFFERENTIAL DIAGNOSIS OF RECURRENT DISEASE AFTER KIDNEY TRANSPLANTATION

De novo glomerulonephritis
Transplanted glomerulonephritis
Chronic rejection
Acute allograft glomerulopathy
Chronic allograft glomerulopathy
Cyclosporine toxicity
Acute rejection
Allograft ischemia
Cytomegalovirus infection

FIGURE 6-48

Acute cellular rejection and cyclosporine toxicity usually can be distinguished easily from recurrent glomerular disease. Recurrent hemolytic uremic syndrome, however, can cause a microangiopathy similar to cyclosporine toxicity, with erythrocyte fragments visible both in blood films and within glomerular capillary loops. The major diagnostic difficulty lies with chronic rejection, especially in the form of transplantation glomerulopathy, and *de novo* or transplanted glomerulonephritis. Chronic transplantation glomerulopathy occurs in 4% of renal allografts and usually is associated with proteinuria of more than 1 g/d, beginning a few months after transplantation. Chronic glomerulopathy shares some features with both recurrent mesangiocapillary glomerulonephritis type I and hemolytic uremic syndrome: glomerular capillary wall thickening, mesangial expansion, and double contour patterns of the capillary walls with mesangial cell interposition [43]. Thus, a definitive diagnosis of recurrent nephritis may require histologic characterization of the underlying primary renal disease and a graft biopsy before transplantation.

INVESTIGATING RECURRENT DISEASE AFTER KIDNEY TRANSPLANTATION

Renal biopsy with immunofluorescence and electron microscopy

Cyclosporin A level

Urine microscopy and culture

24-h urine protein

Renal ultrasonography

Anti–glomerular basement membrane autoantibody and antineutrophil cytoplasm antibody

Cytomegalovirus serology and viral antigen detection

Hepatitis C virus serology and RNA detection

FIGURE 6-49

Confirming a diagnosis of recurrent disease requires a renal biopsy. Features that favor recurrence include an active urine sediment with erythrocytes and erythrocyte casts, heavy proteinuria, and normal cyclosporine levels. Serologic testing for anti–glomerular basement membrane antibody is important in patients with Alport's or Goodpasture's syndrome, and blood film examination for patients with previous hemolytic uremic syndrome. Immuno-fluorescence and electron microscopic studies are rarely performed routinely on transplantation biopsies but can be vital in making a diagnosis of recurrent nephritis.

RECURRENT DISEASES AFTER KIDNEY TRANSPLANTATION

Recurrent diseases that commonly cause graft failure	Histologic recurrence only, graft failure uncommon	Histologic recurrence rare
Primary hyperoxaluria type I	Diabetes mellitus	Systemic lupus erythematosus
Focal segmental glomerulosclerosis	IgA disease	Systemic vasculitis
Hemolytic uremic syndrome	Henoch-Schönlein purpura	Idiopathic rapidly progressive GN
Henoch-Schönlein purpura	Membranous GN	Membranous GN
Mesangiocapillary GN type I (and, less commonly, type II)	Mesangiocapillary GN type II	
IgA disease?	Anti–glomerular basement membrane disease	
	Systemic vasculitis (antineutrophil cytoplasm antibody–associated)	
	Fabry's disease	

FIGURE 6-50

The prevalence and incidence of recurrent disease after transplantation is difficult to ascertain. Certainly, systemic lupus erythematosus and idiopathic rapidly progressive glomerulonephritis rarely recur in grafts, whereas in some groups of patients recurrence of focal segmental glomerulosclerosis is universal [44]. There is much debate as to the frequency of recurrence of immunoglobulin A disease and whether there is any association of recurrence with graft dysfunction [45,46]. Recurrence of an underlying primary renal disease may cause changes within the allograft and predispose patients to acute rejection and graft failure, *eg,* upregulation of human leukocyte antigens in parenchymal tissue. Proteinuria and dyslipidemia also can lead to changes in the expression of cell surface proteins critical for antigen presentation and immune regulation.

PATIENT MANAGEMENT IN RENAL OR HEPATORENAL TRANSPLANTATIONS FOR PRIMARY HYPEROXALURIA

Aggressive preoperative dialysis (and possibly continued postoperatively)

Maintenance of high urine output

Low oxalate, low ascorbic acid, diet low in vitamin D

Phosphate supplements

Magnesium glycerophosphate

High-dose pyridoxine (500 mg/d)

Thiazide diuretics

FIGURE 6-51

Daily hemodialysis for at least 1 week before transplantation depletes the systemic oxalate pool to some extent. Some centers continue aggressive hemodialysis after transplantation, regardless of the renal function of the transplanted organ. In patients receiving combined hepatorenal grafts, dietary measures to reduce oxalate production are not as important as they are in patients receiving isolated kidney grafts. In these patients, excess production of oxalate from glyoxylate still occurs. Magnesium and phosphate supplements are powerful inhibitors of calcium oxalate crystallization and should be used in all recipients, whereas thiazide diuretics may reduce urinary calcium excretion. Pyridoxine is a cofactor for alanine–glyoxylate aminotransferase and can increase the activity of the enzyme in some patients. Pyridoxine has no role in combined hepatorenal transplantation. For most patients, the ideal option is probably a combined transplantation when their glomerular filtration rate decreases below 25 mL/min [47,48].

FEATURES OF RECURRENT SYSTEMIC LUPUS ERYTHEMATOSUS

Rash
Arthralgia
Proteinuria (usually nonnephrotic)
Increasing anti-DNA antibody titers
Increasing antinuclear antibody titers
Decreasing complement levels (C3 and C4)

FIGURE 6-52

Nephritis caused by systemic lupus erythematosus (SLE) rarely recurs in transplantations. SLE accounts for approximately 1% of all patients receiving allografts, and less than 1% of these will develop recurrent renal disease. Time to recurrence has been reported as 1.5 to 9 years after transplantation [49,50]. Cyclosporine therapy does not prevent recurrence. It is reasonable to ensure that serologic test results for SLE are minimally abnormal before transplantation and certainly that patients have no evidence of active extrarenal disease. Patients with lupus anticoagulant and anticardiolipin antibodies are at risk of thromboembolic events, including renal graft vein or artery thrombosis. These patients may require anticoagulation therapy or platelet inhibition with aspirin.

RENAL COMPLICATIONS OF HEPATITIS C VIRUS AFTER KIDNEY TRANSPLANTATION

Clinical
  Proteinuria
  Nephrotic syndrome
  Microscopic hematuria
Histologic and laboratory findings
  Mesangiocapillary glomerulonephritis with or without cryoglobulinemia, hypocomplementemia, rheumatoid factors
  Membranous nephropathy: normal complement, no cryoglobulinemia or rheumatoid factor
  Acute and chronic transplantation glomerulopathy

FIGURE 6-53

Recurrence of both mesangiocapillary glomerulonephritis (MCGN) and, less frequently, membranous nephropathy is well described after transplantation. Nineteen cases of *de novo* or recurrent MCGN after transplantation have been described in patients with hepatitis C virus (HCV) [51]. Almost all had nephrosis and exhibited symptoms 2 to 120 months after transplantation. Eight patients had demonstrable cryoglobulin, nine had hypocomplementemia, and most had normal liver function test results. Membranous GN is the most common *de novo* GN reported in allografts, and it is possible that HCV infection may be associated with its development [51]. Twenty patients with recurrent or *de novo* membranous GN and HCV viremia have been reported. In one study, 8% of patients with membranous GN had HCV antibodies and RNA compared with less than 1% of patients with other forms of GN (excluding MCGN) [52]. Prognosis in these patients was poor, with persistent heavy proteinuria and declining renal function.

DIFFERENTIAL DIAGNOSIS OF SEGMENTAL GLOMERULAR SCARS ON TRANSPLANTATION BIOPSY

Diagnosis	Features
Recurrent FSGS	Recurrent heavy proteinuria within 3 mo
	Original disease caused renal failure in <3 y
Rejection	Insidious onset of proteinuria
	Features of chronic rejection on biopsy, especially vascular sclerosis and glomerulopathy
Cyclosporine-related	Previous thrombotic microangiopathy affecting glomeruli
De novo FSGS	Original disease not FSGS
	Chronic rejection excluded
Other glomerulonephritides	Characteristic immunohistology and electron microscopy, especially in IgA disease

FIGURE 6-54

Segmental glomerular scars in a functioning graft is a common finding. The interpretation of the biopsy requires knowledge of the previous histology in the native kidneys and the clinical course after transplantation. Immunohistology and electron microscopy can be particularly helpful in this setting. Recurrent focal segmental glomerulosclerosis is the most common cause of early massive proteinuria. Both rejection and cyclosporine therapy, however, can cause segmental scars indistinguishable from those of focal segmental glomerulosclerosis (FSGS). Recurrent or *de novo* IgA disease in an allograft also can cause segmental glomerular scarring, but with mesangial hypercellularity, IgA detectable by immunostaining, and paramesangial deposits on electron microscopy.

FEATURES OF RECURRENT AND *DE NOVO* MEMBRANOUS NEPHROPATHY AFTER TRANSPLANTATION

Features	*De novo* membranous	Recurrent membranous
Incidence	2%–5%	3%–57%
Clinical presentation	Often asymptomatic; proteinuria, nephrotic syndrome develops slowly	Proteinuria, nephrotic syndrome develops rapidly
Time of onset	4 mo to 6 y (mean, 22 mo)	1 wk to 2 y (mean, 10 mo)
Histology	Identical to native membranous nephropathy, often shows features of chronic rejection	Identical to native membranous nephropathy; often shows features of chronic rejection
Risk factors for graft failure	None specific	Male gender, aggressive clinical course
Incidence of graft failure	Increased over controls; may be as high as 50% but most patients also have chronic rejection	50%–60%, but some studies have shown no increased graft failure rate compared with other nephritides

FIGURE 6-55

Recurrence of membranous nephropathy in transplantations is variable, with studies reporting incidences from 3% to 57% [44,53]. The major differential diagnosis is *de novo* membranous nephropathy in patients with a different underlying renal pathology. *De novo* allograft membranous glomerulonephritis reported in 2% to 5% of transplantations is often asymptomatic and usually associated with chronic rejection [54]. In contrast, recurrent disease frequently causes nephrotic syndrome, developing within the first 2 years after transplantation. Data on the incidence of graft failure attributable to membranous disease are confusing. Cyclosporine therapy has made no difference in the incidence of the two entities, and hepatitis C virus infection may be associated with membranous disease after transplantation.

MANAGEMENT OF RECURRENT DISEASE AFTER KIDNEY TRANSPLANTATION

Disease	Treatment of recurrence
Focal segmental glomerulosclerosis	Plasma exchange, immunoadsorption, steroids, angiotensin-converting enzyme inhibitors, nonsteroidal anti-inflammatory drugs
IgA nephropathy	With crescents: plasma exchange, cytotoxics
Henoch-Schönlein purpura	Steroids (?)
Mesangiocapillary glomerulonephritis type I	Aspirin, dipyridamole
Mesangiocapillary glomerulonephritis type II	Plasma exchange (?)
Membranous nephropathy	Cytotoxics and steroids (?)
Anti–glomerular basement membrane disease	Plasma exchange, cyclophosphamide
Hemolytic uremic syndrome	Plasma exchange, plasma infusion
Antineutrophil cytoplasm antibody–associated vasculitis	Cyclophosphamide and steroids
Diabetes	Glycemic control
Oxalosis	Aggressive perioperative dialysis, hydration, low oxalate diet, low ascorbic acid diet, phosphate supplements, magnesium glycerophosphate, pyridoxine

FIGURE 6-56

No controlled data exist on the management of recurrent disease after transplantation. For patients with primary hyperoxaluria, measures to prevent further deposition of oxalate have proved successful in controlling recurrent renal oxalosis [48]. In diabetes mellitus, the pathophysiology of recurrent nephropathy undoubtedly reflects the same insults as those causing the initial renal failure, and good evidence exists that glycemic control can slow the development of end-organ damage. Plasma exchange and immunoadsorption are promising therapies for patients with nephrosis who have recurrent focal segmental glomerulosclerosis; however, these therapies do not provide sustained remission [55,56]. In all these cases, establishing a diagnosis of recurrent disease is critical in identifying a possible treatment modality.

References

1. United Network for Organ Sharing: *UNOS Bulletin* 1997, 2.

2. Cecka JM: The role of HLA in renal transplantation. *Human Immunology* 1997, 56:6–16.

3. Gray D, Shepherd H, Daar A, *et al.*: Oral versus intravenous high dose steroid treatment of renal allograft rejection. *Lancet* 1978, 1:117.

4. Chan L, French ME, Beare J, *et al.*: Prospective trial of high dose versus low dose prednisone in renal transplantation. *Transpl Proc* 1980, 12:323.

5. Auphan N, DiDonato JA, Rosette C, *et al.*: Immunosuppression by glucocorticoids: inhibition of NF-kB activation through induction of IkBa. *Science* 1995, 270:286.

6. Ortho Multicenter Study Group: A randomized trial of OKT3 monoclonal antibody for acute rejection of cadaveric renal transplants. *N Engl J Med* 1985, 313:337.

7. Norman DJ, Shield CF, Henell KR, *et al.*: Effectiveness of a second course of OKT3 monoclonal anti-T cell antibody for treatment of renal allograft rejection. *Transplantation* 1988, 46:523.

8. Schroeder TJ, First MR: Monoclonal antibodies in organ transplantation. *Am J Kidney Dis* 1994, 23:138.

9. Rubin RH, Wolfson JS, Cosimi AB, *et al.*: Infection in the renal transplant recipient. *Am J Med* 1981, 70:405–411.

10. Harnett JD, Zeldis JB, Parfrey PS, *et al.*: Hepatitis B disease in dialysis and transplant patients: further epidemiologic and serologic studies. *Transplantation* 1987, 44:369.

11. de Mattos AM, Olyaei AJ, Bennett WMPharmacology of immunosuppressive medications used in renal diseases and transplantation. *Am J Kidney Dis* 1996, 28:631–637.

12. de Mattos AM, Olyaei AJ, Bennett WM: Mechanism and risks of immunosuppressive therapy. In *Immunologic Renal Disease*. Edited by Neilson EG, Couser WG. Philadelphia: Lippincott-Raven; 1996:861–885.

13. Kasiske BL, Ramos EL, Gaston RS, *et al.*: The evaluation of renal transplant candidates: clinical practice guidelines. *J Am Soc Nephrol* 1995, 6:1–34.

14. Kasiske BL, Ravenscraft M, Ramos EL, *et al.*: The evaluation of living renal transplant donors: clinical practice guidelines. *J Am Soc Nephrol* 1996, 7:2288–2313.

15. United States Renal Data System: 1996 Annual Data Report. Bethesda, MD: The National Institutes of Health; 1996.

16. Manske CL, Wilson RF, Wang Y, Thomas W: Atherosclerotic vascular complications in diabetic transplantation candidates. *Am J Kidney Dis* 1997, 29:601–607.

17. Manske CL, Thomas W, Wang Y, Wilson RF: Screening diabetic transplantation candidates for coronary artery disease: identification of a low risk subgroup. *Kidney Int* 1993, 44:617–621.

18. Gaston RS, Curtis JJ: Hypertension in renal transplant recipients. In *Therapy in Nephrology and Hypertension*. Edited by Brady HR, Wilcox CS. Philadelphia: W.B. Saunders Co; 1999:440–443.

19. Curtis JJ, Luke RG, Jones P: Hypertension in cyclosporine-treated renal transplantation recipients is sodium-dependent. *Am J Med* 1988, 85:134–138.

20. Julian BA, Quarles LD, Niemann KMW: Musculoskeletal complications after renal transplantation: pathogenesis and treatment. *Am J Kidney Dis* 1992, 19:99–120.

21. Lin HY, Rocher LL, McQuillan MA, *et al.*: Cyclosporine-induced hyperuricemia and gout. *N Engl J Med* 1989, 321:287–292.

22. Barry JM: Renal transplantation. In *Campbell's Urology*. Edited by Walsh PC, Retik AB, Vaughan ED, Wein AJ. Philadelphia: WB Saunders Co, 1997:505–530.

23. Gruessner A, Sutherland DER: Pancreas transplantation in the United States (US) and Non-US as reported to the United Network for Organ Sharing (UNOS) and the International Pancreas Transplant Registry (IPTR). In *Clinical Transplants 1996*. Edited by Cecka JM, Terasaki PI. Los Angeles: UCLA Tissue Typing Laboratory; 1996:47–67.

24. Brayman KL, Egidi MF, Naji A, *et al.*: Is induction therapy necessary for successful simultaneous pancreas and kidney transplantation in the cyclosporine era? *Transplantation Proc* 1994, 26:2525–2527.

25. Wadstrom J, Brekke B, Wramner L, *et al.*: Triple versus quadruple induction immunosuppression in pancreas transplantation. *Transplantation Proc* 1995, 27:1317–1318.

26. Bartlett ST, Schweitzer EJ, Johnson LB, *et al.*: Equivalent success of simultaneous pancreas kidney and solitary pancreas transplantation. A prospective trial of tacrolimus immunosuppression with percutaneous biopsy. *Ann Surg* 1996, 224:440–449.

27. Gruessner RW, Burke GW, Stratta R, *et al.*: A multicenter analysis of the first experience with FK506 for induction and rescue therapy after pancreas transplantation. *Transplantation* 1996, 61:261–273.

28. Zucker K, Rosen A, Tsaroucha A, *et al.*: Augmentation of mycophenolate mofetil pharmacokinetics in renal transplant patients receiving Prograf® and CellCept®in combination therapy. *Transplantation Proc* 1997, 29:334–336.

29. Harmon WE: Treatment of children with chronic renal failure. *Kidney Int* 1995, 47:951–961.

30. Warady BA, Hebert D, Sullivan EK, *et al.*: Renal transplantation, chronic dialysis and chronic renal insufficiency in children and adolescents: 1995 Annual Report of the North American Pediatric Renal Transplant Cooperative Study. *Pediatr Nephrol* 1997, 11:49–64.

31. Red Book: *Report of the Committee on Infectious Diseases*, edn 24. Edited by Georges Peter. Elk Grove: American Academy of Pediatrics; 1997:18–19.

32. Furth SL, Neu AM, Sullivan EK, *et al.*: Immunization practices in children with renal disease: a report of the North American Pediatric Renal Transplant Cooperative Study. *Pediatr Nephrol* 1997, 11:443–446.

33. McEnery PT, Stablein DM, Arbus G, Tejani A: Renal transplantation in children: a report of the North American Pediatric Renal Transplant Cooperative Study. *N Engl J Med* 1992, 326:1727–1732.

34. Rees L, Rigden SPA, Ward GM: Chronic renal failure and growth. *Arch Dis Child* 1989, 64:573–577.

35. Tejani A, Fine R, Alexander S, *et al.*: Factors predictive of sustained growth in children after renal transplantation: The North American Pediatric Renal Transplant Cooperative Study. *J Pediatr* 1993, 122:397–402.

36. Harmon WE, Jabs K: Factors affecting growth after renal transplantation. *J Am Soc Nephrol* 1992, 2:S295–S303.

37. United States Renal Data System: USRDS 1995 Annual Data Report. Bethesda, MD, The National Institutes of Health, The National Institute of Diabetes and Digestive and Kidney Diseases, 1995. *Am J Kidney Dis* 1995, 26:S1–S186.

38. Najjar MF, Rowland M: Anthropometric reference data and the prevalence of overweight. *Vital Health Stat* 1987, 11:1073.

39. Turenne MN, Port FK, Strawderman RL, *et al.*: Growth rates in pediatric dialysis patients and renal transplant recipients. *Am J Kidney Dis* 1997, 30:193–203.

40. Jabs K, Sullivan EK, Avner ED, Harmon WE: Alternate day steroid dosing improves growth without adversely affecting graft survival or long-term graft function. *Transplantation* 1996, 61:31–36.

41. Yadin O, Grimm PC, Ettenger RB: Renal transplantation in children. *Pediatr Ann* 1991, 20:662–667.

42. Fine RN, Ettenger R: Renal transplantation in children. *Kidney Transplantation: Principles and Practice*, edn 4. Edited by Morris PJ. Philadelphia: WB Saunders Company; 1994:418.

43. Porter KA: Renal transplantation. In *Pathology of the Kidney*. Edited by Heptinstall RH. Boston: Little, Brown; 1992:1799–1934.

44. Kotanko P, Pusey CD, Levy JB: Recurrent glomerulonephritis following renal transplantation. *Transplantation* 1997, 63:1045–1052.

45. Odum J, Peh CA, Clarkson AR, *et al.*: Recurrent mesangial IgA nephritis following renal transplantation. *Nephrol Dial Transplant* 1994, 9:309–312.

46. Ohmacht C, Klicm V, Burg M, *et al.*: Recurrent IgA nephropathy after renal transplantation: a significant contributor to graft loss. *Transplantation* 1997.

47. Watts RWE: Primary hyperoxaluria type 1. *Q J Med* 1994, 87:593–599.

48. Allen AR, Thompson EM, Williams G, *et al.*: Selective renal transplantation in primary hyperoxaluria type 1. *Am J Kidney Dis* 1996, 27:891–895.

49. Montgomery R, Zibari G, Hill GS, *et al.*: Renal transplantation in patients with sickle cell nephropathy. *Transplantation* 1994, 58:618–620.

50. Goss JA, Cole BR, Jendrisak MD: Renal transplantation for systemic lupus erythematosus and recurrent lupus nephritis: a single center experience and review of the literature. *Transplantation* 1991, 52:805–810.

51. Morales JM, Campistol JM, Andres A, *et al.*: Glomerular diseases in patients with hepatitis C virus infection after renal transplantation. *Curr Opinion Nephrol Hypertens* 1997, 6:511–515.

52. Takishita Y, Ishikawa S, Okada K: Two cases of membranous glomerulonephritis associated with hepatitis C virus. *Nippon Jinzo Gakkai Shi* 1994, 36:1203–1207.

53. Couchoud C, Pouteil-Noble C, Colon S, *et al.*: Recurrence of membranous nephropathy after renal transplantation. *Transplantation* 1995, 59:1275–1279.

54. Schwarz A, Krause PH, Offermann G, *et al.*: Impact of *de novo* membranous glomerulonephritis on the clinical course after kidney transplantation. *Transplantation* 1994, 58:650–654.

55. Dantal J, Bigot E, Bogers W, *et al.*: Effect of plasma protein adsorption on protein excretion in kidney-transplant recipients with recurrent nephrotic syndrome. *N Engl J Med* 1994, 330:7–14.

56. Artero ML, Sharma R, Savin VJ, *et al.*: Plasmapheresis reduces proteinuria and serum capacity to injure glomeruli in patients with recurrent focal glomerulosclerosis. *Am J Kidney Dis* 1994, 23:574–581.

Dialysis as Treatment of End-Stage Renal Disease

William L. Henrich

Sivasankaran Ambalavanan, Alfred K. Cheung, Robert W. Hamilton, Toros Kapoian,
Jeffrey L. Kauffman, Ramesh Khanna, Karl D. Nolph, John L. Nosher, Biff F. Palmer,
Gary M. Rabetoy, Richard A. Sherman

CHAPTER

7

Principles of Dialysis: Diffusion, Convection, and Dialysis Machines

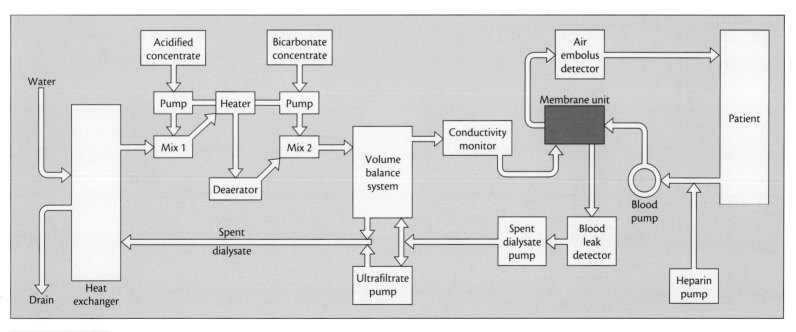

FIGURE 7-1

Simplified schematic of typical hemodialysis system. In hemodialysis, blood from the patient is circulated through a synthetic extracorporeal membrane and returned to the patient. The opposite side of that membrane is washed with an electrolyte solution (dialysate) containing the normal constituents of plasma water. The apparatus contains a blood pump to circulate the blood through the system, proportioning pumps that mix a concentrated salt solution with water purified by reverse osmosis and/or deionization to produce the dialysate, a means of removing excess fluid from the blood (mismatching dialysate inflow and outflow to the dialysate compartment), and a series of pressure, conductivity, and air embolus monitors to protect the patient. Dialysate is warmed to body temperature by a heater.

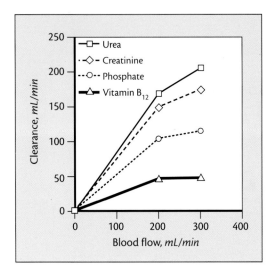

FIGURE 7-2

Effect of blood flow on clearance of various solutes (Fresenius F-5 membrane). The amount of solute cleared by a dialyzer depends on the amount delivered to the membrane. The usual blood flow is 300–400 mL/min, which is adequate to deliver the dialysis prescription. On institution of dialysis to a very uremic patient, the blood flow is decreased to 160 to 180 mL/min to avoid disequilibrium syndrome. As time goes on, blood flow can be increased to standard flows as the patient adjusts to dialysis. Most patients require hemodialysis at least thrice weekly. From this graph it is also evident that small molecules such as urea (molecular weight, 60 D) are cleared more easily than large molecules such as vitamin B$_{12}$ (molecular weight, 1355 D).

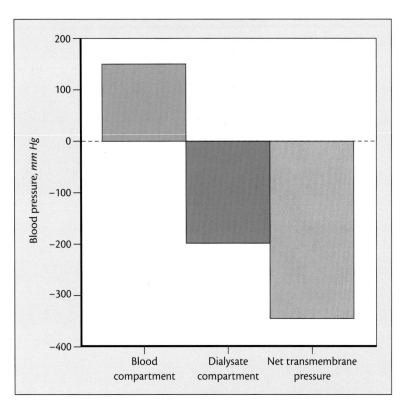

FIGURE 7-3

Hydrostatic ultrafiltration also takes place during hemodialysis. Because the spent dialysate effluent pump (see Fig. 7-1) creates negative pressure on the dialysate compartment of the membrane unit and the blood pump creates positive pressure in the blood compartment, there is a net hydrostatic pressure gradient between the compartments. This causes a flow of water and dissolved substances from blood to the dialysate compartment. The process of solute transfer associated with this flow of water is called "convective transport." In hemodialysis, the amount of low molecular weight solute (*eg*, urea) removed by convection is negligible. In the continuous renal replacement therapies, this is a major mechanism for solute transport.

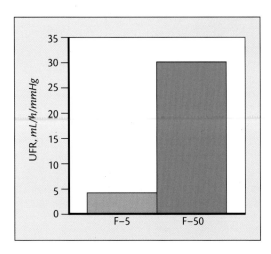

FIGURE 7-4

Dialysis membranes differ in their ability to remove fluid. Differences in ultrafiltration coefficient (UFR) are shown for two different membranes (F-5 and F-50). The F-50 is considered a high-flux membrane.

Dialysate Composition in Hemodialysis and Peritoneal Dialysis

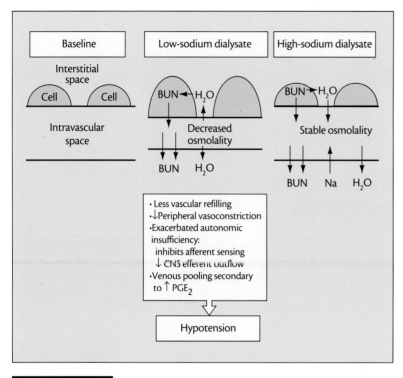

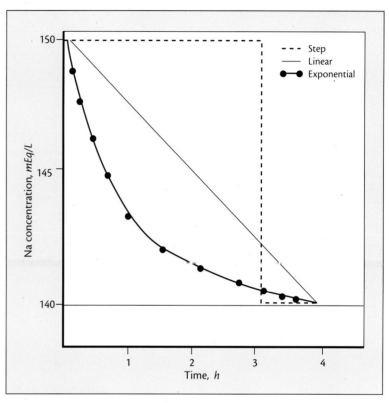

FIGURE 7-5

Use of a low-sodium dialysate is more often associated with intra-dialysis hypotension as a result of several mechanisms [1]. The drop in serum osmolality as urea is removed leads to a shift of water into the intracellular compartment that prevents adequate refilling of the intravascular space. This intracellular movement of water, combined with removal of water by ultrafiltration, leads to contraction of the intravascular space and contributes to the development of hypotension. High-sodium dialysate helps to minimize the development of hypo-osmolality. As a result, fluid can be mobilized from the intracellular and interstitial compartments to refill the intravascular space during volume removal. Other potential mechanisms whereby low-sodium dialysate contributes to hypotension are indicated. BUN—blood urea nitrogen; PGE$_2$—prostaglandin E$_2$.

FIGURE 7-6

There has been interest in varying the concentration of sodium (Na) in the dialysate during the dialysis procedure so as to minimize the potential complications of a high-sodium solution and yet retain the beneficial hemodynamic effects. A high sodium concentration dialysate is used initially, and progressively the concentration is reduced toward isotonic or even hypotonic levels by the end of the procedure. The concentration of sodium can be reduced in a linear, exponential, or step pattern. This method of sodium control allows for a diffusive sodium influx early in the session to prevent a rapid decline in plasma osmolality secondary to efflux of urea and other small molecular weight solutes. During the remainder of the procedure, when the reduction in osmolality accompanying urea removal is less abrupt, the dialysate in sodium level is set lower, thus minimizing the development of hypertonicity and any resultant excessive thirst, fluid gain, and hypertension in the interdialysis period. In some but not all studies, sodium modeling has been shown to be effective in treating intradialysis hypotension and cramps [2–8].

INDICATIONS AND CONTRAINDICATIONS FOR USE OF SODIUM MODELING (HIGH/LOW PROGRAMS)

Indications
  Intradialysis hypotension
  Cramping
  Initiation of hemodialysis in setting of severe azotemia
  Hemodynamic instability (eg, intensive care setting)
Contraindications
  Intradialysis development of hypertension
  Large interdialysis weight gain induced by high-sodium dialysate
  Hypernatremia

FIGURE 7-7

Indications and contraindications for use of sodium modeling (high/low programs). Use of a sodium modeling program is not indicated in all patients. In fact most patients do well with the dialysate sodium set at 140 mEq/L. As a result the physician needs to be aware of the benefits as well as the dangers of sodium remodeling.

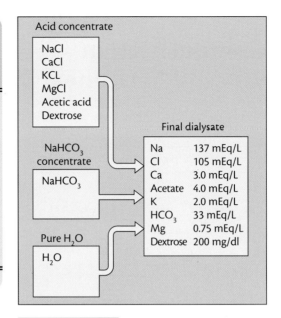

FIGURE 7-8

The current utilization of a bicarbonate dialysate requires a specially designed system that mixes a bicarbonate and an acid concentrate with purified water. The acid concentrate contains a small amount of lactic or acetic acid and all the calcium and magnesium. The exclusion of these cations from the bicarbonate concentrate prevents the precipitation of magnesium and calcium carbonate that would otherwise occur in the setting of a high bicarbonate concentration. During the mixing procedure, the acid in the acid concentrate reacts with an equimolar amount of bicarbonate to generate carbonic acid and carbon dioxide. The generation of carbon dioxide causes the pH of the final solution to fall to approximately 7.0–7.4. The acidic pH and the lower concentrations in the final mixture allow the calcium and magnesium to remain in solution. The final concentration of bicarbonate in the dialysate is approximately 33–38 mmol/L.

High-Efficiency and High-Flux Hemodialysis

DEFINITIONS OF FLUX, PERMEABILITY, AND EFFICIENCY

Flux
  Measure of ultrafiltration capacity
  Low and high flux are based on the ultrafiltration coefficient (K_{uf})
  Low flux: K_{uf} <10 mL/h/mm Hg
  High flux: K_{uf} >20 mL/h/mm Hg
Permeability
  Measure of the clearance of the middle molecular weight molecule (eg, β_2-microglobulin)
  General correlation between flux and permeability
  Low permeability: β_2-microglobulin clearance <10 mL/min
  High permeability: β_2-microglobulin clearance >20 mL/min
Efficiency
  Measure of urea clearance
  Low and high efficiency are based on the urea K_oA value
  Low efficiency: K_oA <500 mL/min
  High efficiency: K_oA >600 mL/min

FIGURE 7-9

Definitions of flux, permeability, and efficiency. The urea value K_oA, as conventionally defined in hemodialysis, is an estimate of the clearance of urea (a surrogate marker of low molecular weight uremic toxins) under conditions of infinite blood and dialysate flow rates. The following equation is used to calculate this value:

$$K_oA = \frac{Q_b Q_d}{Q_b - Q_d} \ln \left[\frac{1 - K_d/Q_b}{1 - K_d/Q_d} \right]$$

where K_o = mass transfer coefficient; A = surface area; Q_b = blood flow rate; Q_d = dialysate flow rate; ln = natural log; K_d = mean of blood and dialysate side urea clearance.

As conventionally defined in hemodialysis, flux is the rate of water transfer across the hemodialysis membrane. Dissolved solutes are removed by convection (solvent drag effect).

Permeability is a measure of the clearance rate of molecules of middle molecular weight, sometimes defined using β_2-microglobulin (molecular weight, 11,800 D) as the surrogate [9,10]. Dialyzers that permit β_2-microglobulin clearance of over 20 mL/min under usual clinical flow and ultrafiltration conditions have been defined as high-permeability membrane dialyzers. Because of the general correlation between water flux and the clearance rate of molecules of middle molecular weight, the term *high-flux membrane* has been used commonly to denote *high-permeability membrane*. A—surface area; K_o—mass tranfer coefficient.

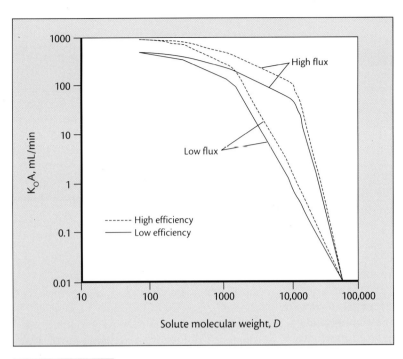

FIGURE 7-10

Theoretic K_oA profile of high- and low-flux dialyzers and high- and low-efficiency dialyzers. Note that here the definition of K_oA applies to the product of the mass transfer coefficient and surface area for solutes having a wide range of molecular weights, and is not limited to urea. Note also the logarithmic scales on both axes [9]. A—surface area; K_o—mass transfer coefficient. (*Adapted from* Cheung and Leypoldt [9].)

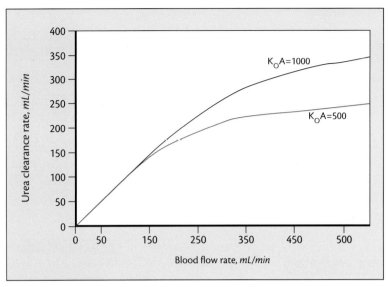

FIGURE 7-11

Comparison of urea clearance rates between low- and high-efficiency hemodialyzers (urea K_oA = 500 and 1000 mL/min, respectively). The urea clearance rate increases with the blood flow rate and gradually reaches a plateau for both types of dialyzers. The plateau value of K_oA is higher for the high-efficiency dialyzer. At low blood flow rates (<200 mL/min), however, the capacity of the high-efficiency dialyzer cannot be exploited and the clearance rate is similar to that of the low-flux dialyzer [9,11]. A—surface area; K_o—mass transfer coefficient. (*Adapted from* Collins [11].)

CHARACTERISTICS OF HIGH-EFFICIENCY DIALYSIS

Urea clearance rate is usually >210 mL/min

Urea K_oA of the dialyzer is usually >600 mL/min

Ultrafiltration coefficient of the dialyzer (K_{uf}) may be high or low

Clearance of middle molecular weight molecules may be high or low

Dialysis can be performed using either cellulosic or synthetic membrane dialyzers

FIGURE 7-12

Characteristics of high-efficiency dialysis. High-efficiency dialysis is arbitrarily defined by a high clearance rate of urea (>210 mL/min). High-efficiency membranes can be made from either cellulosic or synthetic materials. Depending on the membrane material and surface area, the removal of water (as measured by the ultrafiltration coefficient or K_{uf}) and molecules of middle molecular weight (as measured by β_2-microglobulin clearance) may be high or low [9–12]. A—surface area; K_o—mass transfer coefficient.

FIGURE 7-13

Differences between high- and low-efficiency hemodialysis. Conventional hemodialysis refers to low-efficiency low-flux hemodialysis that was the popular modality before the 1980s [9,11]. A—surface area; K_o—mass transfer coefficient.

DIFFERENCES BETWEEN HIGH- AND LOW-EFFICIENCY HEMODIALYSIS

	High efficiency, *mL/min*	Low efficiency, *mL/min*
Dialyzer K_oA	≥600	<500
Blood flow	≥350	<350
Dialysate flow	≥500	<500
Bicarbonate dialysate	Necessary	Optimal

FIGURE 7-14

Technical requirements for high-efficiency dialysis. The K_oA is the theoretic value of the urea clearance rate under conditions of infinite blood and dialysate flow. High blood and dialysate flow rates are necessary to achieve optimal performance of high-efficiency dialyzers. Bicarbonate-containing dialysate is necessary to prevent symptoms associated with acetate intolerance (*ie*, nausea, vomiting, headache, and hypotension), worsening of metabolic acidosis, and cardiac arrhythmia [11,13,14]. K_o—mass transfer coefficient; A—surface area.

FIGURE 7-15

Benefits of high-efficiency dialysis. With improved control of biochemical parameters (such as potassium, hydrogen ions, phosphate, urea, and other nitrogenous compounds), the potential exists for reduced morbidity and mortality without increasing dialysis treatment time [12,15].

FIGURE 7-16

Limitations of high-efficiency dialysis. Removal of a large volume of fluid over a short time period (2–2.5 h) increases the likelihood of hypotension, especially in patients with poor cardiac function or autonomic neuropathy. The loss of a fixed amount of treatment time has a proportionally greater impact during a short treatment time than during a long treatment time. Thus, the margin of safety is narrower if a short treatment time is used in conjunction with high-efficiency dialysis compared with conventional hemodialysis with a longer treatment time. Although unproved, high blood flow rates may predispose patients to vascular access damage. Rapid solute shifts potentially precipitate the dialysis disequilibrium syndrome in those patients with a very high blood urea nitrogen concentration, especially during the first treatment [9,12,14].

Principles of Peritoneal Dialysis

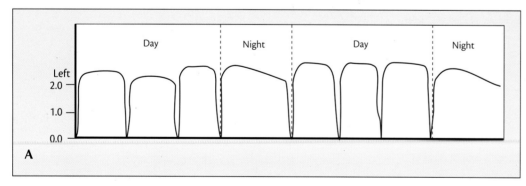

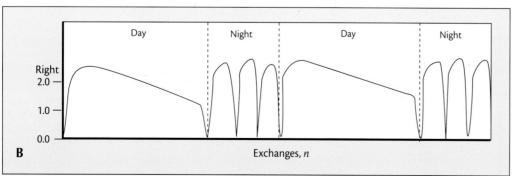

FIGURE 7-17

Continuous peritoneal dialysis regimens. **A,** Continuous ambulatory peritoneal dialysis (CAPD). **B,** continuous cyclic peritoneal dialysis (CCPD). Multiple sequential exchanges are performed during the day and night so that dialysis occurs 24 hours a day, 7 days a week.

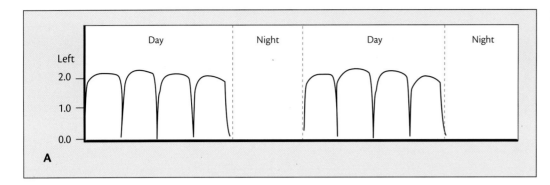

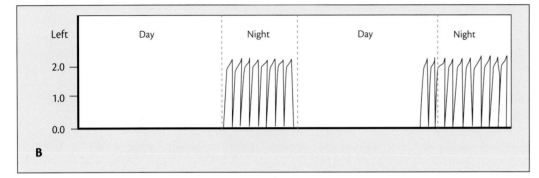

FIGURE 7-18

Intermittent peritoneal dialysis regimens. Peritoneal dialysis is performed every day but only during certain hours. **A,** In daytime ambulatory peritoneal dialysis (DAPD), multiple manual exchanges are performed during the waking hours. **B,** Nightly peritoneal dialysis (NPD) is also performed while patients are asleep using an automated cycler machine. One or two additional daytime manual exchanges are added to enhance solute clearances.

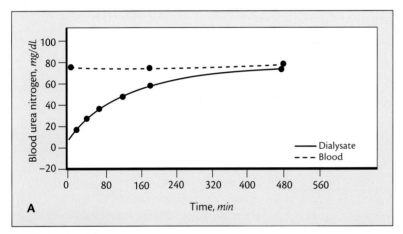

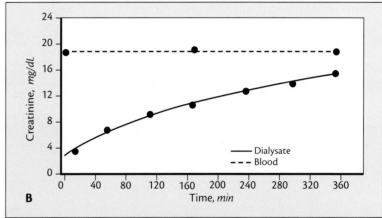

FIGURE 7-19

Solute removal. Solute concentration gradients are at maximum at the beginning of dialysis and diminish gradually as dialysis progresses. As the gradients diminish, the solute removal rates decrease. Solute removal can be enhanced by increasing the dialysate flow rate by either increasing the intraperitoneal dialysate volume per exchange or increasing the frequency of exchange. By convection or enhanced diffusion, solutes are able to accompany the bulk flow of water. (*Adapted from* Nolph *et al.* [16].)

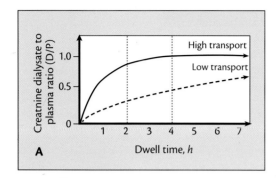

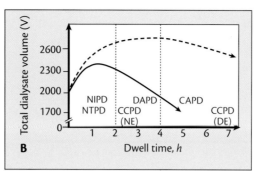

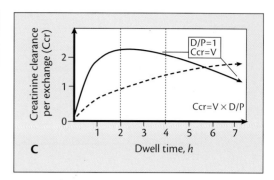

FIGURE 7-20

Solute removal continued. In a highly permeable membrane, smaller molecules (*ie*, urea and creatinine) are transported at a faster rate from the blood to dialysate than are larger molecules, enhancing solute removal. Similarly, glucose (a small solute used in the peritoneal dialysis solution to generate osmotic force for ultrafiltration across the peritoneal membrane) is also transported faster, but in the opposite direction. This high transporter dissipates the osmotic force more rapidly than does the low transporter. Both osmotic and glucose equilibriums are attained eventually in both groups, but sooner in the high transporter group. Intraperitoneal volume peaks and begins to diminish earlier in the high transporter group. When the membrane is less permeable, solute removal is lower, ultrafiltration volume is larger at 2 hours or more, and glucose equilibriums are

attained later. Consequently, intraperitoneal volume peaks later. Ultrafiltration in a low transporter peaks late during dwell time. Therefore, a low transporter continues to generate ultrafiltration even after 8 to 10 hours of dwell. The solute creatinine dialysate to plasma ratio (D/P) increases linearly during the dwell time. Patients with average solute transfer rates have ultrafiltration and mass transfer patterns between those of high and low transporters. NIPD—nightly intermittent peritoneal dialysis; NTPD—nighttime tidal peritoneal dialysis; DAPD—daytime ambulatory peritoneal dialysis; CAPD—continuous ambulatory peritoneal dialysis; CCPD (NE)—continuous cyclic peritoneal dialysis (night exchange); CCPD (DE)—continuous cyclic peritoneal dialysis (day exchange). (*Adapted from* Twardowski [17].)

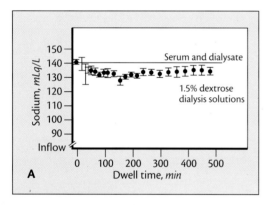

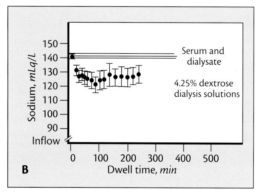

FIGURE 7-21

Solute sieving. **A,** Dialysate sodium concentration is initially reduced and tends to return to baseline later during a long dwell exchange of 6 to 8 hours. **B,** Dialysate sodium concentration decreases, particularly when using 4.25% dextrose dialysis solution, because of the sieving phenomenon. Removal of water during ultrafiltration unaccompanied by sodium, in proportion to its extracellular concentration, is called *sodium sieving* [18,19]. The peritoneum offers greater resistance to the movement of solutes than does water. This probably relates to approximately half the ultrafiltrate being generated by solute-free water movement through aquaporins channels. Therefore, ultrafiltrate is hypotonic compared with plasma. Dialysate chloride is also reduced below simple Gibbs-Donnan equilibrium, particularly during hypertonic exchanges. Patients with a low peritoneal membrane transport type tend to reduce dialysate sodium concentration more than do other patients. Therefore, during a

short dwell exchange of 2 to 4 hours, net electrolyte removal per liter of ultrafiltrate is well below the extracelluar fluid concentration. As a result, severe hypernatremia, excessive thirst, and hypertension may develop. This hindrance can be overcome by lowering the dialysate sodium concentration to 132 mEq/L. In patients who use cyclers with short dwell exchanges and who generate large ultrafiltration volumes, lower sodium concentrations may need to be used (such as 118 mEq/L for 2.5% glucose solutions or 109 mEq/L for 4.25% solutions). In continuous ambulatory peritoneal dialysis with long dwell exchanges of 6 to 8 hours, significant sieving usually does not occur, whereas in automated peritoneal dialysis with short dwell exchanges, sieving may occur. Sieving predisposes patients to thirst and less than optimum blood pressure control, especially in those who have low-normal serum sodium levels, those with low peritoneal membrane transporter rates, or both. (*Adapted from* Nolph *et al.* [16].)

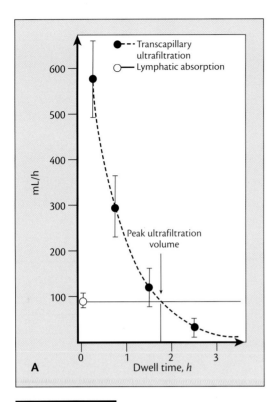

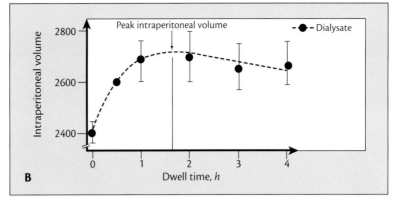

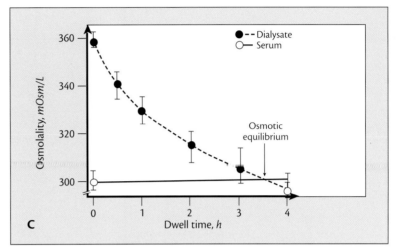

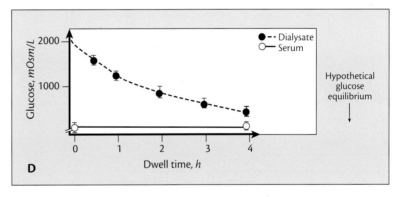

FIGURE 7-22

Fluid removal by ultrafiltration. During peritoneal dialysis, hyperosmolar glucose solution generates ultrafiltration by the process of osmosis. Water movement across the peritoneal membrane is proportional to the transmembrane pressure, membrane area, and membrane hydraulic permeability. The transmembrane pressure is the sum of hydrostatic and osmotic pressure differences between the blood in the peritoneal capillary and dialysis solution in the peritoneal cavity. Net transcapillary ultrafiltration defines net fluid movement from the peritoneal microcirculation into the peritoneal cavity primarily in response to osmotic pressure. Net ultrafiltration would equal the resulting increment in intraperitoneal fluid volume if it were not for peritoneal reabsorption, mostly through the peritoneal lymphatics. Peritoneal reabsorption is continuous and reduces the intraperitoneal volume throughout the dwell. **A,** The net transcapillary ultrafiltration rate decreases exponentially during the dwell time, owing to dissipation of the glucose osmotic gradient secondary to peritoneal glucose absorption and dilution of the solution glucose by the ultrafiltration. Later in the exchange net, ultrafiltration ceases when the transcapillary ultrafiltration is reduced to a rate equal to the peritoneal reabsorption. **B,** When the transcapillary ultrafiltration rate decreases below that of the peritoneal reab-

sorption rate, the net ultrafiltration rate becomes negative. Consequently, the intraperitoneal volume begins to diminish. Thus, peak ultrafiltration and intraperitoneal volumes are observed before osmotic equilibrium during an exchange. **C,** Osmotic equilibrium most likely precedes glucose equilibrium because of both solute sieving and the higher peritoneal reflection coefficient of glucose compared with other dialysate solutes, allowing net transcapillary ultrafiltration to continue at a low rate even after osmotic equilibrium. **D,** Ultrafiltration can be maximized by measures that delay osmotic equilibrium, which can be accomplished by using hypertonic glucose solutions, larger volumes, or both, during an exchange. More frequent exchanges shorten dwell times and increase the dialysate flow rate and thus avert attaining osmotic equilibrium. Additionally, potential exists for enhancing ultrafiltration by measures that reduce the peritoneal reabsorption rate. (*Adapted from* Mactier *et al.* [20].)

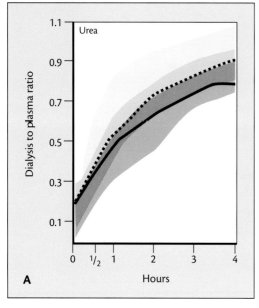

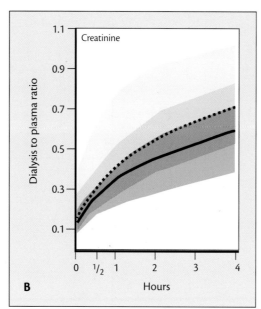

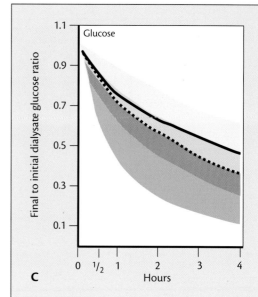

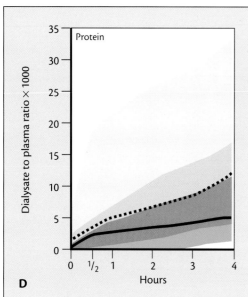

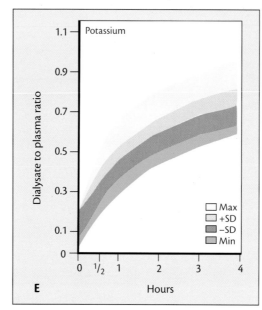

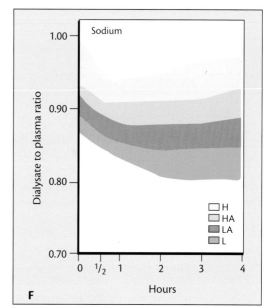

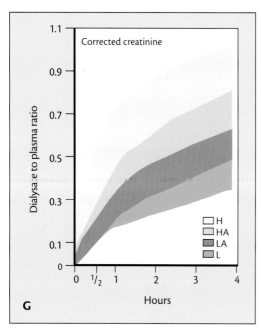

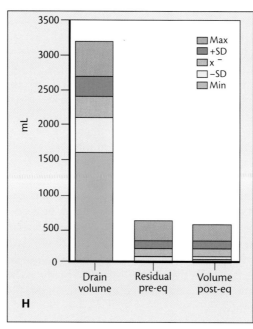

FIGURE 7-23

Classification of peritoneal transport function. Based on the peritoneal equilibrium test results, peritoneal transport function may be classified into average, high (H), and low (L) transport types. The average transport group is further subdivided into high-average (HA) and low-average (LA) types. For the population studied by Twardowski *et al.* [21], the transport classification is based on means; standard deviations (SDs); and minimum and maximum dialysate to plasma ratio (D/P) values over 4 hours for urea, creatinine, glucose, protein, potassium, sodium, and corrected creatinine (*panels A–G*). The volume of drainage correlates positively with dialysate glucose and negatively with D/P creatinine values at 4-hour dwell times (*panel H*). (*Adapted from* Twardowski *et al.* [21].)

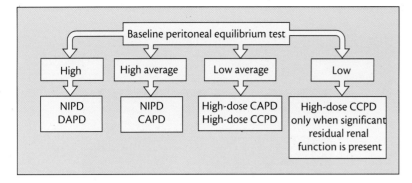

FIGURE 7-24

Using transport type to select a peritoneal dialysis regimen. Because clearance rates continue to increase with time, patients with low transport rates are treated with long dwell exchanges, *ie,* continuous cyclic peritoneal dialysis (CCPD). Owing to the low rate of increase in the dialysate to plasma ratio (D/P), the clearance rate per unit of time is augmented relatively little by rapid exchange techniques such as nightly intermittent peritoneal dialysis (NIPD). On the contrary, the clearance per exchange rate over long dwell exchanges would be less in patients with high transport rates. During the short dwell time, patients with high transport rates capture maximum ultrafiltration and small solutes are completely equilibrated. Therefore, these patients are best treated with techniques using short dwell exchanges, *ie,* NIPD or daytime ambulatory peritoneal dialysis (DAPD). Patients with average transport rates can be effectively treated with either short or long dwell exchange techniques. CAPD—continuous ambulatory peritoneal dialysis.

Dialysis Access and Recirculation

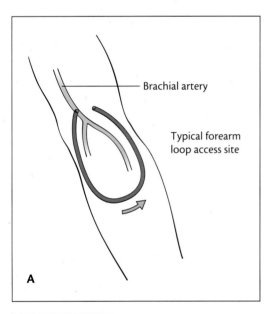

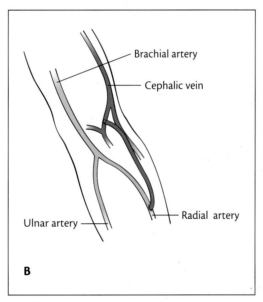

FIGURE 7-25

Polytetrafluoroethylene (PTFE) vein graft. The most common synthetic material used for dialysis access construction is the PTFE conduit. This material replaced bovine heterografts; alternative materials such as the umbilical vein graft have not yet made much headway. Because of the infection risk, Dacron bypass grafts have never functioned well for dialysis. PTFE is an inert material that is formed into a pliable conduit. Its ultramicroscopic structure is a series of nodes connected by tiny filaments, leaving pores whose size can be varied during manufacture. The process of healing after implantation involves ingrowth of fibroblasts into the pore structure, giving a final graft-tissue amalgam that is "incorporated" when encountered by the surgeon for revision. There is virtually no neovascularization through the pores, which are too small for capillary ingrowth. In humans, neointima grow along the graft for no more than 3 cm from the anastomosis. In animal models, neointima can be much more robust, growing along most of the length of the graft and providing it with greater resistance to thrombosis. Typical layouts for the construction of a PTFE access site are **A**, the forearm loop, and **B**, linear forearm graft, respectively. Alternative sites include upper arm loop grafts, groin grafts, axillary artery-to-vein grafts, and a variety of other constructions. The sites of choice are limited by the requirements of hemodialysis: delivery of a high rate of blood flow and accessibility to the dialysis staff for cannulation with an adequate length of graft to keep the needles sufficiently separated and allow rotation of cannulation sites.

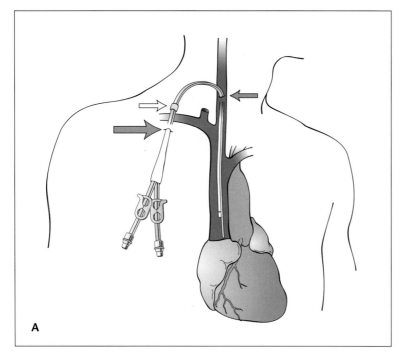

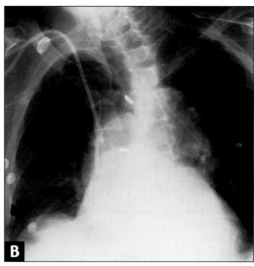

FIGURE 7-26

Right internal jugular vein catheters. The use of central vein catheters has grown significantly over the past several years. These catheters were at one time used only on a temporary basis and served as a "bridge" to permanent vascular access. Improvements in catheter design and function combined with ease of insertion have increased use of central vein catheters in dialysis units. To minimize the risk of central vein stenosis and subsequent thrombosis, central vein catheters should be inserted preferentially into the right internal jugular vein, regardless of whether they are being used for temporary or more permanent purposes. **A,** The typical positioning of a double-lumen catheter is with its tip at the junction of the right atrium and the superior vena cava. The catheter has been "tunneled" underneath the skin so that the exit site (*large arrow*) is located just beneath the right clavicle and distant from the insertion site (*small arrow*). This catheter also has a cuff into which endothelial cells will grow and produce a biologic barrier to bacterial migration. **B,** Chest radiograph showing a dialysis central vein catheter that is composed of two separate single-lumen catheters that have been inserted into the right internal jugular vein. The distal tip of the venous catheter is positioned just above the right atrium. Care must be taken, however, to ensure proper placement of catheters with this type of design, because the two single lumens are radiographically indistinguishable.

The Dialysis Prescription and Urea Modeling

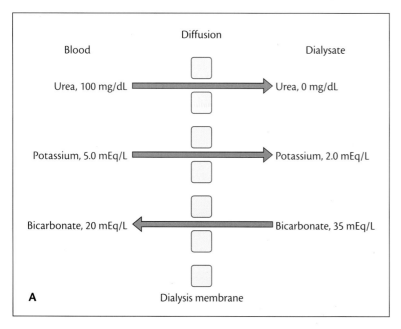

FIGURE 7-27

Diffusional and convective flux in hemodialysis. Dialysis is a process whereby the composition of blood is altered by exposing it to dialysate through a semipermeable membrane. Solutes are transported across this membrane by either diffusional or convective flux. **A,** In diffusive solute transport, solutes cross the dialysis membrane in a direction dictated by the concentration gradient established across the membrane of the hemodialyzer. For example, urea and potassium diffuse from blood to dialysate, whereas bicarbonate diffuses from dialysate to blood. At a given temperature, diffusive transport is directly proportional to both the solute concentration gradient across the membrane and the membrane surface area and inversely proportional to membrane thickness.

(*Continued on next page*)

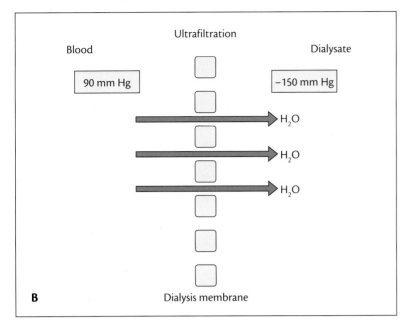

FIGURE 7-27 (*continued*)

B, During hemodialysis water moves from blood to dialysate driven by a hydrostatic pressure gradient between the blood and dialysate compartments, a process referred to as ultrafiltration. The rate of ultrafiltration is determined by the magnitude of this pressure gradient. Movement of water tends to drag solute across the membrane, a process referred to as convective transport or solvent drag. The contribution of convective transport to total solute transport is only significant for average-to-high molecular weight solutes because they tend to have a smaller diffusive flux.

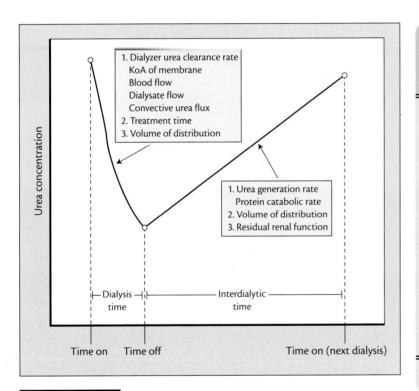

FIGURE 7-28

Delivering an adequate dose of dialysis in hemodialysis. Providing an adequate amount of dialysis is an important part of the dialysis prescription. During the dialytic procedure, a sharp decrease in the concentration of urea occurs followed by a gradual increase during the interdialytic period. The decrease in urea during dialysis is determined by three main parameters: dialyzer urea clearance rate (K), dialysis treatment time (t), and the volume of urea distribution (V). The dialyzer urea clearance rate (K) is influenced by the characteristics of the dialysis membrane (KoA), blood flow rate, dialysate flow rate, and convective urea flux that occurs with ultrafiltration. The gradual increase in urea during the interdialytic period depends on the rate of urea generation that, in an otherwise stable patient, reflects the dietary protein intake, distribution volume of urea, and presence or absence of residual renal function.

FACTORS RESULTING IN A REDUCTION OF THE PRESCRIBED DOSE OF HEMODIALYSIS DELIVERED

Compromised urea clearance
    Access recirculation
    Inadequate blood flow from the vascular access
    Dialyzer clotting during dialysis (reduction of effective surface area)
    Blood pump or dialysate flow calibration error
Reduction in treatment time
    Premature discontinuation of dialysis for staff or unit convenience
    Premature discontinuation of dialysis per patient request
    Delay in starting treatment owing to patient or staff tardiness
    Time on dialysis calculated incorrectly
Laboratory or blood sampling errors
    Dilution of predialysis BUN blood sample with saline
    Drawing of predialysis BUN blood sample after start of the procedure
    Drawing postdialysis BUN >5 minutes after the procedure

FIGURE 7-29

Each of the factors listed may play a major role in the reduction of delivered dialysis dose. Particular attention should be paid to the vascular access and to a reduction in the effective surface area of the dialyzer. Perhaps the most important cause for reduction in dialysis time has to do with premature discontinuation of dialysis for the convenience of the patient or staff. Delays in starting dialysis treatment are frequent and may result in a significant loss of dialysis prescription. Finally, particular attention should be paid to the correct sampling of the blood urea nitrogen level and the site from which the sample is drawn. BUN—blood urea nitrogen.

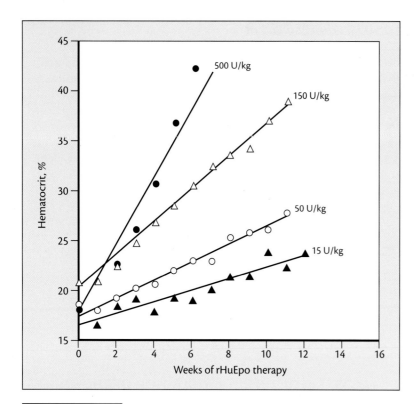

FIGURE 7-30

Correction of anemia in chronic renal failure. Anemia is a predictable complication of chronic renal failure that is due partly to reduction in erythropoietin production. Use of recombinant erythropoietin to correct the anemia in patients with chronic renal failure has become standard therapy. The rate of increase in hematocrit is dose-dependent. The indicated doses were given intravenously three times per week. Current guidelines for the initiation of intravenous therapy suggest a starting dosage of 120 to 180 U/kg/wk (typically 9000 U/wk) administered in three divided doses. Administration of erythropoietin subcutaneously has been shown to be more efficient than is intravenous administration. That is, on average, any given increment in hematocrit can be achieved with less erythropoietin when it is given subcutaneously as compared with intravenously. In adults, the subcutaneous dosage of erythropoietin is 80 to 120 U/kg/wk (typically 6000 U/wk) in two to three divided doses. rHuEpo—recombinant human erythropoietin. (*Data from* Eschbach *et al.* [22].)

MAJOR COMPONENTS OF DIALYSIS PRESCRIPTION

Choose a biocompatible membrane

Prescribe a Kt/V ≥1.3 or a URR ≥70%

Rigorously ensure that the delivered dose equals the amount prescribed

When the delivered dose is less than that prescribed do the following:

   Increase blood flow rate ≥400 mL/min

   Increase dialysate flow rate to ≥800 mL/min

   Use a high-efficiency dialyzer

   Increase treatment time

Choose dialysate composition: sodium, potassium, bicarbonate, and calcium

Adjust ultrafiltration rate to achieve patients' dry weight (assess dry weight regularly)

Adjust recombinant erythropoietin to maintain hematocrit between 33% and 36%

When indicated, use 1,25(OH)$_2$ vitamin D for treatment of secondary hyperparathyroidism

Use normal saline, hypertonic saline, or mannitol for treatment of intradialytic hypotension

FIGURE 7-31

All these components are important as contributors to a successful dialysis prescription. The Dialysis Outcomes Quality Initiative (DOQI) recommendations should be followed to achieve an adequate dialysis prescription, and the time on dialysis should be monitored carefully. When the delivered dialysis dose is less that prescribed, the reversible factors listed in Figure 6-10 should be addressed first. Subsequently, an increase in blood flow to 400 mL/min should be attempted. Increases in dialyzer surface area and treatment time also may be attempted. In addition, attention should be paid to the correct dialysis composition and to the ultrafiltration rate to make certain that patients achieve a weight as close as possible to their dry weight. Hematocrit should be sustained at 33% to 36%. Finally, vitamin D supplementation to prevent secondary hyperparathyroidism and use of normal saline or other volume expanders are encouraged to treat hypotension during dialysis. KoA—constant indicating the efficiency of the dialyzer in removing urea; URR—urea reduction ratio.

Complications of Dialysis

COMPLICATIONS OF HEMODIALYSIS

Complication	Differential diagnosis
Fever	Bacteremia, water-borne pyrogens, overheated dialysate
Hypotension	Excessive ultrafiltration, cardiac arrhythmia, air embolus, pericardial tamponade; hemorrhage (gastrointestinal, intracranial, retroperitoneal); anaphylactoid reaction
Hemolysis	Inadequate removal of chloramine from dialysate, failure of dialysis concentrate delivery system
Dementia	Incomplete removal of aluminum from dialysate water, prescription of aluminum antacids
Seizure	Excessive urea clearance (first treatment), failure of dialysis concentrate delivery system
Bleeding	Excessive heparin or other anticoagulant
Muscle cramps	Excessive ultrafiltration

FIGURE 7-32

Complications associated with hemodialysis.

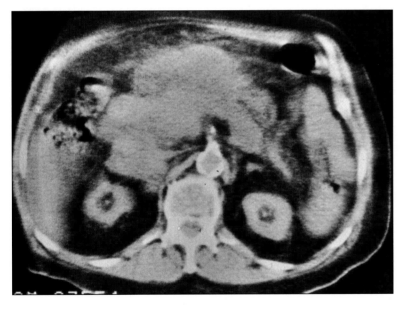

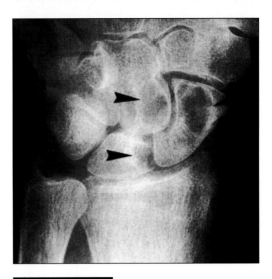

FIGURE 7-33

Dialysis-associated amyloidosis. Multiple carpal bone cysts without joint space narrowing in a patient treated with dialysis for 11 years. This phenomenon has been attributed to inadequate clearance of $\beta_2$microglobulin using low-permeability, cellulose dialysis membranes. (*From* van Ypersele de Strihou *et al.* [23]; with permission.)

FIGURE 7-34

Sclerosing encapsulating peritonitis. This patient had several bouts of peritonitis during the course of her treatment on peritoneal dialysis. She developed partial small bowel obstruction. Abdominal computed tomography revealed a homogeneous mass filling the anterior peritoneum. At laparotomy the mesentery was encased in a "marblelike" fibrotic mass. The patient required long-term home parenteral hyperalimentation for recovery. (*From* Pusateri *et al.* [24]; with permission.)

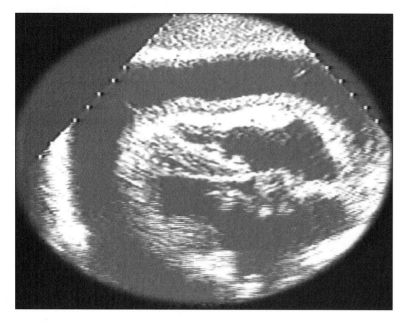

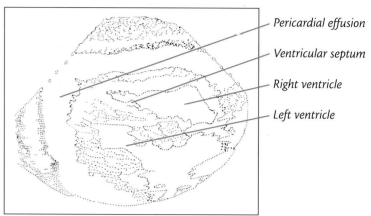

- *Pericardial effusion*
- *Ventricular septum*
- *Right ventricle*
- *Left ventricle*

FIGURE 7-35

Pericardial tamponade. Narrow pulse pressure and a pericardial friction rub suggest pericarditis (a frequent complication of uremia) especially in patients with chest pain. Pericardial tamponade may present as dialysis-induced hypotension. (*Courtesy of* T. Pappas, MD, Medical College of Ohio.)

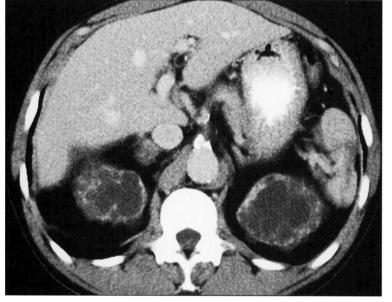

FIGURE 7-36

Acquired cystic disease of the kidney. Abdominal computed tomography demonstrates cystic disease in this patient, who had focal segmental glomerulosclerosis complicated by protein C deficiency and renal vein thrombosis. Eleven years after the initial diagnosis, he developed renal failure requiring hemodialysis. Two years after starting dialysis, he developed hematuria, and these cysts were found. The appearance and clinical course are consistent with acquired cystic disease of the kidney. These cysts carry some risk of malignant transformation.

References

1. Palmer BF: The effect of dialysate composition on systemic hemodynamics. *Semin Dial* 1992, 5:54—60.

2. Dumler F, Grondin G, Levin NW: Sequential high/low sodium hemodialysis: An alternative to ultrafiltration. *Trans Am Soc Artif Intern Organs* 1979, 25:351–353.

3. Raja R, Kramer M, Barber K, Chen S: Sequential changes in dialysate sodium (D_{Na}) during hemodialysis. *Trans Am Soc Artif Intern Organs* 1983, 24:649–651.

4. Daugirdas JT, Al-Kudsi RR, Ing TS, Norusis MJ: A double-blind evaluation of sodium gradient hemodialysis. *Am J Nephrol* 1985, 5:163–168.

5. Acchiardo SR, Hayden AJ: Is Na modeling necessary in high flux dialysis. *Trans Am Soc Artif Organs* 1991, 37:M135–M137.

6. Sadowski RH, Allred EN, Jabs K: Sodium modelling ameliorates intradialytic and interdialytic symptoms in young hemodialysis patients. *J Am Soc Nephrol* 1993, 4:1192–1198.

7. Levin A, Goldstein MB: The benefits and side effects of ramped hypertonic sodium dialysis. *J Am Soc Nephrol* 1996, 7:242–246.

8. Sang GLS, Kovithavongs C, Ulan R, Kjellstrand CM: Sodium ramping in hemodialysis: A study of beneficial and adverse effects. *Am J Kidney Dis* 1997, 29:669–677.

9. Cheung AK, Leypoldt JK: The hemodialysis membranes: a historical perspective, current state and future prospect. *Sem Nephrol* 1997, 17:196–213.

10. Leypoldt JK, Cheung AK, Agodoa LY, *et al.*: Hemodialyzer mass transfer–area coefficients for urea increase at high dialysate flow rates. *Kidney Int* 1997, 51:2013–2017.

11. Collins AJ: High-flux, high-efficiency procedures. In *Principles and Practice of Hemodialysis*. Edited by Henrich W. Norwalk, CT: Appleton & Large; 1996:76–88.

12. von Albertini B, Bosch JP: Short hemodialysis. *Am J Nephrol* 1991, 11:169–173.

13. Keshaviah P, Luehmann D, Ilstrup K, Collins A: Technical requirements for rapid high-efficiency therapies. *Artificial Organs* 1986, 10:189–194.

14. Shinaberger JH, Miller JH, Gardner PW: Short treatment. In *Replacement of Renal Function by Dialysis*, edn 3. Edited by Maher JF. Norwell, MA: Kluwer Academic Publishers; 1989:360–381.

15. Collins AJ, Keshaviah P: High-efficiency, high flux therapies in clinical dialysis. In *Clinical Dialysis*, edn 3. Edited by Nissenson AR. 1995:848–863.

16. Nolph KD, Twardowski ZJ, Popovich RP, *et al.*: Equilibration of peritoneal dialysis solutions during long dwell exchanges. *J Lab Clin Med* 1979, 93:246–256.

17. Twardowski ZJ: Nightly peritoneal dialysis (why? who? how? and when?). *Trans Am Soc Artif Intern Organs* 1990, 36:8–16.

18. Ahearn DJ, Nolph KD: Controlled sodium removal with peritoneal dialysis. *Trans Am Soc Artif Intern Organs* 1972, 28:423.

19. Nolph KD, Hano JE, Teschan PE: Peritoneal sodium transport during hypertonic peritoneal dialysis: physiologic mechanisms and clinical implications. *Ann Intern Med* 1969; 70:931.

20. Mactier RA, Khanna R, Twardowski ZJ, *et al.*: Contribution of lymphatic absorption to loss of ultrafiltration and solute clearances in continuous ambulatory peritoneal dialysis. *J Clin Invest* 1987, 80:1311–1316.

21. Twardowski ZJ, Nolph KD, Khanna R, *et al.*: Peritoneal equilibration test. *Peritoneal Dial Bull* 1987, 7:138–147.

22. Eschbach JW, Egrie JC, Downing MR, *et al.*: Correction of the anemia of end-stage renal disease with recombinant human erythropoietin. *N Engl J Med* 1987, 316:73–78.

23. van Ypersele de Strihou C, Jadoul M, Malghem J, *et al.*: Effect of dialysis membrane and patient's age on signs of dialysis-related amyloidosis. The working party on dialysis amyloidosis. *Kidney Int* 1991, 39:1012–1019.

24. Pusateri R, Ross R, Marshall R, *et al.*: Sclerosing encapsulating peritonitis: report of a case with small bowel obstruction managed by long-term home parenteral hyperalimentation and a review of the literature. *Am J Kidney Dis* 1986, 8:56–60.

Systemic Diseases and the Kidney

Saulo Klahr

Karel J.M. Assmann, Phyllis August, Rashad S. Barsoum,
Jo H.M. Berden, Jacques S. Bourgoignie, Guiseppe D'Amico,
Garabed Eknoyan, Ronald J. Falk, Franco Ferrario, Magdi R. Francis,
Eli A. Friedman, Marc B. Garnick, Morie A. Gertz, J. Charles Jennette,
Robert A. Kyle, A. Vishnu Moorthy, Richard E. Reiselbach,
David Roth, T.K. Sreepada Rao, Visith Sitprija, L.W. Statius van Eps

Diabetic Nephropathy: Impact of Comorbidity

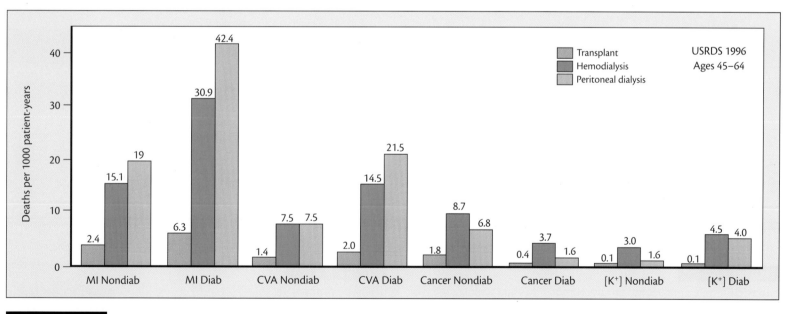

FIGURE 8-1

Comorbidity in ESRD. Death of diabetic patients with end-stage renal disease (ESRD) relates to comorbidity, as shown in this table abstracted from the 1997 report of the United States Renal Data System (USRDS) [1]. Representative subsets of patients with ESRD with and without diabetes treated by peritoneal dialysis, hemodialysis, or renal transplantation are shown. Note that for each comorbid cause of death, rates are higher in patients receiving peritoneal dialysis than in those receiving hemodialysis and are lowest in renal transplant recipients. For undetermined reasons, deaths due to cancer are less frequent in diabetic than in nondiabetic patients with ESRD. CVA—cerebrovascular accident; Diab—diabetes; K+—potassium; MI—myocardial infarction.

OPTIONS IN DIABETES WITH ESRD

	CAPD/CCPD	Hemodialysis	Transplantation
First-year survival	75%	75%	>90%
Survival >10 y	<5%	<5%	>25%
Diabetic complications	Progress	Progress	Slow progression
Rehabilitation	Poor	Poor	Fair to excellent
Patient acceptance	Fair	Fair	Good to excellent

FIGURE 8-2

Options in diabetes with end-stage renal disease (ESRD). Comparing outcomes of various options for uremia therapy in diabetic patients with ESRD is flawed by the differing criteria for selection for each treatment. Thus, if younger, healthier subjects are offered kidney transplantation, then subsequent relative survival analysis will be adversely affected for the residual pool treated by peritoneal dialysis or hemodialysis. Allowing for this caveat, the table depicts usual outcomes and relative rehabilitation results for continuous ambulatory peritoneal dialysis (CAPD), continuous cyclic peritoneal dialysis (CCPD), hemodialysis, and transplantation.

Vasculitis

SELECTED CATEGORIES OF VASCULITIS

Large vessel vasculitis
   Giant cell arteritis
   Takayasu arteritis
Medium-sized vessel vasculitis
   Polyarteritis nodosa
   Kawasaki disease
Small vessel vasculitis
   ANCA small vessel vasculitis
      Microscopic polyangiitis
      Wegener's granulomatosis
      Churg-Strauss syndrome
   Immune complex small vessel vasculitis
      Henoch-Schönlein purpura
      Cryoglobulinemic vasculitis
      Lupus vasculitis
      Serum sickness vasculitis
      Infection-induced immune complex vasculitis
   Anti–GBM small vessel vasculitis
      Goodpasture's syndrome

RENAL INJURY CAUSED BY DIFFERENT CATEGORIES OF VASCULITIS

Large vessel vasculitis
   Ischemia causing renovascular hypertension (uncommon)
Medium-sized vessel vasculitis
   Renal infarcts (frequent)
   Hemorrhage (uncommon) and rupture (rare)
ANCA small vessel vasculitis
   Pauci-immune crescentic glomerulonephritis (common)
   Arcuate and interlobular arteritis (occasional)
   Medullary angiitis (uncommon)
   Interstitial granulomatous inflammation (rare)
Immune complex small vessel vasculitis
   Immune complex proliferative or membranoproliferative glomerulonephritis with or without crescents (common)
   Arteriolitis and interlobular arteritis (rare)
Anti–GBM small vessel vasculitis
   Crescentic glomerulonephritis (common)
   Extraglomerular vasculitis (only with concurrent ANCA disease)

FIGURE 8-3

Many different approaches to categorizing vasculitis exist. We use the approach adopted by the Chapel Hill International Consensus Conference on the Nomenclature of Systemic Vasculitis [3]. The Chapel Hill System divides vasculitides into those that have a predilection for large arteries (ie, the aorta and its major branches), medium-sized vessels (ie, main visceral arteries), and small vessels (predominantly capillaries, venules, and arterioles, and, occasionally, small arteries). However, there is so much overlap in the size of the vessel involved by different vasculitides that other criteria are very important for precise diagnosis, especially when distinguishing among the different types of small vessel vasculitis. ANCA—antineutrophil cytoplasmic antibody.

FIGURE 8-4

The type of renal vessel involved by a vasculitis determines the resultant renal dysfunction. Large vessel vasculitides cause renal dysfunction by injuring the renal arteries and the aorta adjacent to the renal artery ostia. These injuries result in reduced renal blood flow and resultant renovascular hypertension. Medium-sized vessel vasculitis most often affects lobar, arcuate, and interlobular arteries, resulting in infarction and hemorrhage. Small vessel vasculitides most often affect the glomerular capillaries (ie, cause glomerulonephritis), but some types (especially the antineutrophil cytoplasmic antibody vasculitides) may also affect extraglomerular parenchymal arterioles, venules, and capillaries. Anti-GBM disease is a form of vasculitis that involves only capillaries in glomeruli or pulmonary alveoli, or both.

NAMES AND DEFINITIONS FOR LARGE VESSEL VASCULITIS

Giant cell arteritis	Granulomatous arteritis of the aorta and its major branches, with a predilection for the extracranial branches of the carotid artery. Often involves the temporal artery. Usually occurs in patients older than age 50 years and often is associated with polymyalgia rheumatica.
Takayasu arteritis	Granulomatous inflammation of the aorta and its major branches. Usually occurs in patients younger than 50 years.

FIGURE 8-5

The two major categories of large vessel vasculitis, giant cell (temporal) arteritis and Takayasu arteritis, are both characterized pathologically by granulomatous inflammation of the aorta, its major branches, or both. The most reliable criterion for distinguishing between these two disease is the younger age of patients with Takayasu arteritis compared with giant cell arteritis [2]. The presence of polymyalgia rheumatica supports a diagnosis of giant cell arteritis. Clinically significant renal disease is more commonly associated with Takayasu arteritis than giant cell arteritis, although pathologic involvement of the kidneys is a frequent finding with both conditions [3,4].

NAMES AND DEFINITIONS FOR MEDIUM VESSEL VASCULITIS

Polyarteritis nodosa	Necrotizing inflammation of medium-sized or small arteries without glomerulonephritis or vasculitis in arterioles, capillaries, or venules.
Kawasaki disease	Arteritis involving large, medium-sized, and small arteries, and associated with mucocutaneous lymph node syndrome. Coronary arteries are often involved. Aorta and veins may be involved. Usually occurs in children.

FIGURE 8-6

The medium-sized vasculitides are confined to arteries by the definitions of the Chapel Hill Nomenclature System [2,5]. By this approach the presence of evidence for involvement of vessels smaller than arteries (*ie,* capillaries, venules, arterioles), such as glomerulonephritis, purpura, or pulmonary hemorrhage, would point away from these diseases and toward one of the small vessel vasculitides. Both polyarteritis nodosa and Kawasaki disease cause acute necrotizing arteritis that may be complicated by thrombosis and hemorrhage. The presence of mucocutaneous lymph node syndrome distinguishes Kawasaki disease from polyarteritis nodosa.

NAMES AND DEFINITIONS FOR SMALL VESSEL VASCULITIS

Henoch-Schönlein purpura	Vasculitis with IgA-dominant immune deposits affecting small vessels, *ie,* capillaries, venules, or arterioles. Typically involves skin, gut and glomeruli, and is associated with arthralgias or arthritis.
Cryoglobulinemic vasculitis	Vasculitis with cryoglobulin immune deposits affecting small vessels, *ie,* capillaries, venules, or arterioles, and associated with cryoglobulins in serum. Skin and glomeruli are often involved.
Wegener's granulomatosis	Granulomatous inflammation involving the respiratory tract, and necrotizing vasculitis affecting small to medium-sized vessels, *eg,* capillaries, venules, arterioles, and arteries. Necrotizing glomerulonephritis is common.
Churg-Strauss syndrome	Eosinophil-rich and granulomatous inflammation involving the respiratory tract and necrotizing vasculitis affecting small to medium-sized vessels, and associated with asthma and blood eosinophilia
Microscopic polyangiitis	Necrotizing vasculitis with few or no immune deposits affecting small vessels, *ie,* capillaries, venules, or arterioles. Necrotizing arteritis involving small and medium-sized arteries may be present. Necrotizing glomerulonephritis is very common. Pulmonary capillaritis often occurs.

FIGURE 8-7

The small vessel vasculitides have the highest frequency of clinically significant renal involvement of any category of vasculitis. This is not surprising given the numerous small vessels in the kidneys and their critical roles in renal function. The renal vessels most often involved by all small vessel vasculitides are the glomerular capillaries, resulting in glomerulonephritis. Glomerular involvement in immune complex vasculitis typically results in proliferative or membranoproliferative glomerulonephritis, whereas ANCA disease usually causes necrotizing glomerulonephritis with extensive crescent formation. Involvement of renal vessels other than glomerular capillaries is rare in immune complex vasculitis but common in ANCA vasculitis.

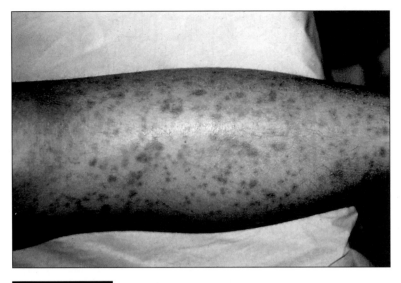

FIGURE 8-8

Cutaneous purpura in a patient with Henoch-Schönlein purpura. This clinical appearance could be caused by any of the small vessel vasculitides, and thus is not specific for Henoch-Schönlein purpura. Henoch-Schönlein purpura is the most common small vessel vasculitis in children [6]. In a young child with purpura, nephritis and abdominal pain, the likelihood of Henoch-Schönlein purpura is approximately 80%; however, in an older adult with the same clinical presentation, the likelihood of Henoch-Schönlein purpura is very low and the patient has an approximately 80% chance of having an ANCA-associated vasculitis.

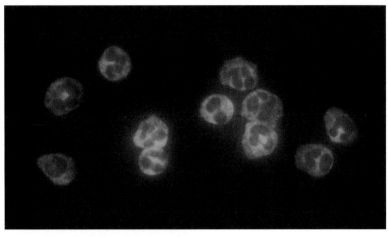

FIGURE 8-9 (*see* Color Plate)

The C-ANCA staining pattern of ethanol-fixed normal human neutrophils in an indirect immunofluorescence assay of serum. Approximately 90% of C-ANCA are specific for proteinase 3 (PR3-ANCA) in specific immunochemical assays, such as enzyme immunoassay [7–9].

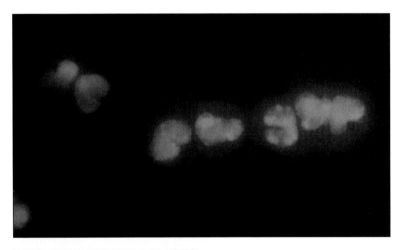

FIGURE 8-10 (*see* Color Plate)

The P-ANCA staining pattern of ethanol-fixed normal human neutrophils in an indirect immunofluorescence assay of serum. Approximately 90% of P-ANCA in patients with nephritis or vasculitis are specific for myeloperoxidase (MPO-ANCA) in specific immunochemical assays, such as EIA. P-ANCA in patients with other types of inflammatory disease, such as inflammatory bowel disease, are typically not specific for MPO. Using ethanol-fixed neutrophils as substrate, nuclear staining caused by antinuclear antibodies (ANA) cannot be distinguished confidently from nuclear staining caused by P-ANCA. Using formalin-fixed neutrophils as substrate, P-ANCA stain the cytoplasm but ANA do not. The difference in staining pattern between ethanol and formalin-fixed cells is due to the artifactual diffusion of solubilized cationic ANCA-antigens to the nucleus during substrate preparation of the ethanol-fixed cells, as opposed to immobilization of the antigens in the cytoplasm by covalent crosslinking during formalin fixation.

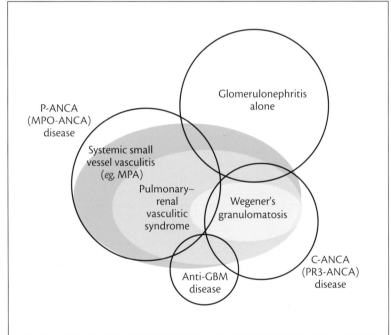

FIGURE 8-11

Categorization of patients with crescentic glomerulonephritis with respect to both the immunopathologic category of disease (immune complex versus anti-GBM versus ANCA) and the clinicopathologic expression (glomerulonephritis alone versus Wegener's granulomatosis versus Goodpasture's syndrome versus other small vessel vasculitis) [10]. Note that most patients with ANCA have some expression of systemic vasculitis rather than glomerulonephritis alone. Most patients with Wegener's granulomatosis have C-ANCA/PR3-ANCA but some have P-ANCA/MPO-ANCA. Also note that some patients with anti-GBM and some patients with immune complex disease also are ANCA positive. (*Adapted from* Jennette [10]).

Amyloidosis

CLASSIFICATION OF AMYLOIDOSIS

Amyloid type	Classification	Major protein component
Primary amyloidosis (AL)	Primary, including multiple myeloma	κ or λ light chain
Secondary amyloidosis (AA)	Secondary	Protein A
Familial amyloidosis (AF)	Familial	
	Neuropathic: Portugal, Sweden, Japan, and other countries	Transthyretin mutant (prealbumin)
	Cardiopathic: Denmark and Appalachia in the United States	Transthyretin mutant (prealbumin)
	Nephropathic: familial Mediterranean fever	Protein A
Senile systemic amyloidosis (AS)	Senile cardiac	Transthyretin normal (prealbumin)
Dialysis amyloidosis (AD)	Dialysis arthropathy	β_2-microglobulin

FIGURE 8-12

Classification of amyloidosis. The fibrils in primary amyloidosis consist of monoclonal κ or λ light chains. Rarely, monoclonal heavy chains are responsible. The major component of the amyloid fibril in secondary amyloidosis is protein A. It has a molecular weight of 8.5 kD and contains 76 amino acids. It is derived from serum amyloid A, which is an acute-phase protein. The level of serum amyloid A is increased in patients with rheumatoid arthritis and Crohn's disease. In familial amyloidosis, the Portuguese, Swedish, and Japanese variants are characterized by substitution of methionine for valine at residue 30 (Met-30) in the transthyretin molecule. This mutation is characterized by the development of peripheral neuropathy. Cardiomyopathy from a transthyretin mutation has been reported in Denmark (Met-111) and in the Appalachian area of the United States (Ala-60). Familial renal amyloid from a mutation of the fibrinogen α-chain (Leu-554 or Glu-526) or mutations of lysozyme have been reported. Amyloidosis associated with familial Mediterranean fever consists of protein A. Senile systemic amyloidosis involving the heart results from the deposition of normal transthyretin. Long-term dialysis often results in systemic amyloidosis from β_2-microglobulin deposition.

SYSTEMIC AMYLOIDOSIS

Amyloid type	Amyloid stains				
	Congo red	κ or λ	Serum amyloid A	β_2-microglobulin	Transthyretin (prealbumin)
Primary (AL)	+	+	-	-	-
Secondary (AA)	+	-	+	-	-
FMF	+	-	+	-	-
Associated with long-term hemodialysis	+	-	-	+	-
Familial (AF)	+	-	-	-	+
Senile systemic (AS)	+	-	-	-	+

FIGURE 8-13

Systemic amyloidosis. Types of proteins constituting the amyloid fibrils. In primary amyloidosis the fibrils consist of monoclonal κ or λ light chains. In secondary amyloidosis the fibrils consist of protein A. Systemic amyloidosis associated with long-term hemodialysis consists of β_2-microglobulin. The amyloid fibrils consist of mutated transthyretin or, rarely, fibrinogen-α or lysozyme in familial amyloidosis. Senile systemic amyloidosis is characterized by the deposition of normal transthyretin in the heart. (*Adapted from* Kyle [11].)

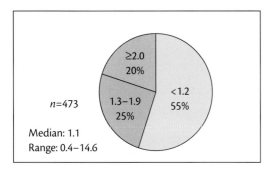

FIGURE 8-14

Serum creatinine (mg/dL) in patients at diagnosis of primary systemic amyloidosis. Renal insufficiency was present in almost half of patients. Proteinuria was present in about 75% of patients.

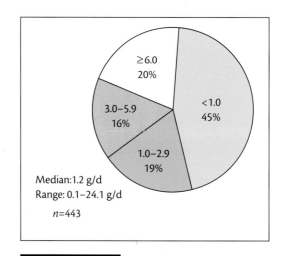

FIGURE 8-15

Urine total protein values in patients at diagnosis of primary systemic amyloidosis in an 11-year study at the Mayo Clinic. More than one third of patients exhibited 24-hour urine total protein values of 3.0 g/d or more. Over half of patients had a urine protein value of more than 1 g/d. The electrophoretic pattern showed mainly albumin. (*Adapted from* Kyle [11].)

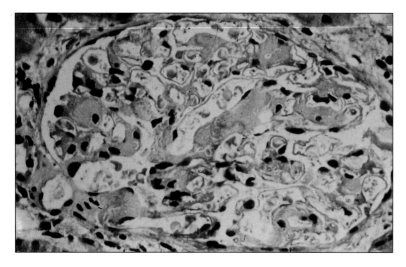

FIGURE 8-16 (*see* Color Plate)

Photomicrograph showing a renal biopsy specimen stained with Congo red dye taken from a patient with primary systemic amyloidosis. Note the homogeneous deposition of amyloid in the glomerulus. Results of kidney biopsy are positive in about 95% of patients.

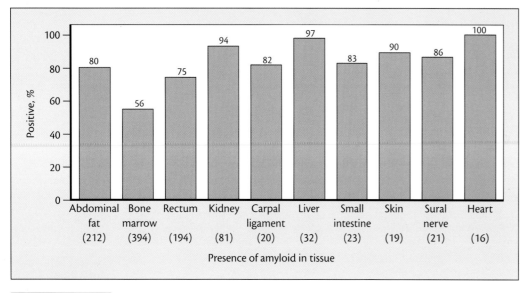

FIGURE 8-17

Diagnosis of primary systemic amyloidosis based on the presence of amyloid in tissue in an 11-year study at the Mayo Clinic. The initial diagnostic procedure should be an abdominal fat aspirate [12]. The diagnosis will be confirmed in 80% of patients. Experience in the staining technique and interpretation of the fat aspirate is important before routine use. A bone marrow aspirate and bone marrow biopsy specimen should be obtained to determine the degree of plasmacytosis, and results of amyloid stains are positive in more than half of patients. Either the abdominal fat aspirate or bone marrow biopsy specimen is positive in 90% of patients. When amyloid is still suspected and the test results of these tissues are negative, one should proceed to performing a rectal biopsy, which is positive in approximately 80% of patients. The specimen must include the submucosa. When the test results for these sites are negative, tissue should be obtained from an organ with suspected involvement. (Numbers in parentheses indicate number of patients.)

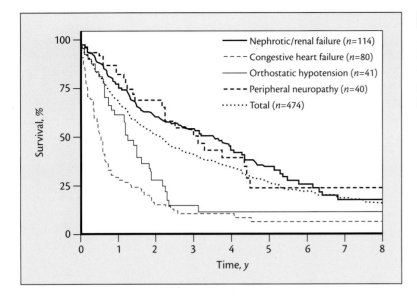

FIGURE 8-18

Analysis of median survival in patients with primary systemic amyloidosis in an 11-year study at the Mayo Clinic. The median survival of 474 patients seen within 1 month of diagnosis was 13.2 months. The median duration of survival was 4 months for the 80 patients who exhibited congestive heart failure on presentation.

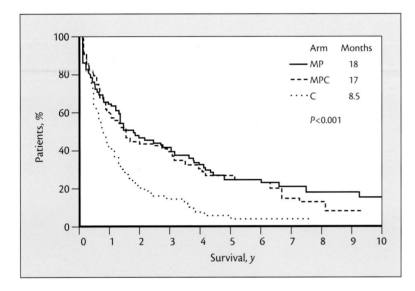

FIGURE 8-19

Survival curves in patients with primary systemic amyloidosis. Because amyloid fibrils consist of monoclonal immunoglobulin light chains, treatment with alkylating agents that are effective against plasma cell neoplasms is warranted. We treated 220 patients who had positive results on biopsy. The patients were randomized to receive colchicine (C, 72 patients), melphalan and prednisone (MP, 77), or melphalan, prednisone, and colchicine (MPC, 71). Patients were stratified according to their chief clinical manifestations: renal disease (105 patients), cardiac involvement (46), peripheral neuropathy (19), or other (50). The median duration of survival after randomization was 8.5 months in the colchicine group; 18 months in the group assigned to melphalan and prednisone; and 17 months in the group assigned to melphalan, prednisone, and colchicine ($P < 0.001$). In patients who had a reduction in serum or urine monoclonal protein at 12 months, the overall duration of survival was 50 months; whereas among those without a reduction in monoclonal protein at 12 months, the duration of survival was 36 months ($P < 0.003$). Thirty-four patients (15%) survived for 5 years or longer. (*Adapted from* Kyle *et al.* [12].)

CAUSES OF SECONDARY AMYLOIDOSIS

Cause	Patients, n
Rheumatic disease	
Rheumatoid arthritis	31
Ankylosing spondylitis	5
Other	6
Total	42
Infection	
Inflammatory bowel disease	6
Bronchiectasis	5
Osteomyelitis	5
Other	3
Total	19
Malignancy	2
None	1

FIGURE 8-20

Causes of secondary amyloidosis. Rheumatoid arthritis is the most frequent cause of secondary amyloidosis. In our study of 64 patients, rheumatoid arthritis was present for a median of 18 years before the diagnosis was made [13]. Inflammatory bowel disease, bronchiectasis, and osteomyelitis are not uncommon causes of secondary amyloidosis. (*Adapted from* Gertz and Kyle [13].)

PRESENTING CLINICAL FEATURES OF SECONDARY AMYLOIDOSIS

Feature	Patients, %
Proteinuria or renal insufficiency	91
Diarrhea, obstipation, or malabsorption	22
Goiter	9
Hepatomegaly	5
Neuropathy or carpal tunnel syndrome	3
Lymphadenopathy	2
Hematuria	2
Cardiac amyloidosis	0

FIGURE 8-21

Presenting features of secondary amyloidosis. Proteinuria is the most frequent laboratory finding in patients with secondary amyloidosis. Involvement of the gastrointestinal tract as manifested by diarrhea, obstipation, or malabsorption occurred in one fifth of our patients. Treatment of secondary amyloidosis depends on the underlying disease. Familial Mediterranean fever frequently is associated with secondary amyloidosis unless the patient is treated with colchicine. (*Adapted from* Gertz and Kyle [13].)

Sickle Cell Disease

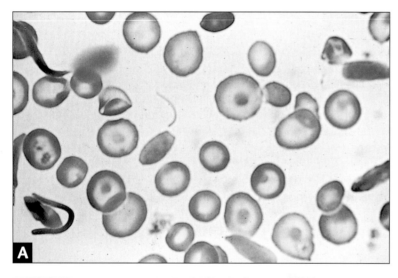

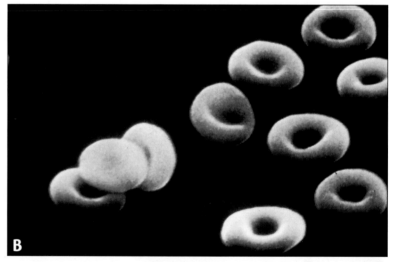

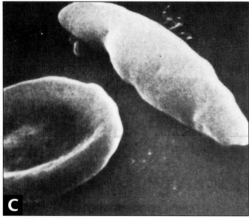

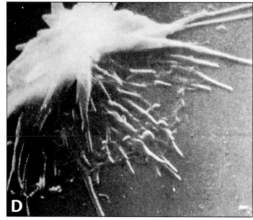

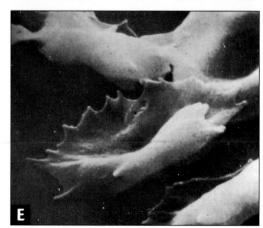

FIGURE 8-22

Polymerization of hemoglobin S. Polymerization of deoxygenated hemoglobin S is the primary event in the molecular pathogenesis of sickle cell disease, resulting in a distortion of the shape of the erythrocyte and a marked decrease in its deformability. These rigid cells are responsible for the vaso-occlusive phenomena that are the hallmark of the disease [14]. Interesting shapes of variable forms result depending on the localization of the polymers in the cell. A collection of electron microscopy scans of sickle cells undergoing intracellular polymerization is shown here. The slides were created in different laboratories. **A,** Characteristic peripheral blood smear from a patient with sickle cell anemia. Extreme sickled forms and target cells are seen. **B,** Electron microscopy scan of normal erythrocytes. **C,** Electron microscopy scan of a normal erythrocyte and a sickle cell. **D–L,** This series of sickle cells show many possible formations of sickled erythrocytes.

(*continued on next page*)

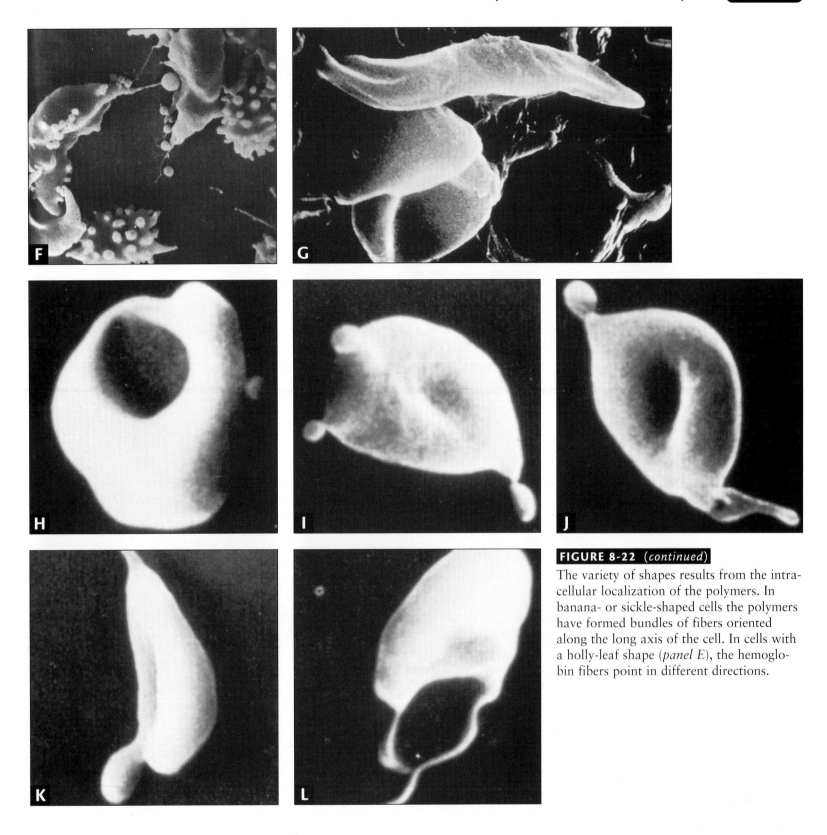

FIGURE 8-22 (*continued*)
The variety of shapes results from the intracellular localization of the polymers. In banana- or sickle-shaped cells the polymers have formed bundles of fibers oriented along the long axis of the cell. In cells with a holly-leaf shape (*panel E*), the hemoglobin fibers point in different directions.

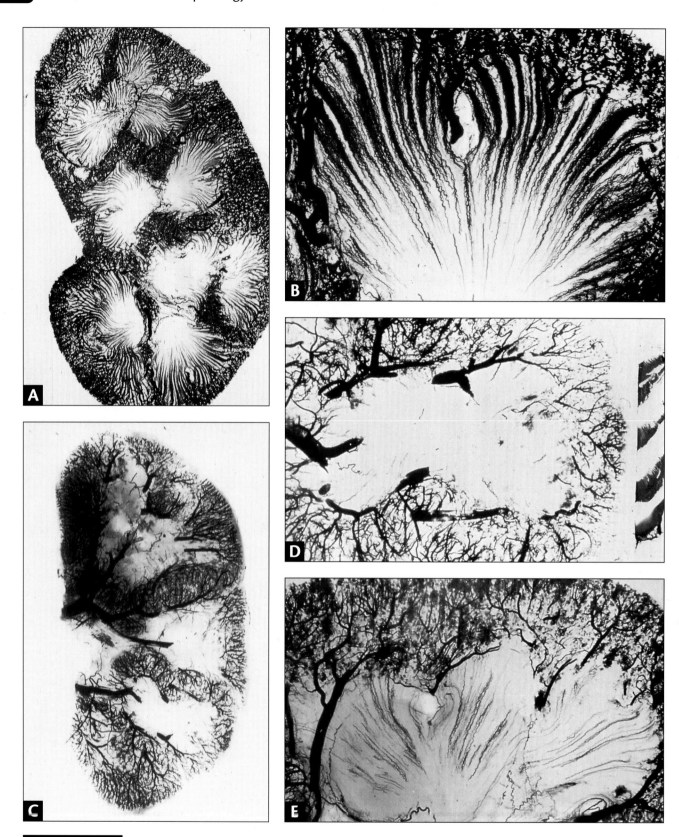

Macroscopy and microradioangiographs of sickle cell kidneys. The kidneys of patients with sickle cell disease usually are of near normal size, and most kidneys show no significant gross alterations. Abnormalities can be expected in the renal medulla as erythrocytes form sickles more readily in the relatively hypoxic and hyperosmotic renal medulla than in other capillary circulations. Formation of microthrombi causes further impairment of the vasa recta circulation. **A** and **B**, Injection microradioangiographs of the kidney in a person without hemoglobinopathy are shown: the entire kidney (*panel A*) and a detailed view (*panel B*). **C** and **D**, Injection microradioangiographs of the kidney in a patient with sickle cell disease are shown: the entire kidney (*panel C*) and a detailed view (*panel D*). **E**, Injection microradioangiograph of a kidney in a patient with sickle cell hemoglobin C disease. In the normal kidney (*panel A*), vasa recta are visible radiating into the renal papilla. In sickle cell anemia (*panel D*), vasa recta are virtually absent. Those vessels that are present show abnormalities: they are dilated, form spirals, end bluntly, and many appear to be obliterated. In the patient with hemoglobin SC (*panel E*) changes are seen intermediately between patients with hemoglobin SC and normal persons. (*From* van Eps *et al.* [15]; with permission.)

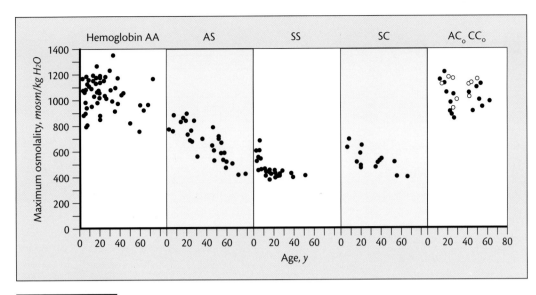

FIGURE 8-24

Relationship between maximal urinary osmolality and age in normal subjects and in patients with hemoglobinopathies. Results of an investigation into a large group of normal persons and those with homozygotous hemoglobin disease (Hb SS; Hb SS + Hb F), heterozygotous

hemoglobin disease (Hb AS), sickle cell hemoglobin C disease (SC), hemoglobin C trait (AC), and hemoglobin C disease (Hb CC). Normal persons have a mean maximal urinary osmolality of 1058 ±SD 128 mOsm/kg H_2O. The most marked impairment in concentrating capacity occurs in Hb SS disease. Maximal urinary osmolality decreases significantly in the first decade of life and stabilizes in patients over 10 years of age at a mean of 434 ±SD 21 mOsm/kg H_2O. The measurement has been designated the fixed maximum of sickle cell nephropathy. In patients with Hb AS and Hb SC, a progressive decrease in maximal urinary osmolality can be observed with age. C hemoglobin alone (AC or CC) does not impair the concentrating ability of the kidneys. The renal concentrating capacity of the heterozygote (Hb AS) also is affected, but only later in life. (*Adapted from* van Eps *et al.* [16].)

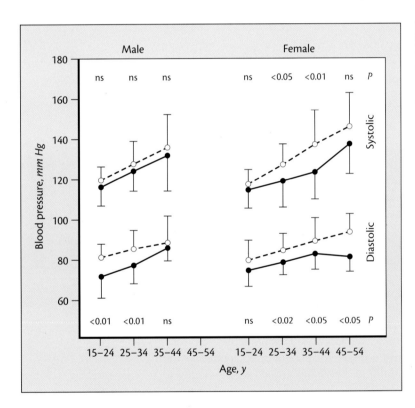

FIGURE 8-25

Blood pressure and sickle cell anemia. Mean standard deviation of systolic and diastolic blood pressure in control subjects (*dotted lines*) and patients with sickle cell anemia (*closed lines*) who are matched for age and gender. (*From* De Jong and van Eps [17].)

Renal Involvement in Malignancy

CAUSES OF PRERENAL ACUTE RENAL FAILURE

Clinical syndrome	Cause
ECF volume contraction (hypovolemia)	External fluid loss (skin, gastrointestinal, renal, hemorrhage)
	Internal fluid loss (peritonitis, bowel obstruction, acute pancreatitis, hemorrhage, malignant effusion)
Peripheral vasodilation	Sepsis
	Anaphylaxis
	Anesthesia
	Drug overdose
Impaired cardiac function	Myocardial infarct, failure
	Arrhythmia
	Pericardial tamponade
	Pulmonary embolus
Bilateral extrarenal vascular occlusion	Arterial
	Venous
Functional disorders of intrarenal circulation	Hepatorenal syndrome
	Drugs that inhibit prostaglandin synthesis

FIGURE 8-26

Causes of prerenal failure (ARF). Prerenal ARF is encountered frequently in the cancer patient, particularly in association with depletion of the extracellular fluid (ECF) volume, which is caused by excessive loss from the gastrointestinal tract due to vomiting or diarrhea induced by cancer or its therapy. Also, hypovolemia may occur owing to internal fluid loss due to translocation of ECF volume with sequestration in third spaces, as seen in peritonitis, bowel obstruction, malignant effusion, or interleukin-2 therapy [18].

A decrease in effective intravascular volume may occur owing to peripheral vasodilation, as frequently noted in sepsis. A decrease in cardiac output due to cardiac tamponade secondary to malignant pericardial disease also may produce prerenal ARF. Hepatobiliary disease may cause alterations in intrarenal hemodynamics with resultant hepatorenal syndrome, as seen in hepatic veno-occlusive disease following bone marrow transplantation. The administration of nonsteroidal anti-inflammatory agents for analgesia in the cancer patient may lead to ARF by elimination of the prostaglandin-mediated intrarenal vasodilatation. This homeostatic mechanism represents a critical hemodynamic adjustment necessary for maintaining glomerular filtration rate in a patient with cancer in whom renal blood flow may be decreased owing to a variety of causes.

CAUSES OF INTRINSIC ACUTE RENAL FAILURE

Glomerular abnormalities	Glomerulonephritis
	Hemolytic-uremic syndrome
Tubular abnormalities	Ischemic acute tubular necrosis (ATN)
	Exogenous nephrotoxins
	Antineoplastic agents
	Antimicrobials
	Radiocontrast media
	Anesthetic agents
	Endogenous nephrotoxins
	Myoglobin
	Hemoglobin
	Immunoglobulins and light chains
	Calcium and phosphorus
	Uric acid and xanthine
Interstitial abnormalities	Drug-induced acute tubulointerstitial nephritis
	Acute pyelonephritis
	Tumor infiltration
	Radiation nephropathy
Abnormalities of intrarenal blood vessels	Disseminated intravascular coagulation
	Hemolytic-uremic syndrome
	Malignant hypertension
	Vasculitis

FIGURE 8-27

The four major causes of malignancy-associated intrinsic acute renal failure (ARF). With glomerular abnormalities, the pathologic process most frequently involves diffuse proliferative or crescentic glomeru-

lonephritis. Although immune-complex–mediated glomerular disease is not uncommon in patients with cancer [19], glomerular disease causing ARF in the cancer patient has been reported in only a few cases [20]. Hemolytic-uremic syndrome with vascular endothelial injury in both the glomeruli and the intrarenal blood vessels may occur in patients with disseminated malignancy or after chemotherapy for malignancy.

With respect to tubular abnormalities, ARF may arise either on the basis of ischemia or as a result of exposure to exogenous or endogenous nephrotoxins. Renal ischemia is usually the initiating factor when ATN follows sepsis or shock or when it arises as a postsurgical complication. Cancer patients are particularly vulnerable to ARF induced by exogenous nephrotoxins in view of their frequent exposure to a wide variety of nephrotoxic drugs. The indicated nephrotoxins of endogenous origin are encountered with increasing frequency in the cancer patient.

The most frequent cause of interstitial abnormalities is acute tubulointerstitial nephritis, which may be induced in cancer patients via hypersensitivity to various drugs. These patients frequently receive the analgesics and antimicrobials associated with this form of ARF. Immunosuppressed cancer patients may be particularly vulnerable to severe acute bacterial pyelonephritis. ARF may occur in this setting, even in the absence of urinary tract obstruction or another underlying renal disease [21]. Tumor infiltration of the kidney may involve the interstitium but rarely causes ARF [22]. Finally, radiation nephropathy may occur following radiation therapy for cancer and has been associated with ARF [23], although when it occurs, it more frequently produces chronic renal failure.

The fourth major cause of intrinsic ARF is abnormalities of intrarenal blood vessels. Disseminated intravascular coagulation may occur in association with sepsis in the cancer patient [24]. In addition, because the cancer patient is more often older, atheroembolic disease or malignant hypertension must be considered as a possible cause of intrarenal vascular occlusion in the presence of ARF. Finally, vasculitis is a consideration, particularly in the presence of hepatitis B antigenemia.

CAUSES OF RENAL FAILURE IN MULTIPLE MYELOMA

Cause	Pathogenesis
Light-chain cast nephropathy	Intratubular precipitation of light chains
AL amyloidosis	Deposition of amyloid fibers composed of light chains (Congo red positive)
Light-chain deposition disease	Nodular glomerulosclerosis with granular deposits (Congo red negative) of light chains along the basement membrane
Plasma cell infiltration of the kidney	Often incidental finding at autopsy
	Rare cause of renal dysfunction
Fanconi's syndrome and other tubular dysfunction	Tubular toxicity of light chains
Hypercalcemic nephropathy	Bone resorption causing hypercalcemia
Acute uric acid nephropathy	Renal tubular precipitation of uric acid following tumor lysis
Radiocontrast nephropathy	Interaction between light chains and radiocontrast agents

FIGURE 8-28

Renal failure in multiple myeloma. The patient with multiple myeloma is at increased risk for the development of acute renal failure [25]. In up to 25% of patients with multiple myeloma,

acute renal failure may be present at the time of initial diagnosis. In others, it may occur at any time during the disease. Renal failure can be due to diverse mechanisms. The light chains produced by the monoclonal B lymphocytes may be nephrotoxic [26]. While the toxicity of the light chains leads to a variety of tubular transport disorders, including Fanconi's syndrome, the intratubular precipitation of these proteins causes light-chain cast nephropathy and acute renal failure. The light chains (usually lambda) may be transformed into Congo-red–positive amyloid fibrils and deposited diffusely throughout the body [27]. Deposition of amyloid in renal tissue results in the nephrotic syndrome and, often, renal failure. Biopsy of the kidney, abdominal fat pad, or rectal mucosa is useful in the diagnosis of AL amyloidosis. Light chains may also be deposited in a granular pattern along the basement membranes of blood vessels in a variety of organs. In the kidney, these deposits are noted in the glomeruli, causing an expansion of the mesangium, and appear as nodular glomerulosclerosis. This condition is referred to as light-chain deposition disease (LCDD) [28].

Other causes of renal failure in a patient with multiple myeloma include metabolic disturbances such as hypercalcemia and hyperuricemia. Hypercalcemia may be due to direct bone erosion by the malignant cells or to the elaboration of cytokines, which activate osteoclasts. The administration of radiocontrast agents to patients with multiple myeloma may lead to interaction with light chains and tubular precipitation, thereby causing acute renal failure. The prognosis for recovery from acute renal failure in a patient with multiple myeloma is generally poor unless reversible factors such as hypercalcemia or dehydration are responsible [25].

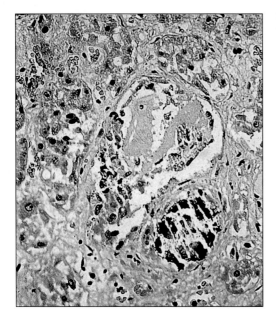

FIGURE 8-29

Nephrocalcinosis in a patient with multiple myeloma. Irregular fractured hematoxylinophilic deposits of calcium are seen in this fibrotic renal tissue. Hypercalcemia may produce serious structural changes in the kidney, resulting in acute or chronic renal failure.

Hypercalcemia is a relatively common complication of malignancy. Increased bone reabsorption is most often responsible owing to bone metastases or to the release of humoral substances such as parathyroid hormone–like peptide or cytokines such as transforming growth factor-α [29]. Secretion of calcitriol, the active form of vitamin D, also may occur in some lymphomas [30]. Renal dysfunction in the setting of hypercalcemia results from both calcium-induced constriction of the afferent arteriole and the deposition of calcium in the tubules and interstitium, leading to intratubular obstruction and secondary tubular atrophy and interstitial fibrosis [31]. Prompt treatment generally restores renal function, but irreversible damage can occur with long-standing hypercalcemia [32]. Recovery of the glomerular filtration rate varies inversely with the extent of nephrocalcinosis, interstitial scarring, associated obstructive uropathy, infection, and hypertension. All the foregoing reflect the duration and severity of hypercalcemia. (*From* Skarin [33]; with permission.)

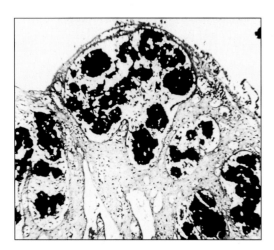

FIGURE 8-30

Acute uric acid nephropathy (AUAN). Intrarenal obstruction caused by uric acid precipitation in collecting ducts produces severe tubular dilatation (DeGalantha stain). This patient, who received chemotherapy for acute lymphocytic leukemia before allopurinol was available, had a plasma urate concentration of 44 mg/dL at the time of death.

Acute uric acid nephropathy is most frequently encountered in patients with a large tumor burden (often due to rapidly proliferating lymphoma or leukemia) in whom aggressive radiation or chemotherapy has been recently initiated. If rapid lysis of tumor cells occurs, massive quantities of uric acid precursors (and often other tumor products) are released. This induces a marked increase in synthesis of uric acid and thus acute hyperuricemia. The subsequent renal uricosuric response may be of sufficient magnitude to exceed solubility limits for uric acid in the distal nephron, particularly in the presence of dehydration or metabolic acidosis. The resultant intrarenal obstruction produces a characteristic pattern of acute renal failure [34]. In the setting of particularly extensive disease with rapid cell lysis, profound hyperkalemia, hyperphosphatemia, and hypocalcemia (due to precipitation of calcium phosphate) may be observed. This is termed acute tumor lysis syndrome [35]. This syndrome usually occurs after treatment of poorly differentiated lymphoma or leukemia; if it arises spontaneously, hyperphosphatemia is not prominent because phosphate is incorporated into rapidly proliferating tumor cells.

Rarely, xanthine nephropathy can occur during tumor lysis when allopurinol is used to prevent the production of uric acid. The resultant xanthine oxidase inhibition can produce a marked increase in blood and urine xanthine and hypoxanthine concentrations. Xanthine, like uric acid, is poorly soluble in an acidic urine; xanthine crystalluria occurs when its concentration exceeds its solubility, thereby causing obstructive nephropathy [36].

CAUSES OF POSTRENAL ACUTE RENAL FAILURE

Anatomic site	Cause
Urethral obstruction	Prostatic hypertrophy
Bladder neck obstruction	Prostatic or bladder cancer
	Functional: neuropathy or drugs
Bilateral ureteral obstruction (or unilateral obstruction with single kidney)	Extraureteral
	Cancer of prostate or uterine cervix
	Periureteral fibrosis
	Accidental ureteral ligation during pelvic surgery for cancer
	Intraureteral
	Uric acid crystals or stones
	Blood clots
	Pyogenic debris
	Edema
	Necrotizing papillitis

FIGURE 8-31

The etiology of postrenal failure involves obstruction at various anatomic sites by tumors of the urinary tract or surrounding tissues. Some of the more common causes of bladder neck obstruction in the cancer patient include prostatic hypertrophy [37] and prostatic or bladder cancer [38]. Postrenal acute renal failure may also be produced by bilateral obstruction of both ureters (or unilateral ureteral obstruction in the presence of a single kidney). This may be caused by invasion of the ureters by bladder neoplasms or, more commonly, by retroperitoneal spread of malignancies, particularly of colon, prostate, bronchus, or breast origin.

CAUSES OF HEMATURIA AND/OR THE NEPHROTIC SYNDROME

Paraneoplastic glomerulonephritis
  Membranous glomerulonephritis
  Minimal change nephrotic syndrome
  Crescentic glomerulonephritis
  Membranoproliferative glomerulonephritis
Primary or metastatic renal cancer
Chemotherapy agents causing nephrotic syndrome
  Mitomycin C
  Gemcitabine
  Interferon

FIGURE 8-32

Causes of hematuria and/or the nephrotic syndrome. Hematuria and/or the nephrotic syndrome may occur in association with malignancy without causing acute or chronic renal failure. Causes may include one of the many paraneoplastic types of glomerulonephritis, with proteinuria and often the nephrotic syndrome resulting from the glomerular injury; hematuria is also noted in some cases. In contrast, isolated hematuria is the predominant feature when primary or metastatic renal cancer erodes the intrarenal vasculature. Proteinuria, and in some cases the nephrotic syndrome, may be the presenting nephrotoxicity of cancer chemotherapy agents.

A. COMPARISON OF PARAPROTEINEMIAS

Diagnosis	Frequency*	Clinical Findings	Renal Lesions	Diagnostic Means
Multiple myeloma	Yes	Proteinuria (light chain) Acute renal failure Hypercalcemia	Light-chain cast nephropathy Acute tubular necrosis	Immunoelectrophoresis or bone marrow Light chains in urine
AL amyloidosis	Yes	Proteinuria Nephrotic syndrome	Deposits of amyloid fibrils in the kidney	Renal or rectal biopsy Immunoelectrophoresis
Light-chain deposition disease	No	Proteinuria Nephrotic syndrome Chronic renal failure	Nodular glomerulosclerosis with granular deposition of light chains along the glomerular and tubular basement and membrane; usually kappa light chains	Renal biopsy Bone marrow biopsy Immunoelectrophoresis
Waldenström's macroglobulinemia	Rarely	No renal symptoms or minimal proteinuria	Intraglomerular "coagula" of IgM	Immunoelectrophoresis Bone marrow biopsy
Monoclonal gammopathy of unknown significance (MGUS)	Rarely	Proteinuria Nephrotic syndrome	Proliferative glomerulonephritis in some case	Immunoelectrophoresis Bone marrow biopsy Renal biopsy

* Frequency of renal involvement.

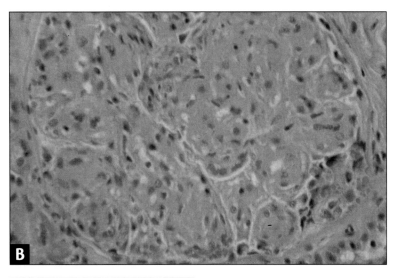

B

FIGURE 8-33 (*see* Color Plate)

Paraproteinemias and multiple myeloma. **A,** Paraprotein abnormalities as a cause of nephrotic syndrome. This table compares the characteristics of various paraproteinemias. Paraproteins are abnormal immunoglobulins or abnormal immunoglobulin fragments produced by B lymphocytes. They are monoclonal, appear in the serum or urine (or both), and cause renal damage by several different mechanisms. Paraproteinemias comprise a group of disorders characterized by overproduction of different paraproteins.

Multiple myeloma is a common type of paraproteinemia. The overproduction of immunoglobulins or light chains, or both, causes renal toxicity, directly affecting the tubular cells or forming casts after precipitation in the tubular lumen. The light chains may be transformed into amyloid fibrils and deposited in various tissues, including the kidney. Amyloidosis is diagnosed by performing a biopsy of the involved organ and staining the tissue with Congo red stain. On occasion, the light chains do not form fibrils but are deposited as granules along the basement membrane of blood vessels and glomeruli. Kappa chains often behave in this manner. This entity is called light-chain deposition disease [39] (*panel B*).

Paraproteins composed of IgM are noted in Waldenström's macroglobulinemia. Renal dysfunction is uncommon in this condition [40]. Hyperviscosity is present. On rare occasions, thrombi composed of IgM may be noted in the glomeruli of these patients.

In the most common form of paraproteinemia, monoclonal protein is detected in the serum of an otherwise healthy person. This condition is referred to as monoclonal gammopathy of unknown significance (MGUS) and may on occasion progress to multiple myeloma or amyloidosis [41].

B, Light-chain deposition disease (LCDD) in a patient with multiple myeloma. A light microscopic study of a renal biopsy specimen from a 65-year-old man with recently diagnosed multiple myeloma who was found to have an elevated serum creatinine concentration (2.6 mg/dL) and proteinuria of 3 g/d. Note the nodular mesangial lesions, capillary wall thickening, and hypercellularity resembling diabetic nodular glomerulosclerosis. Immunofluorescence staining was positive for kappa light chains but negative for lambda light chains.

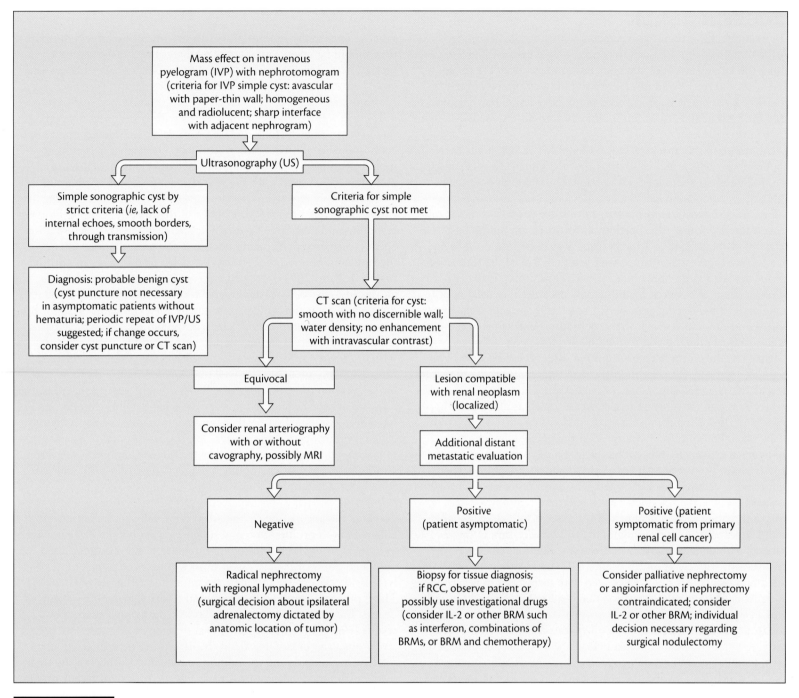

Diagnostic evaluation of and therapeutic approach to primary renal cancer. The discovery of evidence during the history or physical examination that suggests a renal abnormality should be followed by either an intravenous pyelogram or an abdominal ultrasound. With increasing frequency, however, evidence of a space-occupying lesion in the kidney is found incidentally during radiographic testing for other unrelated conditions. Renal ultrasonography may help distinguish simple cysts from more complex abnormalities. A simple cyst is defined sonographically by the lack of internal echoes, the presence of smooth borders, and the transmission of the ultrasound wave. If these three features are present, the cyst is most likely benign. At one time, cyst puncture was used, but it seems to be unnecessary today in the asymptomatic patient without hematuria. Periodic repetition of the ultrasound is suggested for follow-up. If a change in the lesion occurs, cyst puncture, needle aspiration, or CT scanning should be considered to evaluate the lesion further.

If the sonographic criteria for a simple cyst are not met or the intravenous pyelogram suggests a solid or complex mass, a CT scan should be performed. If a renal neoplasm is demonstrated on CT scanning, renal vein or vena caval involvement should be assessed with CT scanning or magnetic resonance imaging. Although used frequently in the past, selective renal arteriography has assumed a more limited use, mainly in further evaluating the renal vasculature in patients who are to undergo partial nephrectomy (nephron-sparing surgery). CT scanning is also very helpful in determining the presence of lymphadenopathy.

The differential diagnosis of a renal mass detected on CT scanning includes primary renal cancers, metastatic lesions of the kidney, and benign lesions. The latter include angiomyolipomas (renal hamartomas), oncocytomas, and other rare or unusual growths. If a renal cancer is considered based on the radiographic studies of the kidney, the patient should undergo a preoperative staging evaluation to assess the presence of metastases in the lung, bone, or brain. The operative and diagnostic approach is dictated according to the preoperative stage of the patient.

(continued on next page)

FIGURE 8-34 (*continued*)

For example, the patient who presents with stage IV disease by virtue of a positive bone scan may need only a needle biopsy of either the kidney lesion or the bone lesion to establish the tissue diagnosis and thus avoid more extensive surgery on the kidney. In contrast, a patient with an isolated pulmonary lesion may be considered for both nephrectomy and pulmonary nodulectomy at one operative intervention.

The standard therapy for localized renal cell carcinoma is radical nephrectomy, which includes removal of the kidney, Gerota's fascia, the ipsilateral adrenal gland, and regional hilar lymph nodes. The value of an extended hilar lymphadenectomy seems to be its ability to provide prognostic information, since there is rarely a therapeutic reason for performing this portion of the operation. In the past, the removal of the ipsilateral adrenal gland was done routinely; today, most data suggest that it is involved less than 5% of the time, more frequently with large upper-pole lesions. Thus, today, ipsilateral adrenalectomy is reserved for those patients with abnormal-appearing glands or enlarged glands on CT scan or those with large upper-pole lesions, in which the probability of direct extension of the tumor to the adrenal gland is more likely [42].

Partial nephrectomy (nephron-sparing surgery) has become more popular, especially for patients with small tumors, for those at risk for developing bilateral tumors, or for patients in whom the contralateral kidney is at risk for other systemic diseases, such as diabetes or hypertension [43]. The main concern associated with partial nephrectomy is the likelihood of tumor recurrence in the operated kidney, since many renal cancers may be multicentric. Local recurrence rates of 4% to 10% have been reported; lower rates have been reported when partial nephrectomy was performed for smaller lesions (< 3 cm) with a normal contralateral kidney. Lesions that are centrally located, however, still require radical nephrectomy. Frequent follow-up, usually with CT scanning or ultrasonography, will be necessary in those patients who undergo partial nephrectomy. Inferior vena caval involvement with renal cancer occurs more frequently with right-sided tumors and is usually associated with metastases in nearly 50% of patients. Vena caval obstruction may lead to the diagnosis; it may present with abdominal distention from ascites, hepatic dysfunction, nephrotic syndrome, abdominal wall venous collaterals, varicocele, malabsorption, or pulmonary embolus. The anatomic location of the caval thrombus is important prognostically; supradiaphragmatic lesions, which may involve the heart, can be resected, but the prognosis is poor. Subdiaphragmatic lesions enjoy a better 5-year survival, but the survival rate is usually less than 50% [44]. In the surgical management of these patients, a team of specialists is required, especially if a cardiac tumor thrombectomy is contemplated.

The role of surgery in the management of metastatic disease either at initial presentation or later remains controversial. Although most data that support nephrectomy plus metastatectomy are anecdotal, many patients with synchronous renal cell cancer and an isolated pulmonary nodule may be considered for surgical resection of both lesions. Likewise, patients who develop an isolated lesion in the liver or lung some time following the removal of the kidney also may be considered for surgical removal of the metastasis. Nevertheless, even when such vigorous surgery is carried out, most patients do poorly. Additional controversy surrounds the practice of performing nephrectomy in patients with widespread metastatic disease as a means of potentially improving their response to systemic therapy. Many investigative programs require such resection, but at this writing, the practice should be considered investigational. A patient who does experience an excellent response to systemic therapy should be considered for nephrectomy following the response, however.

Finally, since many renal tumors can become quite large, consideration should be given to palliative nephrectomy (in the setting of metastatic disease), especially if the patient experiences uncontrollable hematuria or pain or is catabolic secondary to the sheer mass of the tumor.

The medical management of patients with either locally advanced renal cancer or metastatic disease provides a great challenge to physicians and clinical investigators. Although chemotherapy and hormonal treatments have been studied extensively in patients with metastatic renal cancer, no single treatment protocol or program has been uniformly effective. Therefore, most physicians treating the disease usually rely on novel modalities of treatment, including biologic response modifiers, investigational anticancer agents, differentiation agents (such as retinoic acid), vaccines, and gene therapy. Interferon therapy with interferon-α, -β, or -γ has led to responses in approximately 15% to 20% of treated patients [64]. Interferons demonstrate antiproliferative activity against renal cell cancers in vitro, stimulate immune cell function, and can modulate the expression of major histocompatibility complex molecules. Although responses have been seen in cancers involving many different anatomic areas, patients who have had a prior nephrectomy with isolated pulmonary metastases and who are otherwise well may enjoy a higher response rate [65]. Duration of response is usually less than 2 years; longer lasting remissions have been noted in a few selected patients. Interferons have been combined with other immune modifiers as well as with chemotherapy agents with no real improvement in patient outcome in larger-scale trials. Several smaller trials have combined interferon with interleukin-2 or chemotherapy agents (*eg*, 5-fluorouracil) with some encouraging preliminary results.

Interleukin 2 (IL-2) has received a great deal of attention as a potential advance in the treatment of renal cell cancer. This agent enhances both proliferation and functioning of lymphocytes involved in antigen recognition and tumor elimination. Initial studies used very high doses of IL-2 in association with ex vivo populations of lymphoid cells grown and matured under the influence of IL-2 [66]. These programs resulted in substantial toxicity, including patient deaths, but nevertheless had early and encouraging therapeutic results. Unfortunately, the initial encouraging results were not consistently observed in larger-scale trials. Efforts are now directed at selectively manipulating the immune-enhancing features of the treatment, with modification of the toxic effects. In several recent studies, the use of lower doses of IL-2 *without* the cellular components has resulted in comparable results with less toxicity.

The toxicity of IL-2 is related to alterations in vascular permeability, leading to a capillary leak type of syndrome. Although the drug is approved by the Food and Drug Administration for the management of patients with metastatic renal cell cancer, its use should be restricted to those patients who can tolerate the side effect profile and those patients with acceptable cardiac, renal, pulmonary, and hepatic function.

Investigational therapies continue to be studied for renal cell cancer. These include novel cytokines such as interleukin-12, combinations of biologics with or without chemotherapeutic agents, circadian timing of chemotherapy administration, vaccine therapy, various forms of cellular therapy, and gene therapy [67]. Although all these approaches have a solid scientific preclinical rationale, none, unfortunately, can be considered standard treatment. The sobering fact still remains that nearly 50% of all patients diagnosed with renal cell cancer die of their disease within 5 years of diagnosis, and a substantial proportion have advanced stages of cancer spread at initial presentation.

POTENTIALLY NEPHROTOXIC CHEMOTHERAPEUTIC AGENTS

Drug	Risk			Type of renal failure			Time course	
	High	Intermediate	Low	Acute	Chronic	Specific tubular damage	Immediate	Delayed
Alkylating agents								
Cisplatin	X			X	X	X	X	X
Carboplatin			X	X	X	X	X	X
Cyclophosphamide			X			X	X	
Ifosfamide			X	X		X	X	
Streptozotocin	X			X		X		X
Semistine (methyl-CCAU)		X			X			X
Carmustine (BCNU)			X		X			X
Antimetabolites								
Methotrexate†	X			X			X	
Cytosine arabinoside (Ara-A)			X	X			X	
5-Fluorouracil (5-FU)‡			X	X	X		X	
5-Azacitidine			X	X		X	X	
6-Thiognanine			X	X			X	
Antitumor antibiotics								
Mitomycin§			X		X			X
Mithramycin¶	X			X			X	
Doxorubicin			X	X			X	
Biologic agents								
Interferons			X	X	X		X	X
Interleukin-2	X			X			X	

*Fanconi's syndrome as the most severe manifestation.

†Only seen with intermediate to high dose regimens.

‡Only seen when given in combination with mitomycin C.

§Hemolytic-uremic syndrome as the most severe manifestation.

¶Frequent with antineoplastic doses, rare in doses used for hypercalcemia.

FIGURE 8-35

Toxic therapeutic agents. Nephrotoxicity due to antineoplastic agents may result in chronic renal failure but also may manifest as acute renal failure, specific tubular dysfunction, or the nephrotic syndrome. Nephrotoxicity has been observed with use of alkylating agents, antimetabolites, antitumor antibiotics, and biologic agents, as outlined in the table. These neoplastic agents may induce nephrotoxicity soon after initiation of therapy or only after long-term administration. The risk of nephrotoxicity varies with each agent. This table summarizes the risk of nephrotoxicity, time of onset, and type of functional impairment produced by each agent. (*Adapted from* Massry and Glassock [45].)

Renal Involvement in Tropical Diseases _____

CLINICAL MANIFESTATIONS OF TROPICAL BACTERIAL NEPHROPATHIES

Disease	Abnormal sediment	Proteinuria	ARF	CRF	HUS	Hemolysis	DIC	Jaundice	Commonly associated features
Salmonellosis	+++	++++	+	-	+	+	+	+	Gastrointestinal
Shigellosis			+	-	++*	+	+	+	Neurologic[†]
Leptospirosis	++++	++++	++++	-	+	+	+	++++	Hemorrhagic tendency
									Polyuria[‡]
Melioidosis	+++++	+	++	-					Hyponatremia[§]
Cholera		+	-						Hypokalemia, acidosis
Tetanus	+	++++	+++	-					Sympathetic overflow
Scrub typhus	+	++	+	-		+		+	
Diphtheria	+	+	+	-					Myocarditis, polyneuritis
Tuberculosis	++	+/+++		+					Retroperitoneal nodes
Leprosy	++	+++	+	+					Lepromas

*Associated with *Shigella* serotype I endotoxin [46].

[†]Visual disturbances, drowsiness, seizures, and coma in 40% of cases [47].

[‡]In 90% of cases [49].

[§]Nephrogenic diabetes insipidus [48].

One plus sign indicates < 10%; *two plus signs* indicate 10%–24%; *three plus signs* indicate 25%–49%; *four plus signs* indicate 50%–80%; *five plus signs* indicate > 80%.

Dash indicates not reported.

FIGURE 8-36

Clinical manifestations of tropical bacterial nephropathies. Note the wide spectrum of clinical manifestations that may ultimately reflect on the kidneys [46–48]. ARF—acute renal failure; CRF—chronic renal failure; DIC—disseminated intravascular coagulation; HUS—hemolytic uremic syndrome.

SPECTRUM OF RENAL PATHOLOGY IN TROPICAL BACTERIAL INFECTIONS

Disease	Glomerulonephritis								Vasculitis	AIN	ATN	Other tubular changes
	MPGN	EXGN	MCGN	MN	NG	CGN	Amyloid	Deposits of immunoglobulins, complement, and antigen				
Salmonellosis	++	++*						G,M,A,C3,Ag[†]		++	+	Cloudy swelling
Shigellosis	+								+		+	Cloudy swelling
Leptospirosis	+				+			M,C3	+	++	+++	
Melioidosis	+									+++	+	Cloudy swelling
Cholera											++	Vacuolation[‡]
Tetanus											++	
Scrub typhus	+									+	+	Cloudy swelling
Diphtheria										++	+/++	Degeneration[§]
Tuberculosis						+				+		
Leprosy	+/+++		+	+		+[¶]	+	G,M,A,C3		+	+/+++**	Functional defects

*When associated with *Schistosoma mansoni* infection in Egypt [53].

[†]Vi antigen deposits [54].

[‡]Hypokalemic nephropathy [50].

[§]Exotoxin-induced inhibition of protein synthesis in tubule cells [51].

[¶]Usually complicates amyloidosis: 2.4%–8.4% [18].

**63% in lepromatous leprosy; 2% in nonlepromatous types [55].

One plus sign indicates <10%; *two plus signs* indicate 10%–24%; *three plus signs* indicate 25%–50%.

FIGURE 8-37

Spectrum of renal pathology in tropical bacterial infections [50–52]. AIN—acute interstitial nephritis; ATN—acute tubular necrosis; CGN—crescentic glomerulonephritis; EXGN—exudative glomerulonephritis; MCGN—mesangiocapillary glomerulonephritis; MN—membranous glomerulopathy; NG—necrotizing glomerulitis.

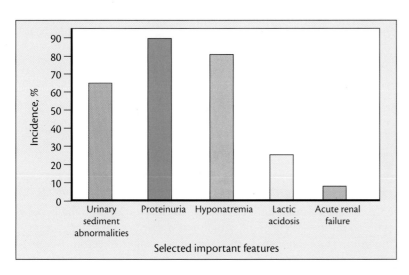

FIGURE 8-38

Clinical manifestations of renal involvement in dengue hemorrhagic fever. Note that proteinuria and abnormal urinary sediment are the most common manifestations. Also note the high incidence of hyponatremia, as with many other tropical infections [56,57].

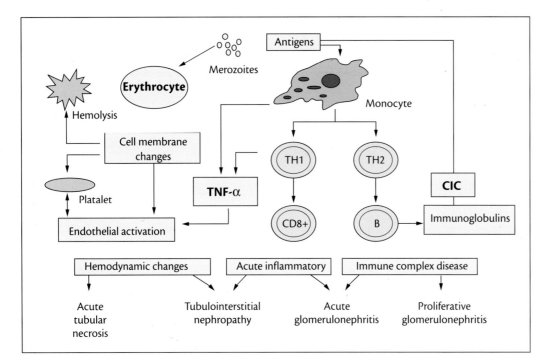

FIGURE 8-39

The pathogenesis of falciparum malarial renal complications. Note the infection triggers two initially independent pathways: red cell parasitization and monocyte activation. These subsequently interact, as the infected red cells express abnormal proteins that induce an immune reaction by their own right, in addition to providing sticky points (knobs) for clumping and adherence to platelets and capillary endothelium. TNF-α released from the activated monocytes shares in the endothelial activation. As both pathways proceed and interact, a variety of renal complications develop, including acute tubular necrosis, acute interstitial nephritis and acute glomerulonephritis. B—B-lymphocyte; CD8—cytotoxic T cell; CIC—circulating immune complexes; TH—T-helper cells (1 and 2); TNF-α—tumor necrosis factor-α.

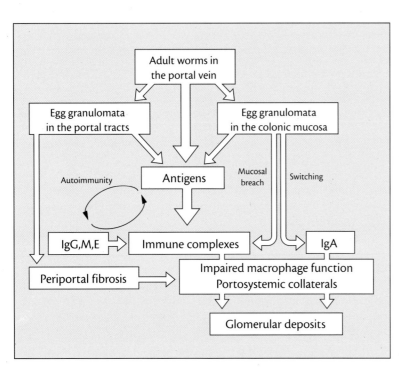

FIGURE 8-40

Pathogenesis of *Schistosoma mansoni* glomerulopathy. Note the crucial role of hepatic fibrosis, which 1) induces glomerular hemodynamic changes; 2) permits schistosomal antigens to escape into the systemic circulation, subsequently depositing in the glomerular mesangium; and 3) impairs clearance of IgA, which apparently is responsible for progression of the glomerular lesions. IgA synthesis seems to be augmented through B-lymphocyte switching under the influence of interleukin-10, a major factor in late schistosomal lesions [58].

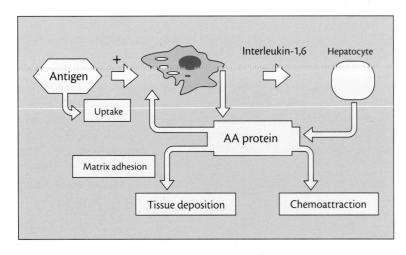

FIGURE 8-41

Pathogenesis of schistosoma-associated amyloidosis. The monocyte continues to release interleukin-1 and interleukin-6 under the influence of schistosomal antigens. These antigens stimulate the hepatocytes to release AA protein, which has a distinct chemoattractant function. The monocyte is the normal scavenger of serum AA protein, a function that is impaired in hepatosplenic schistosomiasis. Serum AA protein accumulates and tends to deposit in tissue.

FIGURE 8-42

NEPHROPATHIES ASSOCIATED WITH EXPOSURE TO ANIMAL TOXINS

	Acute renal failure	Vasculitis	Subnephrotic proteinuria	Nephrotic syndrome
Snake bite	+++	+	+ (MPGN)	
Scorpion sting	+			
Insect stings	+			++ (MCD, MPGN, MN)
Jelly fish sting	+			
Spider bite	+			
Centipede bite	+			
Raw carp bile	++			

One plus sign indicates < 10%; *two plus signs* indicate 10%–24%; *three plus signs* indicate 25%–50%.

Nephropathies associated with exposure to toxins of animal origin. Note that acute renal failure is the most common and important renal complication. Vascular and glomerular lesions are occasionally encountered with specific exposures [59–65]. MCD—minimal change disease; MN—membranous glomerulonephritis; MPGN—mesangial proliferative glomerulonephritis.

Renal Disease in Patients with Hepatitis and HIV

FIGURE 8-43

RENAL DISEASE ASSOCIATED WITH HEPATITIS B VIRUS INFECTION

Lesion	Clinical presentations	Pathogenesis
Membranous nephropathy	Nephrotic syndrome	Deposition of HBeAg with anti-HBeAb
Polyarteritis nodosa	Vasculitis, nephritic	Deposition of circulating antigen-antibody complexes
Membranoproliferative glomerulonephritis	Nephrotic, nephritic	Deposition of complexes containing HBsAg and HBeAg

Renal disease associated with hepatitis B. Infection with hepatitis B virus (HBV) may be associated with a variety of renal diseases [66,67]. Many patients are asymptomatic, with plasma serology positive for hepatitis B surface antigen (HBsAg), hepatitis B core antibody (HBcAb), and hepatitis B antigen (HBeAg). The pathogenetic role of HBV in these processes has been documented primarily by demonstration of hepatitis B antigen-antibody complexes in the renal lesions [66,68,69]. Three major forms of renal disease have been described in HBV infection. In membranous nephropathy, it is proposed that deposition of HBeAg and anti-HBe antibody forms the classic subepithelial immune deposits [66,68–70]. Polyarteritis nodosa is a medium-sized vessel vasculitis in which antibody-antigen complexes may be deposited in vessel walls [66,67]. Finally, membranoproliferative glomerulonephritis is characterized by deposits of circulating antigen-antibody complexes in which both HBsAg and HBeAg have been implicated [68].

RENAL DISEASE ASSOCIATED WITH HEPATITIS C VIRUS INFECTION

Disease	Renal manifestations	Serologic testing
Mixed cryoglobulinemia [71–76]	Hematuria, proteinuria (often nephrotic), variable renal insufficiency	Positive cryoglobulins; rheumatoid factor often present
Membranoproliferative glomerulonephritis [78]	Hematuria, proteinuria (often nephrotic)	Hypocomplementemia; rheumatoid factor and cryoglobulins may be present
Membranous nephropathy [79,80]	Proteinuria (often nephrotic)	Complement levels normal; rheumatoid factor negative

FIGURE 8-44

Renal disease associated with hepatitis C. Hepatitis C virus (HCV) infection is associated with parenchymal renal disease. Chronic HCV infection has been associated with three different types of renal disease. Type II or essential mixed cryoglobulinemia has been strongly linked with HCV infection in almost all patients with this disorder [71–76]. The clinical manifestations of this renal disease include hematuria, proteinuria that is often in the nephrotic range, and a variable degree of renal insufficiency. Essential mixed cryoglobulinemia had been considered an idiopathic disease; however,

recent studies have noted one or more of the following features in over 95% of patients with this disorder: circulating anti-HCV antibodies; polyclonal IgG anti-HCV antibodies within the cryoprecipitate; and HCV RNA in the plasma and cryoprecipitate [71,72]. Furthermore, evidence exists suggesting direct involvement of HCV-containing immune complexes in the pathogenesis of this renal disease [71]. Sansono *et al.* [77] demonstrated HCV-related proteins in the kidneys of eight of 12 patients with cryoglobulinemia and membranoproliferative glomerulonephritis (MPGN) by indirect immunohistochemistry. Convincing clinical data exist suggesting that HCV is responsible for some cases of MPGN and possibly membranous nephropathy [78–80]. In one report of eight patients with MPGN, purpura and arthralgias were uncommon and cryoglobulinemia was absent in three patients [78]. Circulating anti-HCV antibody and HCV RNA along with elevated transaminases provided strong evidence of an association with HCV infection. Establishing the diagnosis of HCV infection in these diseases is important because of the potential therapeutic benefit of α-interferon treatment [78]. A number of reports exist that demonstrate a beneficial response to chronic antiviral therapy with α-interferon [71,78,81,82]. Even more compelling evidence for a beneficial effect of α-interferon in HCV-induced mixed cryoglobulinemia was demonstrated in a randomized prospective trial of 53 patients given either conventional therapy alone or in combination with α-interferon [83]. Because of the likely recurrence of viremia and cryoglobulinemia with cessation of α-interferon therapy after conventional treatment (3×10^6 U three times weekly for 6 mo), extended courses of therapy (up to 18 mo) and higher dosing regimens are being studied [84–86].

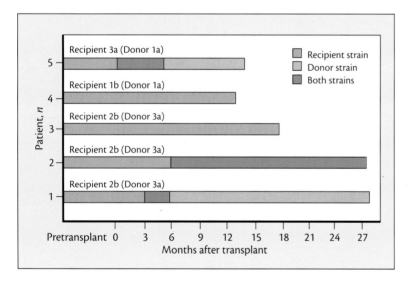

FIGURE 8-45

Patterns of hepatitis C virus (HCV) infection after transplantation of a kidney from a positive donor into a positive recipient. In a simple but important study, Widell *et al.* [87] demonstrated three differing virologic patterns of HCV infection emerging after kidney transplantation from a donor infected with HCV into a recipient infected with HCV. Superinfection with the donor strain, persistence of the recipient strain, or long-term coinfection with both the donor and recipient strain may result. The clinical significance of infection with more than one HCV strain has not been determined in the transplantation recipient with immunosuppression, although no data exist to suggest that coinfection confers a worse outcome. For this reason, many centers will transplant a kidney from a donor who was infected with HCV into a recipient infected with HCV rather than discard the organ. (*Data from* Widell *et al.* [87].)

GLOMERULAR DISEASE IN KIDNEY RECIPIENTS INFECTED WITH HEPATITIS C VIRUS

Reference	Number of anti–HCV-positive patients	Histologic diagnosis				Total cases of GN
		MGN	MPGN	DPGN	CGN	
Cockfield and Prieksaitis [88]	51	–	–	–	–	11*
Huraib et al. [89]	30	0	5	1	1	7
Morales et al. [90]	166	7	0	0	0	7
Roth et al. [91]	98	0	5	0	0	5
Morales et al. [92]	409	15	0	0	0	15

*No specific diagnosis.

FIGURE 8-46

Glomerular disease in HCV-positive recipients. Chronic hepatitis C virus (HCV) infection has been associated with several different immune-complex–mediated diseases in the renal allograft, including membranous and membranoproliferative glomerulonephritis (MPGN) [88–92]. From a cohort of 98 renal allograft recipients with HCV, Roth et al. [91] detected de novo membranoproliferative glomerulonephritis in the biopsies of five of eight patients with proteinuria of over 1 g/24 h [91]. Compared with a control group of nonproteinuric kidney recipients infected with HCV, patients with MPGN had viral particles present in greater amounts in the high-density fractions of sucrose density gradients associated with significant amounts of IgG and IgM. Thus, deposition of immune complexes containing HCV genomic material may be involved in the pathogenesis of this form of MPGN. The differential diagnosis for significant proteinuria in a patient infected with HCV after transplantation should include immune-complex glomerulonephritis. Similarly, if the renal allograft biopsy shows immune-complex glomerulonephritis, the patient should be tested for HCV infection without regard to serum alanine aminotransferase levels. CGN—crescentic glomerulonephritis; DPGN—diffuse proliferative GN; MGN—membranous GN; MPGN—membranoproliferative GN.

RENAL COMPLICATIONS OF HIV INFECTION

Acid-base and electrolyte disturbances

Acute renal failure

HIV–associated nephropathies

Renal infections and tumors

FIGURE 8-47

Renal complications of HIV. Renal complications are frequent, and these rates are expected to increase as patients with HIV live longer. Many renal diseases are incidental and are the consequences of opportunistic infections, neoplasms, or the treatment of these infections and tumors. The renal diseases include a variety of acid-base and electrolyte disturbances, acute renal failure having various causes, specific HIV-associated nephropathies, and renal infections and tumors.

MANAGEMENT OF SEVERE ACUTE RENAL FAILURE

	HIV	Non-HIV
Conservative	20 (14%)	42 (14%)
Recovered	85%	83%
Needing dialysis	126	264
Not initiated	42%	22%
Initiated	73	207
Recovered	56%	47%

FIGURE 8-48

Acute renal failure management. Rao and Friedman [93] compared the course of 146 patients with severe acute renal failure (serum creatinine >6 mg/dL) infected with HIV with a group of 306 contemporaneous persons not infected with HIV but with equally severe acute renal failure. The patients infected with HIV were younger than those in the group not infected (mean age 38.4 and 55.2 years, respectively; $P<0.001$) and were more often septic (52% and 24%, respectively; $P<0.001$). Over 80% of patients in each group recovered renal function when conservative therapy alone was sufficient. When dialysis intervention was needed, it was not initiated more often in the group with HIV than in the control group (42% and 24%, respectively; $P<0.003$). In those patients in whom dialysis was initiated, recovery occurred in about half in each group. Overall, the mortality in patients with severe acute renal failure was not significantly different in those with HIV infection from those in the group not infected with HIV (immediate mortality, 60% and 56%, respectively; mortality at 3 months, 71% and 60%, respectively).

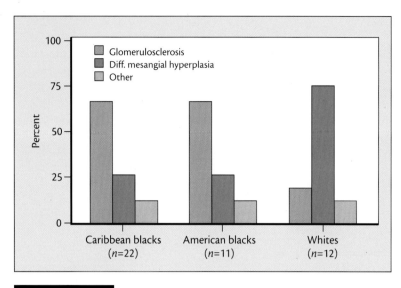

FIGURE 8-49

Glomerulosclerosis associated with HIV. In the United States, HIV-associated focal segmental or global glomerulosclerosis was described originally in 1984 in large East Coast cities, particularly New York and Miami [94–96]. This entity initially was considered with skepticism because it was not seen in San Francisco, where most patients testing seropositive were white homosexuals [97,98]. In New York, patients with glomerulosclerosis were

largely black intravenous (IV) drug abusers, a group of patients in whom heroin nephropathy was prevalent. Thus, concern existed that this entity merely represented the older heroin nephropathy now seen in HIV-infected IV drug abusers. However, in a Miami-based population of adult non-IV drug users with glomerular disease and HIV infection, 55% of Caribbean and American blacks had severe glomerulosclerosis, 9% had mild focal glomerulosclerosis, and 27% had diffuse mesangial hyperplasia. In contrast, two of 12 (17%) whites had a mild form of focal glomerulosclerosis, 75% had diffuse mesangial hyperplasia, and none had severe glomerulosclerosis. These morphologic differences were reflected in more severe clinical presentations, with blacks more likely to manifest proteinuria in the nephrotic range (>3.5 g/24 h) and renal insufficiency (serum creatinine concentration (>3 mg/dL). Whites often had proteinuria under 2 g/24 h and serum creatinine values less than 2 mg/dL [99]. In blacks, glomerulosclerosis has been described in all groups at risk for HIV infection, including IV drug users, homosexuals, patients exposed to heterosexual transmission or to contaminated blood products, and children infected perinatally [100,101]. Subsequent reports confirmed the unique clinical and histopathologic manifestations of HIV-associated glomerulosclerosis and its striking predominance in blacks independent of IV drug abuse [102]. Racial factors explain the absence of HIV-associated glomerulosclerosis in whites and Asians. The cause of this strong racial predilection is unknown.

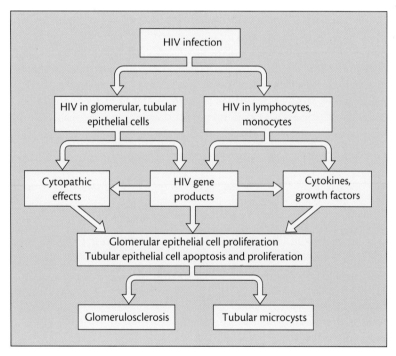

FIGURE 8-50

Possible pathogenic mechanisms of glomerulosclerosis associated with HIV infection. HIV-associated glomerulosclerosis is not the result of opportunistic infections. Indeed, the nephropathy may be the first manifestation of HIV infection and often occurs in patients before opportunistic infections develop. HIV-associated glomerulosclerosis also is not an immune-complex–mediated glomerulopathy because immune deposits are generally absent. Three mechanisms have been proposed: direct injury of renal epithelial cells by infective HIV, although direct renal cell infection has not been demonstrated conclusively and systematically; injury by HIV gene products; or injury by cytokines and growth factors released by infected lymphocytes and monocytes systemically or intrarenally or released by renal cells after uptake of viral gene products. The variable susceptibility to glomerulosclerosis also suggests that unique viral-host interactions may be necessary for expression of the nephropathy [103–108].

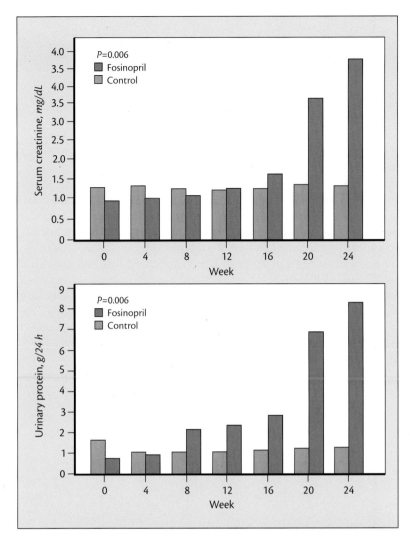

FIGURE 8-51

Effect of angiotensin-converting enzyme (ACE) inhibitors on progression of glomerulosclerosis associated with HIV infection. Serum ACE levels are increased in patients with HIV infection [109]. Kimmel *et al.* [110], using captopril, and Burns *et al.* [111], using fosinopril, demonstrated a renoprotective effect of ACE inhibitors in patients with biopsy-proven HIV-associated glomerulosclerosis. In the former study, the median time to end-stage renal disease was increased from 30 to 74 days in nine patients given 6.25 to 25 mg captopril three times a day. In the latter study, 10 mg of fosinopril was given once a day to 11 patients with early renal insufficiency (serum creatinine <2 mg/dL). Serum creatinine and proteinuria remained stable during 6 months of treatment with fosinopril. In contrast, patients not treated with fosinopril exhibited progressive and rapid increases in serum creatinine and proteinuria. Similar outcomes prevailed in patients with proteinuria in the nephrotic range and serum creatinine levels less than 2 mg/dL. Captopril also is beneficial to the progression of the nephropathy in HIV-transgenic mice [112]. The mechanism(s) of the renoprotective effects of ACE inhibitors are unclear and may include hemodynamic effects, decreased expression of growth factors, or an effect on HIV protease activity. Renal biopsy early in the course of the disease is important to define the renal lesion and guide therapeutic intervention.

OTHER NEPHROPATHIES ASSOCIATED WITH HIV INFECTION

Immune-complex glomerulopathies
   Proliferative glomerulonephritis
   Membranous glomerulonephritis
   Lupus-like nephropathy
   IgA nephropathy
Hemolytic-uremic syndrome, thrombotic
   thrombocytopenic purpura

FIGURE 8-52

Other nephropathies associated with HIV. A variety of immune-complex-mediated glomerulopathies have been documented in patients with HIV infection. Some represent glomerular diseases associated with HIV infection, whereas others may be incidental or manifestations of associated diseases.

Renal Involvement in Sarcoidosis _____

RENAL INVOLVEMENT IN SARCOIDOSIS

Calcium metabolism
    Hypercalciuria (50–60)*
    Hypercalcemia (10–20)
    Nephrolithiasis (≈10)
    Nephrocalcinosis (5–10)
Tubulointerstitial nephritis
    Granulomatous (15–40)
    Fibrotic (10–20)
Glomerulopathy (rare)
    Membranous
    Proliferative
    Focal segmental glomerulosclerosis
Arteritis (rare)
    Granulomatous angiitis
Obstructive nephropathy (rare)
    Retroperitoneal lymphadenopathy
    Retroperitoneal fibrosis

· Numbers in parentheses indicate percentage of patients.

FIGURE 8-53

Renal involvement in sarcoidosis. The principal manifestations of renal involvement in sarcoidosis are the functional abnormalities resulting from the altered metabolism of calcium as a result of the increased synthesis of 1,25-dihydroxy-vitamin D_3 by the macrophages of the granulomatous lesions. The consequent increased calcium absorption from the gastrointestinal tract results in the hypercalciuria that can be detected in more than half of patients. The frequency of hypercalciuria depends on the extent of granulomatous lesions and on the time of the year, being more common in spring and summer when exposure to the sun is greatest. Hypercalcemia is less common and usually depends on coexistent deterioration of renal function when the capacity of the kidney to excrete calcium is compromised. In most patients, hypercalciuria is asymptomatic. Its principal manifestations are inability to concentrate the urine, and polyuria. Nephrolithiasis occurs in about 10% of patients; another 10% develop nephrocalcinosis.

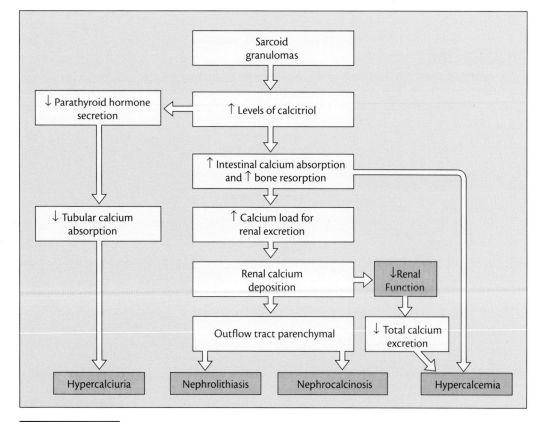

FIGURE 8-54

Abnormal calcium metabolism and pathophysiology of renal involvement in sarcoidosis. Increased synthesis of calcitriol (1,25-dihydroxy-vitamin D_3) by the macrophages of the granulomatous lesions of sarcoidosis are at the core of the abnormal calcium metabolism that accounts for the principal manifestations of renal involvement of sarcoidosis (*gray boxes*). Patients with hypercalciuria, which by far is the most common, may remain asymptomatic, and the disease may go undetected. Polyuria and a reduced capacity to concentrate the urine are its main manifestations. Either of these two features may be the result of tubulointerstitial nephritis caused by sarcoidosis, and can be present in the absence of any altered calcium metabolism. Nephrocalcinosis also may be asymptomatic. In contrast, nephrolithiasis presents as renal colic or hematuria. Hypercalcemia develops only when the load of calcium to be excreted exceeds the ability of the kidneys to excrete the calcium load, either because of reduced renal function or, less commonly, when the amount of calcium absorbed is excessive. The magnitude of hypercalcemia determines its symptomatology. The circulating level of parathyroid hormone should be determined in patients with hypercalcemia. An increase in the prevalence of parathyroid adenomas seems to occur in sarcoidosis. In hypercalcemia caused by elevated levels of calcitriol and by reduced renal excretion of calcium, parathyroid hormone levels should be negligible. Detection of elevated levels of parathyroid hormone should lead to the search for an adenoma. Patient management is directed at reducing calcitriol synthesis by treating the granulomatous lesions with steroids. Equally important measures in the management of such patients are restriction of calcium intake, avoidance of dietary supplements that contain vitamin D, shunning exposure to sunlight, and increased fluid intake.

Renal Involvement in Essential Mixed Cryoglobulinemia

CLASSIFICATION OF CRYOGLOBULINEMIAS AND ASSOCIATED DISEASES

Type I: single monoclonal IgA, IgG, or IgM	Type II: polyclonal IgG bound to monoclonal anti-IgG rheumatoid factor*	Type III: polyclonal IgG bound to polyclonal anti-IgG rheumatoid factor*
Multiple myeloma	B-lymphocytic neoplasm	Autoimmune diseases: SLE, polyarteritis nodosa, rheumatoid arthritis, scleroderma, Sjögren's syndrome, and Henöch-Schonlein purpura
Waldenström's macroglobulinemia	Diffuse lymphoma	Infectious diseases: mononucleosis, cytomegalovirus, hepatitis B, subacute bacterial endocarditis, leprosy, malaria, schistosomiasis, toxoplasmosis, AIDS
Chronic lymphocytic leukemia	Chronic lymphocytic leukemia	Miscellaneous diseases: primary proliferative glomerulonephritis, lymphoma, chronic hepatitis, biliary cirrhosis
Idiopathic monoclonal gammopathy	Sjögren's syndrome	Essential
	Essential	

*Usually IgM.

FIGURE 8-55

Classification of cryoglobulinemias and associated diseases as proposed by Brouet *et al.* in 1974 [113]. Up to the end of the 1980s, the cause of about 30% of both types II and III mixed cryoglobulins was not clear, and this group of mixed cryoglobulinemias was called *essential* [114,115]. It now is evident that most essential mixed cryoglobulinemias are associated with hepatitis C virus infection. (*Adapted from* Brouet *et al.* [113].)

DETECTION OF CIRCULATING CRYOGLOBULINS AND DETERMINATION OF CRYOPRECIPITATE

Prewarm syringe, needle, and tubes at 37°C

Take 20 mL of whole blood and put it immediately at 37°C

Incubate for 2 h at 37°C to allow clotting

Centrifuge twice at 1700 g X 10 at 37°C to discard platelets and erythrocytes

Cryoglobulins precipitate reversibly from cooled serum

Keep serum at 4°C in a conical graduate tube

Look at the serum after 7 d

Centrifuge serum at 400 g X 10 at 4°C and calculate the cryocrit as the percentage of packed cryoglobulins and serum ratio

FIGURE 8-56

Correct methodology for detecting circulating cryoglobulins. Cryoglobulins are immunoglobulins that precipitate reversibly from cooled serum.

DISTINCTIVE FEATURES OF MEMBRANOPROLIFERATIVE GLOMERULONEPHRITIS, OR CRYOGLOBULINEMIC GLOMERULONEPHRITIS

Exudative component
The major constituent of intracapillary proliferation is an infiltration of leukocytes, mainly monocytes, that sometimes is massive.

Intraluminal thrombi
Huge deposits of cryoglobulins called *intraluminal thrombi* sometimes fill the capillary lumen.

Interposition of monocytes in the double contour of the capillary wall
Monocytes, in close contact with the subendothelial deposits of cryoglobulins, are interposed between the glomerular basement membrane and the newly formed membranelike material, to give the double-contoured appearance of the capillary wall, whereas peripheral interposition of mesangial matrix and cells is moderate.

Structured crystalloid deposits on electron microscopy
Intraluminal and subendothelial deposits of cryoglobulins sometimes show a specific fibrillar structure on electron microscopy.

Vasculitis of small and medium-sized arteries
Necrotizing arteritis, without concomitant features of segmental necrotizing glomerulonephritis, is found in one third of patients.

FIGURE 8-57

The distinctive features of the membranoproliferative glomerulonephritis. This disorder, called *cryoglobulinemic glomerulonephritis*, occurs only in patients with type II mixed cryoglobulinemia, especially in the acute stage of the disease [116,117]. In about 20% of patients with type II mixed cryoglobulinemia, a less distinctive picture of lobular membranoproliferation is found, whereas an additional 20% exhibit mild mesangial proliferation. These various types of histologic lesions can be found by repeat biopsies in the same patient during different stages of the disease.

RENAL SYNDROME AT PRESENTATION IN PATIENTS WITH CRYOGLOBULINEMIC GLOMERULONEPHRITIS AND ASSOCIATED HISTOLOGIC LESION

Renal syndrome	Patients, %	Frequent histologic features
Isolated proteinuria with microscopic hematuria, sometimes associated with moderate chronic renal insufficiency	≈55	Membranoproliferative glomerulonephritis (MPGN), with moderate infiltration of monocytes Lobular MPGN Mesangioproliferative glomerulonephritis
Acute nephritic syndrome, sometimes complicated by acute oliguric renal failure	≈25	MPGN with leukocytic infiltration, or intraluminal thrombi owing to abrupt massive precipitation of cryoglobulins, usually associated with renal and systemic vasculitis, or both
Nephrotic syndrome	≈20	MPGN, frequently of lobular type, with some infiltration of monocytes

FIGURE 8-58

Renal syndrome at presentation in patients with cryoglobulinemic glomerulonephritis and associated histologic lesion. During the course of this disease, both the systemic and renal signs may vary remarkably, with periods of exacerbation alternating with periods of quiescence. Very often, exacerbation of the extrarenal signs is associated with exacerbation of renal disease (recurrent episodes of nephritic or nephrotic syndrome); however, a flare-up of renal disease may occur even in the absence of exacerbation of the extrarenal signs. Partial or total prolonged remission occurs spontaneously or after treatment in 10% to 15% of patients. Arterial hypertension frequently is severe and is present in most patients with cryoglobulinemic nephropathy.

LABORATORY ABNORMALITIES IN ESSENTIAL MIXED CRYOGLOBULINEMIA

Circulating cryoglobulins
Cryocrits ranging from 2% to 70%, with large variations during the course of the disease

Hypocomplementemia
Very low levels of early C components (C1q and C4) and CH50; slightly low levels of C3; and high levels of late C components, C5 and C9

FIGURE 8-59

Relevant laboratory abnormalities in "essential" mixed cryoglobulinemia. During the course of this disease, cryoglobulins may temporarily become undetectable. Low levels of serum C4 cannot be corrected by treatment. Low levels of C3 frequently are found during clinical flare-ups and can be corrected by treatment.

TREATMENT OF ACUTE RENAL EXACERBATIONS OF CRYOGLOBULINEMIC GLOMERULONEPHRITIS AND VASCULITIS

Steriods are used to control inflammatory renal and systemic involvement

Cytotoxic drugs are used to block production of new cryoglobulins by the specific lymphocytic clone that produces the monoclonal immunoglobulin Mk RF and, therefore, the precipitating cryoglobulins

Plasma exchange is used to remove circulating cryoglobulins from the blood before they deposit in the glomerulus and arterial walls

FIGURE 8-60

This approach to treatment of the acute renal exacerbations of cryoglobulinemia and vasculitis used previously when the viral cause of the disease was unknown is still valid now that the viral cause is evident. It is a common experience that the antiviral agent interferon-α, when given alone, does not control renal complications in the acute stage of the disease [118].

PROPOSED TREATMENT FOR MIXED CRYOGLOBULINEMIA ASSOCIATED WITH HEPATITIS C VIRUS INFECTION

Drug	Dosage	Duration
Interferon-α	3.0–6.0 MU, 3 times weekly	6–12 mo
Steroids	Methylprednisolone, 0.75–1.0 g/d, intravenously	3 d
	Prednisone, 0.5 mg/kg of body weight tapered over a few weeks until maintenance dose of 10–15 mg/d is achieved	6 mo
Cyclophosphamide	2 mg/kg of body weight	3–4 mo
Plasmapheresis	Exchanges of 3 L of plasma, 3 times weekly	2–3 wk

FIGURE 8-61

The proposed treatment for mixed cryoglobulinemia associated with hepatitis C virus infection in the presence of severe acute signs of renal involvement, ie, glomerulonephritis and vasculitis. Plasma exchange is used only when acute renal insufficiency caused by massive precipitation of cryoglobulins is present. Interferon-α is given for more than 6 months only when negation of hepatitis C virus RNA is achieved in the first months, suggesting a beneficial effect on the viremia. Only the antiviral treatment with interferon-α eventually associated with low doses of steriods to control the systemic signs of mixed cryoglobulinemias should be given if renal involvement is mild. The association of interferon-α with another antiviral agent (ribavirin, 0.6 to 1.0 g/d orally), now is being tested in patients with hepatitis C virus infection, with promising results [118].

Kidney Disease and Hypertension in Pregnancy

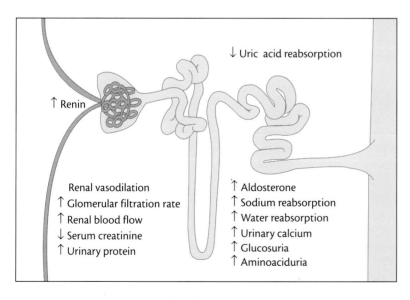

↓ Uric acid reabsorption

↑ Renin

Renal vasodilation
↑ Glomerular filtration rate
↑ Renal blood flow
↓ Serum creatinine
↑ Urinary protein

↑ Aldosterone
↑ Sodium reabsorption
↑ Water reabsorption
↑ Urinary calcium
↑ Glucosuria
↑ Aminoaciduria

FIGURE 8-62

Changes in renal function during pregnancy. Marked renal hemodynamic changes are apparent by the end of the first trimester. Both the glomerular filtration rate (GFR) and effective renal plasma flow (ERPF) increase by 50%. ERPF probably increases to a greater extent, and thus, the filtration fraction is decreased during early and mid pregnancy. Micropuncture studies performed in animals suggest that the basis for the increase in GFR is primarily the increase in glomerular plasma flow [119]. The average creatinine level and urea nitrogen concentration are slightly lower in pregnant women than in those who are not pregnant (0.5 mg/d and 9 mg/dL, respectively). The increased filtered load also results in increased urinary protein excretion, glucosuria, and aminoaciduria. The uric acid clearance rates increase to a greater extent than does the GFR. Hypercalciuria is a result of increased GFR and of increases in circulating 1,25-dihydroxy-vitamin D_3 in pregnancy (*absorptive hypercalciuria*). The renin-angiotensin system is stimulated during gestation, and cumulative retention of approximately 950 mEq of sodium occurs. This sodium retention results from a complex interplay between natriuretic and antinatriuretic stimuli present during gestation [120].

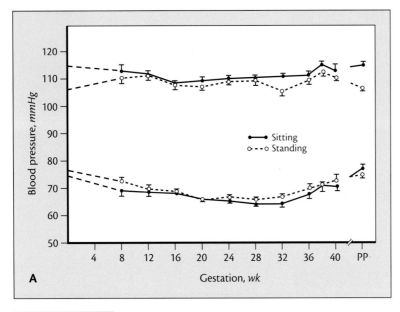

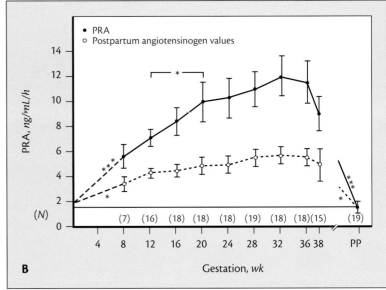

FIGURE 8-63

Blood pressure and the renin-aldosterone system in pregnancy. Normal pregnancy is associated with profound alterations in cardiovascular and renal physiology. These alterations are accompanied by striking adjustments of the renin-angiotensin-aldosterone system. **A,** Blood pressure and peripheral vascular resistance decrease during normal gestation. The decrease in blood pressure is apparent by the end of the first trimester of pregnancy and often approaches prepregnancy levels at term. **B,** Despite the decrease in blood pressure, plasma renin activity (PRA) increases during the first few weeks of pregnancy; on average, close to a fourfold increase in PRA occurs by the end of the first trimester, with additional increases until at least 20 weeks. The source of the increased renin is thought to be the maternal renal release of renin.

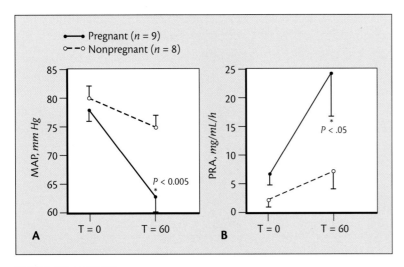

FIGURE 8-64

Functional significance of the stimulated renin-angiotensin system (RAS) in pregnancy. We determine whether changes in the RAS in pregnancy are primary, and the cause of the increase in plasma volume, or whether these changes are secondary to the vasodilation and changes in blood pressure. To do so, we administered a single dose of captopril to normotensive pregnant women in their first and second trimesters and age-matched normotensive women who were not pregnant. We then measured mean arterial pressure (MAP) and plasma renin activity (PRA) before and 60 minutes after the dose.

A, Despite similar baseline blood pressures, blood pressure decreased more in pregnant women compared with those who were not pregnant in response to captopril. This observation suggests that the RAS plays a greater role in supporting blood pressure in pregnancy. **B,** Baseline PRA was higher in pregnant women compared with those who were not pregnant, and pregnant women had a greater increase in renin after captopril compared with those who were not pregnant. T—time. (*Adapted from* August *et al.* [121].)

INTERRELATIONSHIPS BETWEEN PREGNANCY AND RENAL DISEASE

Impact of pregnancy on renal disease	Impact of renal disease on pregnancy
Hemodynamic changes → hyperfiltration	Increased risk of pre-eclampsia
Increased proteinuria	Increased incidence of prematurity, intrauterine growth retardation
Intercurrent pregnancy-related illness, *eg*, pre-eclampsia	
Possibility of permanent loss of renal function	

FIGURE 8-65

Pregnancy may influence the course of renal disease. Some women with intrinsic renal disease, particularly those with baseline azotemia and hypertension, suffer more rapid deterioration in renal function after gestation. In general, as kidney disease progresses and function deteriorates, the ability to sustain a healthy pregnancy decreases. The presence of hypertension greatly increases the likelihood of renal deterioration [120]. Although hyperfiltration (increased glomerular filtration rate) is a feature of normal pregnancy, increased intraglomerular pressure is not a major concern because the filtration fraction decreases. Possible factors related to the pregnancy-related deterioration in renal function include the gestational increase in proteinuria and intercurrent pregnancy-related illnesses, such as pre-eclampsia, that might cause irreversible loss of renal function. Women with renal disease are at greater risk for complications related to pregnancy such as pre-eclampsia, premature delivery, and intrauterine growth retardation.

MANAGEMENT OF CHRONIC RENAL DISEASE DURING PREGNANCY

Preconception counseling

Multidisciplinary approach

Frequent monitoring of blood pressure (every 1–2 wk) and renal function (every mo)

Balanced diet (moderate sodium, protein)

Maintain blood pressure at 120–140/80–90 mm Hg

Monitor for signs of pre-eclampsia

FIGURE 8-66

Management of chronic renal disease during pregnancy is best accomplished with a multidisciplinary team of specialists. Preconception counseling permits the explanation of risks involved with pregnancy. Patients should understand the need for frequent monitoring of blood pressure and renal function. Protein restriction is not advisable during gestation. Salt intake should not be severely restricted. When renal function is impaired, modest salt restriction may help control blood pressure. Blood pressure should be maintained at a level at which the risk of maternal complications owing to elevated blood pressure is low. Patients should be monitored closely for signs of pre-eclampsia, particularly in the third trimester.

RENAL EVALUATION DURING PREGNANCY

Serology

Function

Ultrasonography

Biopsy: <32 wk

　Deteriorating function

　Morbid nephrotic syndrome

FIGURE 8-67

Investigation of the cause of renal disease during pregnancy can be conducted with serologic, functional, and ultrasonographic testing. Renal biopsy is rarely performed during gestation. Renal biopsy usually is reserved for situations in which renal function suddenly deteriorates without apparent cause or when symptomatic nephrotic syndrome occurs, particularly when azotemia is present. Almost no role exists for renal biopsy after gestational week 32 because at this stage the fetus will likely be delivered, independent of biopsy results [122].

INTRINSIC RENAL DISEASE VERSUS PRE-ECLAMPSIA

	Renal disease	Pre-eclampsia
Serum creatinine	>1.0 mg/dL	0.8–1.2 mg/dL
Urinary protein	Variable	>300 mg/d
Uric acid	Variable	>5.5 mg/dL
Blood pressure	Variable	>140/90 mm Hg
Liver function test results	Normal	May be increased
Platelet count	Normal	May be decreased
Urine analysis	Variable	Protein, with or without erythrocytes, leukocytes

FIGURE 8-68

New-onset azotemia, proteinuria, and hypertension occurring in the second half of pregnancy should be distinguished from pre-eclampsia. Most cases of pre-eclampsia are associated with only mild azotemia; significant azotemia is more suggestive of renal disease. Azotemia in the absence of proteinuria or hypertension would be unusual in pre-eclampsia, and thus, would be more suggestive of intrinsic renal disease. Thrombocytopenia, elevated liver function test results, and significant anemia are not typical features of renal disease (except for thrombotic microangiopathic syndromes) and are features of the variant of preeclampsia known as the hemolysis, elevated liver enzymes, and low platelet count (HELLP) syndrome.

DIFFERENTIAL DIAGNOSIS OF MICROANGIOPATHIC SYNDROMES DURING PREGNANCY

	HELLP	AFLP	TTP	HUS
Hypertension	80%	25–50%	Occasional	Present
Renal insufficiency	Mild to moderate	Moderate	Mild to moderate	Severe
Fever, neurologic symptoms	0	0	++	0
Onset	3rd trimester	3rd trimester	Any time	Postpartum
Platelet count	Low to very low	Low to very low	Low to very low	Low to very low
Liver function test results	High to very high	High to extremely high	Usually normal	Usually normal
Partial thromboplastin time	Normal to high	High	Normal	Normal
Antithrombin III	Low	Low	Normal	Normal

FIGURE 8-69

Clinical and laboratory features of the HELLP (hemolysis, elevated liver enzymes, and low platelet count) syndrome, acute fatty liver of pregnancy (AFLP), thrombotic thrombocytopenic purpura (TTP), and hemolytic uremic syndrome (HUS). (*Adapted from* Saltiel *et al.* [123].)

Preconception

Screen for secondary hypertension (pheo, renovascular hypertension)
Counseling: Increased risk of pre-eclampsia (25%)
           Lifestyle adjustments: increase rest, decrease exercise
           Adjust medications: discontinue ACE inhibitors

First trimester

Diastolic BP, *mm Hg*

<90	90–100	≥ 100
Consider careful decrease in BP medication	Adjust medications: Stop ACE and angiotensin II β-blockers Decrease diuretic dose	Increase medication

Baseline evaluation for secondary hypertension if clinically suspected

Second trimester

Nonpharmacologic treatment
Home BP monitoring
Adequate rest

Diastolic BP, *mm Hg*

<90	90–100	≥ 100
Consider careful decrease in BP medication	Continue treatment	Indicates significant hypertension: consider stopping work; close surveillance for pre-eclampsia

Third trimester

Increased surveillance for pre-eclampsia
Check BP every 2 weeks

FIGURE 8-70

Treatment algorithm for chronic hypertension. Ideally, patients with chronic hypertension should be evaluated before pregnancy so that secondary hypertension can be diagnosed and treated appropriately. Women can be counseled regarding the need for possible lifestyle adjustments, and medications can be adjusted. Blood pressure (BP) medications may require adjustment, depending on the magnitude of the pregnancy-related changes in blood pressure. In the latter half of pregnancy, close surveillance for early signs of pre-eclampsia increases the likelihood that the condition will be diagnosed before it progresses to a severe stage.

Renal Involvement in Collagen Vascular Diseases and Dysproteinemias

EPIDEMIOLOGIC AND GENETIC CHARACTERISTICS OF SYSTEMIC LUPUS ERYTHEMATOSUS

Epidemiology	Genetics

Prevalence: between 25 and 250 per 100,000 persons, depending on racial and geographic background	Concordancy in twins
	  Monozygotic: 50%–60%
	  Dizygotic: 5%–10%

Race: more prevalent in Asians and blacks	Familial aggregation in 10%

Gender: female preponderance; gender ratio between 20 and 40 years; male:female, 1:9	Association with the following:
	  HLA: B7, B8, DR2, DR3, DQ$_W$1
	  Complement:
	    C4A Q0
	    C1q or C4 deficiency
	  Fc γ receptor IIA low-affinity phenotype
	  X chromosome ?

Age: onset mainly between 20–40 y	

FIGURE 8-71

The major epidemiologic characteristics of systemic lupus erythe-matosus are listed. The prevalence of the disease depends on ethnic background. The highest prevalence is seen in Asians and blacks. As in other systemic autoimmune diseases, there is a striking prepon-derance in women, especially during childbearing age. This prepon-derance is related to hormonal status. Animal studies have shown that estrogens have a facilitating effect on disease expression, where-as androgens have a suppressive effect. The importance of estrogens is further substantiated by the fact that changes in the hormonal homeostasis (*eg*, at onset of puberty, during use of oral anticontra-ceptives, and during pregnancy and puerperium) are associated with an increased frequency of lupus onset and disease flare-up. The genetic susceptibility is illustrated by the concordance of the disease in twins, occurrence of familial aggregation, and association with certain genes, mainly human leukocyte antigens (HLAs).

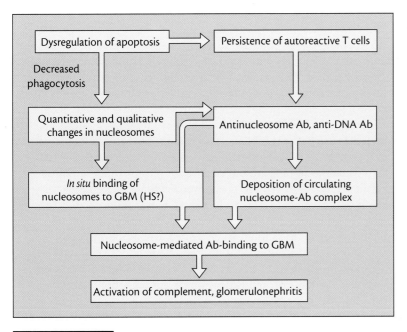

FIGURE 8-72

Hypothesis for the pathophysiology of lupus nephritis. In recent years, evidence has emerged that the process of apoptosis is dis-turbed in systemic lupus erythematosus (SLE). The first indication was found in the MRL/l lupus mouse model, in which a deficiency of the Fas receptor was identified [124]. Activation of this Fas receptor induces apoptosis. Transgenic correction of the Fas-receptor defect prevents development of lupus [125]. In human SLE, Fas receptor expression is normal; however, a number of other observations indi-cate abnormalities in apoptosis [126,127]. Alterations in apoptosis can lead to the persistence of autoreactive T and B cells, because apoptosis is the major mechanism for the elimination of autoreactive cells. In addition, these alterations can lead to quantitative and quali-tative differences in the release of nucleosomes.

Nucleosomes are the basic structures of chromatin. They consist of pairs of the core histones H2A, H2B, H3, and H4 around which double-stranded DNA (dsDNA) is wrapped twice. DNA in the cir-culation of patients with SLE is present in the form of oligonucleo-somes [128]; the only way to generate these oligonucleosomes is by the process of apoptosis. Presently, ample evidence exists that the autoimmune response in SLE is T-cell–dependent and autoantigen-driven [129]. However, dsDNA is very poorly immunogenic, which is in line with the fact that antigen-presenting cells cannot present DNA-derived oligonucleotides to T cells by way of their major his-tocompatibility complex class II molecules. However, recently it has become evident that the nucleosome is the driving autoantigen in SLE.

In murine lupus, T cells specific for nucleosomes have been identi-fied. These T cells not only drive the formation of nucleosome-specif-ic autoantibodies (*ie*, antibodies that react with the intact nucleo-some but not with its constituent DNA and histones) but also the formation of anti-DNA and antihistone antibodies [130]. The his-tone-derived epitopes that drive these responses recently have been identified [131]. These nucleosome-specific autoantibodies precede the emergence of anti-dsDNA and antihistone antibodies, suggesting that the loss of tolerance for nucleosomes is an initial key event in SLE [132,133]. Both in human and murine lupus, nucleosome-specif-ic antibodies are detected in up to 80% of cases [133–135].

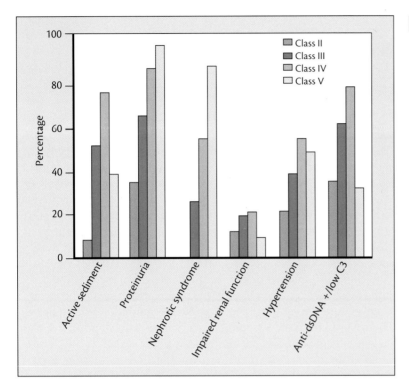

FIGURE 8-73

Incidence of renal manifestations and serologic abnormalities in the different forms of lupus nephritis. The clinical manifestations of lupus nephritis are not different from other forms of glomerulonephritis and include a nephritic sediment (dysmorphic erythrocytes and erythrocyte casts), proteinuria or nephrotic syndrome, impaired renal function, and hypertension. Although certain clinical manifestations are more prevalent in certain forms (nephrotic syndrome for WHO class V, nephritic sediment for WHO class IV), it is clear that on the basis of clinical symptoms it is not possible to classify the form of nephritis correctly. This inability underlines the necessity for obtaining a renal biopsy specimen. In addition, listed are the occurrence of both a positive result on performing a Farr assay and a low complement 3 level for the different forms of lupus nephritis. Anti-dsDNA—anti–double-stranded DNA. (*Adapted from* Appel *et al.* [136]).

TREATMENT OF THE DIFFERENT FORMS OF LUPUS NEPHRITIS

WHO classification	Treatment options
I	Treatment guided by extrarenal lesions
II	Corticosteroids:
III, IV	Cyclophosphamide pulses, oral prednisone Methylprednisolone pulses, azathioprine, low doses of oral prednisone
V	Corticosteroids (and azathioprine or cyclophosphamide)
VI	No further immunosuppression ? Supportive treatment

FIGURE 8-74

Treatment options for the different forms of lupus nephritis are summarized. Only for World Health Organization (WHO) classes III, IV, and V are a limited number of prospective studies available. For the other forms, a balanced compilation is made from the literature and personal experience. Berden [129] provides a more detailed analysis of the therapeutic options. For class I lupus nephritis, no specific renal therapy is necessary; treatment is dictated by the presence of extrarenal symptoms.

In general, patients with class II lupus nephritis respond satisfactorily to monotherapy with oral corticosteroids. The patient, however,

must be monitored for transition to a more severe form, which is generally heralded by worsening of clinical renal symptoms.

For patients with classes III and IV lupus nephritis, corticosteroid monotherapy is not sufficient. Cytotoxic immunosuppressive therapy, either cyclophosphamide or azathioprine, should be added to the treatment.

According to a recent analysis [137], patients with a pure membranous lupus nephritis without a proliferative component (class V, according to the 1995 revised WHO classification) respond satisfactorily to corticosteroid monotherapy. Patients who have a membranous nephropathy with a proliferative component (formerly classified as WHO class VC or VD) have a much worse prognosis and should be treated as are patients with a class IV lupus nephritis. When a patient with class V (A or B) lupus nephritis does not respond to corticosteroids, addition of azathioprine or cyclophosphamide should be considered (as in idiopathic membranous glomerulonephritis, in which oral treatment seems to be superior over monthly intravenous pulses [138–140]). When cyclophosphamide treatment is initiated the therapeutic response should be evaluated after 6 months, and the drug should be discontinued if no improvement has occurred [141].

Treatment of WHO class VI nephritis should be balanced on weighing the risks of intensification of immunosuppressive treatment and the expected benefits. When renal function already is strongly impaired and the renal biopsy specimen shows predominantly chronic irreversible lesions, further deterioration of renal function may be unavoidable. Therefore, an increase in immunosuppressive therapy is questionable. This approach is strengthened by the fact that lupus disease activity mostly subsides during renal replacement therapy. Results of renal transplantation are good, and the disease rarely recurs after transplantation [129].

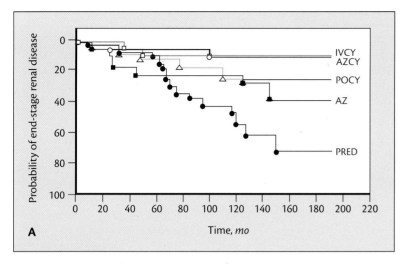

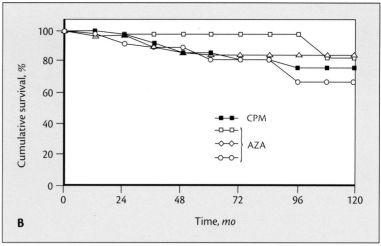

FIGURE 8-75

Probability of end-stage renal disease (ESRD) and renal survival in patients with two forms of lupus nephritis. **A,** The probability of ESRD in patients with proliferative lupus nephritis treated with different drug regimens. This update of the prospective trial by the National Institutes of Health (NIH) on the treatment of these patients clearly demonstrates that prednisone monotherapy, in a significantly greater proportion of patients, leads to the development of ESRD compared with patients on regimens containing cytotoxic drugs. The results between azathioprine (AZ) and drug regimens containing cyclophosphamide (CPM) are not significantly different, Note that in up to 7 years the results do no differ between the different treatment groups. From these studies it is clear that although the therapeutic efficacy is equal for the three treatment regimens containing CPM, fewer side effects occurred in patients treated with intravenous pulses of CPM.
B, Renal survival in patients with World Health Organization (WHO) class IV lupus nephritis treated with either CPM or AZ. The NIH trial [142,143] did not reveal a significant difference between the therapeutic efficacy of CPM and AZ (see *part A*). However, the side effects of both drugs are not identical. CPM has a greater bone marrow toxicity, leads to amenorrhea in many patients, is teratogenic, and displays a unique urothelial toxicity (hemorrhagic cystitis and bladder carcinoma). Therefore, prospective studies comparing CPM with AZ are warranted but not available. The results of the NIH trial are compared with those reported for AZ [144,145–147]. This analysis, carried out by Cameron [144], does not reveal a significant difference between CPM and AZ. A recent meta-analysis [148] again showed that monotherapy with prednisone was inferior to treatment with cytotoxic drugs in combination with steroids. However, as in the NIH trial and the analysis by Cameron, no differences were found between CPM and AZ in preserving renal function. AZCY—combined therapy with azathioprine and cyclophosphamide; IVCY—intravenous pulses of cyclophosphamide; POCY—oral cyclophosphamide. (*Part A adapted from* Steinberg and Steinberg [143]; *part B adapted from* Cameron [144].)

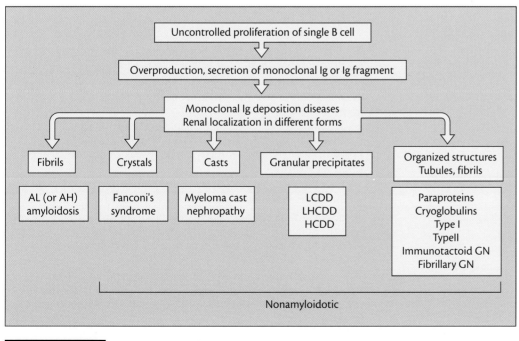

FIGURE 8-76

Types of renal involvement in dysproteinemias. The uncontrolled proliferation of a B-cell clone leads to overproduction of a monoclonal immunoglobulin (Ig), either an intact molecule or fragments thereof (light or heavy chains). These molecules can deposit in the kidney and other vital organs, depending on the immunoglobulin class, light or heavy chain isotype, and other only partly understood physiochemical properties. The terminology used in these disorders is sometimes confusing and inconsistent. We use the definitions proposed by Gallo and Kumar [149]. All diseases characterized by deposits of monoclonal immunoglobulin–related material are named *monoclonal immunoglobulin deposition diseases*. These deposits can occur in several forms, as outlined in the figure, and are identified by specific stains (such as Congo red) and on immunofluorescence and electron microscopy. The histologic and clinical manifestations are dependent on the type of deposition. Included in this overview are fibrillary and immunotactoid glomerulonephritis, which in certain cases also show deposits containing monoclonal immunoglobulins. AH—heavy chain amyloidosis; AL—light chain amyloidosis; GN—glomerulonephritis; HCDD—heavy chain deposition disease; LCDD—light chain deposition disease; LHCDD—light and heavy chain deposition disease.

CLINICAL PRESENTATION, FREQUENCY, AND CAUSES OF RENAL INVOLVEMENT IN DYSPROTEINEMIAS

Acute deterioration of renal function (5%–10%)
  Dehydration
  Hypercalcemia
  Cast nephropathy
  Crescentic glomerulonephritis
Chronic renal insufficiency (45%–75%)
  Myeloma cast nephropathy
  Light chain (AL) amyloidosis
  Interstitial plasma cell infiltration (rare)
Proteinuria-nephrotic syndrome (50%–80%)
  Light chain (AL) amyloidosis
  Light chain deposition disease
  Heavy chain deposition disease
  Cryoglobulinemic glomerular lesions
Fanconi's syndrome (1%)
Secondary lesions (20%–30%)
  Pyelonephritis
  Nephrocalcinosis
  Hyperuricemic nephropathy

FIGURE 8-77

Renal involvement in dysproteinemias can lead to different clinical manifestations: acute renal failure, progressive deterioration of renal function, proteinuria (which very often is in the nephrotic range), or, seldom, Fanconi's syndrome. Furthermore, a number of secondary conditions may occur that can induce additional renal damage. Certain features are associated with particular clinical symptoms. The type of clinical lesion that develops is predominantly determined by the so-called nephrotoxic characteristics of the excreted light chains, as demonstrated by infusion of light chains into mice. These infusions led to the same type of renal lesion as in humans [150,151].

References

1. United States Renal Data System: *USRDS 1997 Annual Data Report.* Bethesda, MD: The National Institutes of Health, National Institute of Diabetes and Digestive and Kidney Diseases; April, 1997.

2. Jennette JC, Falk RJ, Andrassy K, *et al.*: Nomenclature of systemic vasculitides: the proposal of an international consensus conference. *Arthritis Rheum* 1994, 37:187–192.

3. Klein RG, Hunder GG, Stanson AW, *et al.*: Larger artery involvement in giant cell (temporal) arteritis. *Ann Intern Med* 1975, 83:806–812.

4. Arend WP, Michel BA, Bloch DA, *et al.*: The American College of Rheumatology 1990 criteria for the classification of Takayasu arteritis. *Arthritis Rheum* 1990, 33:1129–1134.

5. Lhote F, Guillevin L: Polyarteritis nodosa, microscopic polyangiitis, and Churg-Strauss syndrome. *Rheum Dis Clin North Am* 1995, 21:911–947.

6. Dillon MJ, Ansell BM: Vasculitis in children and adolescents. *Rheum Dis Clin North Am* 1995, 21:1115–1136.

7. Gross WL, Schmitt WH, Csernok E: ANCA and associated diseases: immunodiagnostic and pathogenetic aspects. *Clin Exp Immunol* 1993, 91:1–12.

8. Kallenberg CGM, Brouwer E, Weening JJ, Cohen Tervaert JW: Anti-neutrophil cytoplasmic antibodies: current diagnostic and pathophysiologic potential. *Kidney Int* 1994, 46:1–15.

9. Jennette JC, Falk RJ: Anti-neutrophil cytoplasmic autoantibodies: discovery, specificity, disease associations and pathogenic potential. *Adv Pathol Lab Med* 1995, 8:363–377.

10. Jennette JC: Anti-neutrophil cytoplasmic autoantibody-associated disease: a pathologist's perspective. *Am J Kidney Dis* 1991, 18:164–170.

11. Kyle RA: Amyloidosis. In *Hematology: Basic Principles and Practice.* Edited by Hoffman R, Benz EJ Jr, Shattil SJ, *et al.* New York: Churchill Livingstone; 1991:1038–1047.

12. Kyle RA, Gertz MA, Greipp PR, *et al.*: A trial of three regimens for primary amyloidosis: colchicine alone, melphalan and prednisone, and melphalan, prednisone, and colchicine. *N Engl J Med* 1997, 336:1202–1207.

13. Gertz MA, Kyle RA: Secondary systemic amyloidosis: response and survival in 64 patients. *Medicine* 1991, 70:246–256.

14. Bunn HF: Mechanisms of disease: pathogenesis and treatment of sickle cell disease. *N Engl J Med* 1997, 337:762–769.

15. Statius van Eps LW, Pinedo Veels C, De Vries H, De Koning J: Nature of concentrating defect in sickle cell nephropathy, microradioangiographic studies. *Lancet* 1970, 1:450.

16. Statius van Eps LW, Schouten H, la Porte-Wijsman LW, Struyker Boudier AM: The influence of red blood cell transfusions on the hyposthenuria and renal hemodynamics of sickle cell anemia. *Clin Chim Acta* 1967, 17:449.

17. De Jong PE, Statius van Eps LW: Sickle cell nephropathy: new insights into its pathophysiology. Editorial review. *Kidney Int* 1985, 27:711.

18. Guleria AS, Yang JC, Topalian SL, *et al.*: Renal dysfunction associated with the administration of high-dose interleukin-2 in 199 consecutive patients with metastatic melanoma or renal cell carcinoma. *J Clin Oncol* 1994, 12:2714–2722.

19. Zimmerman SW, Moorthy AV, Burkholder PM, Jenkins PG: Glomerulopathies associated with neoplastic disease. In *Cancer and the Kidney.* Edited by Rieselbach RE, Garnick MB. Philadelphia: Lea & Febiger; 1982.

20. Jenkins PG, Rieselbach RE: Acute renal failure: diagnosis, clinical spectrum, and management. In *Cancer and the Kidney.* Edited by Rieselbach RE, Garnick MB. Philadelphia: Lea & Febiger; 1982.

21. Baker LRJ, Cattell WR, Fry IK, Mallison WJ: Acute renal failure due to bacterial pyelonephritis. *Q J Med* 1979, 48:603.

22. Mayer RJ: Infiltrative and metastatic disease of the kidney. In *Cancer and the Kidney*. Edited by Rieselbach RE, Garnick MB. Philadelphia: Lea & Febiger; 1982.

23. Greenberger JS, Weichselbaum RR, Cassady JR: Radiation nephropathy. In *Cancer and the Kidney*. Edited by Rieselbach RE, Garnick MB. Philadelphia: Lea & Febiger; 1982.

24. Lodish JR, Boxer RJ: Urinary tract hemorrhage. In *Cancer and the Kidney*. Edited by Rieselbach RE, Garnick MB. Philadelphia: Lea & Febiger; 1982.

25. Johnson WJ, Kyle RA, Pineda AA, *et al.*: Treatment of renal failure associated with multiple myeloma. *Arch Intern Med* 1990, 50:863–869.

26. Solomon A, Weiss DT, Kattine AA: Nephrotoxic potential of Bence-Jones proteins. *N Engl J Med* 1991, 324:1845–1851.

27. Kyle RA, Gertz MA: Systemic amyloidosis. *Crit Rev Oncol Hematol* 1990, 10:49–87.

28. Preud'homme JL, Aucouturier P, Striker L: Monoclonal immunoglobulin deposition disease (Randall type): relationship with structural abnormalities of immunoglobulin chains. *Kidney Int* 1994, 46:965–972.

29. Rosol TJ, Capen CC: Mechanisms of cancer-induced hypercalcemia. *Lab Invest* 1992, 67:680–702.

30. Seymour JF, Gagel RF: Calcitriol: the major humoral mediator of hypercalcemia in Hodgkin's disease and non-Hodgkin's lymphomas. *Blood* 1993, 82:1383–1394.

31. Benabe JE, Martinez-Maldonado M: Hypercalcemic nephropathy. *Arch Intern Med* 1978, 138:777–779.

32. Coe FL, Favus MJ, Kathpalia SC, *et al.*: Calcium and phosphorus metabolism in cancer: hypercalcemic nephropathy. In *Cancer and the Kidney*. Edited by Rieselbach RE, Garnick MB. Philadelphia: Lea & Febiger; 1982.

33. Skarin AT: *Atlas of Diagnostic Oncology*. New York: Gower Medical Publishing; 1991.

34. Rieselbach RE, Sorensen LB: Uric acid metabolism in cancer: hyperuricemic nephropathy. In *Cancer and the Kidney*. Edited by Rieselbach RE, Garnick MB. Philadelphia: Lea & Febiger; 1982.

35. Bishop MR, Coccia PF: Tumor lysis syndrome. In *Clinical Oncology*. Edited by Abeloff MD, Armitage JO, Lichter AS, Niederhuber JR. New York: Churchill Livingstone; 1995:557–561.

36. Band PR, Silverberg DS, Henderson JF, *et al.*: Xanthine nephropathy in a patient with lymphosarcoma treated with allopurinol. *N Engl J Med* 1970, 2283:354.

37. Gutmann FD, Boxer RJ: Pathophysiology and management of urinary tract obstruction. In *Cancer and the Kidney*. Edited by Rieselbach RE, Garnick MB. Philadelphia: Lea & Febiger; 1982.

38. Boxer RJ, Garnick MB, Anderson T: Extrarenal cancer of the genitourinary tract. In *Cancer and the Kidney*. Edited by Rieselbach RE, Garnick MB. Philadelphia: Lea & Febiger; 1982.

39. Sanders PW, Herrera GA: Monoclonal immunoglobulin light chain-related renal disorders. *Semin Nephrol* 1993, 13:324–341.

40. Tsuji M, Ochiai S, Taka T, *et al.*: Nonamyloidotic nephrotic syndrome in Waldenstrom's macroglobulinemia. *Nephron* 1990, 54:176–178.

41. Kyle RA: "Benign" monoclonal gammopathy—after 20-35 years of follow-up. *Mayo Clin Proc* 1993, 68:26–36.

42. Shalev M, Cipolla B, Guille F, *et al.*: Is ipsilateral adrenalectomy a necessary component of radical nephrectomy? *J Urol* 1995, 153:1415–1417.

43. Licht MR, Novick AC, Goormastic M: Nephron sparing surgery in incidental versus suspected renal cell carcinoma. *J Urol* 1994, 152:39–42.

44. Thrasher JB, Paulson DF: Prognostic factors in renal cancer. *Urol Clin North Am* 1993, 20:247–262.

45. Massry, Glassock: *Textbook of Nephrology*, edn 3. Baltimore: Williams & Wilkins; 1995.

46. Srivastava RN, Mocedgil A, Bagga A, *et al.*: Hemolytic uremic syndrome in children in northern India. *Pediatr Nephrol* 1991, 5:284–288.

47. O'Riordan T, Kavanagh P, Mellotte G, *et al.*: Haemolytic uraemic syndrome in shigella. *Irish Med J* 1990, 83:72–73.

48. Magaldi AJ, Yasuda PN, Kudo LH, *et al.*: Renal involvement in leptospirosis: a pathophysiologic study. *Nephron* 1992, 62:332–339.

49. Susaengrat W, Dhiensiri T, Sinavatana P, *et al.*: Renal failure in melioidosis. *Nephron* 1987, 46:167–169.

50. Sinniah R, Churg J, Sobin LH (eds.): *Renal Disease: Classification and Atlas of Infectious and Tropical Diseases*. Chicago: ASCP Press; 1988.

51. Melby EI, Jacobsen J, Olsnes S, *et al.*: Entry of protein toxins in polarized epithelial cells. *Cancer Res* 1993, 53:1753–1760.

52. Nigam P, Pant KC, Kapoor KK, *et al.*: Histo-functional status of kidney in leprosy. *Indian J Lepr* 1986, 58:567–575.

53. Bassily S, Farid Z, Barsoum RS, *et al.*: Renal biopsy in schistosoma-salmonella associated nephrotic syndrome. *J Trop Med Hyg* 1976, 79:256–258.

54. Khajehdehi P, Tastegar A, Karazmi A: Immunological and clinical aspects of kidney disease in typhoid fever in Iran. *Q J Med* 1984, 209:101–107.

55. Chugh KS, Damle PB, Kaur S: Renal lesions in leprosy amongst North Indian patients. *Postgrad Med J* 1983, 59:707–711.

56. Baker NM, Mills AE, Rachman I, *et al.*: Hemolytic uremic syndrome in typhoid fever. *Br Med J* 1974, 2:84–87.

57. Sitprija V, Boonpucknavig W: The kidney in dengue. *Proceedings of the 11th Asian Colloquium of Nephrology*. Singapore; 1996:260–265.

58. Barsoum RS, Nabil M, Saady G, *et al.*: Immunoglobulin A and the pathogenesis of schistosomal glomerulopathy. *Kidney Int* 1996, 50:920–928.

59. Chugh KS: Snake bite induced renal failure in India. *Kidney Int* 1989, 194.

60. Waterman J: Some notes on scorpion poisoning in Trinidad. *Trans R Soc Trop Med Hyg* 1993, 32:607.

61. Barss P: Renal failure and death after multiple stings in Papua New Guinea. Ecology, prevention and management of attacks by vespid wasps. *Med J Aust* 1989, 151:659.

62. Spielman FJ, Bowe EA, *et al.*: Acute renal failure as a result of *Physalia physalis* sting. *South Med J* 1982, 75:1425.

63. Kibukamusoke JW, Chugh KS, Sakhuja V: Renal effects of envenomation. In *Tropical Nephrology*. Edited by Kibukamusoke JW. Canberra, Australia: Citforge Pty; 1984:170.

64. Logan JL, Ogden DA: Rhabdomyolysis and acute renal failure following the bite of the giant desert centipede, *Scolopendra heros*. *West J Med* 1985, 142:549.

65. Lin CT, Huang PC, Yen TS, *et al.*: Partial purification and some characteristic nature of a toxic fraction of the grass carp bile. *Clin Biochem Soc* 1977, 6:1.

66. Johnson RJ, Couser WG: Hepatitis B infection and renal disease: clinical, immunopathogenetic and therapeutic considerations. *Kidney Int* 1990, 37:663.

67. Lai KN, Lai FM: Clinical features and natural history of hepatitis B virus–related glomerulopathy in adults. *Kidney Int* 1991, 35(suppl):S40.

68. Takekoshi Y, Tochimaru H, Nagatta Y, Itami N: Immunopathogenetic mechanisms of hepatitis B virus–related glomerulopathy. *Kidney Int* 1991, 35(suppl):S34.

69. Lai KN, Li PK, Lui SF, *et al.*: Membranous nephropathy related to hepatitis B virus in adults. *N Engl J Med* 1991, 324:1457.

70. Lin CY: Clinical features and natural course of HBV-related glomerulopathy in children. *Kidney Int* 1991, 35(suppl):S46.

71. Agnello V, Chung RT, Kaplan LM: A role for hepatitis C virus infection in type II cryoglobulinemia. *N Engl J Med* 1992, 327:1490–1495.

72. Misiani R, Bellavita P, Fenili D, *et al.*: Hepatitis C virus infection in patients with essential mixed cryoglobulinemia. *Ann Intern Med* 1992, 117:573–577.

73. Disdier P, Harle JR, Weiller PJ: Cryoglobulinemia and hepatitis C infection. *Lancet* 1991, 338:1151–1152.

74. Dammacco F, Sansono D: Antibodies to hepatitis C virus in essential mixed cryoglobulinemia. *Clin Exp Immunol* 1992, 87:352–356.

75. Galli M, Monti G, Monteverde A: Hepatitis C virus and mixed cryo-globulinemias. *Lancet* 1992, 1:989.

76. Ferri C, Greco F, Longobardo G: Antibodies to hepatitis C virus in patients with mixed cryoglobulincmia. *Arthritis Rheum* 1991, 34:1606–1610.

77. Sansono D, Gesualdo L, Mano C, *et al.*: Hepatitis C virus related proteins in kidney tissue from hepatitis C virus–infected patients with cryoglobulinemic membranoproliferative glomerulonephritis. *Hepatology* 1997, 25:1237–1244.

78. Johnson RJ, Gretch DR, Yamabe H, *et al.*: Membranoproliferative glomerulonephritis associated with hepatitis C virus infection. *N Engl J Med* 1993, 328:465–470.

79. Rollino C, Roccatello D, Giachino O, *et al.*: Hepatitis C virus infec-tion and membranous glomerulonephritis. *Nephron* 1991, 59:319–320.

80. Davda R, Peterson J, Weiner R, *et al.*: Membranous glomerulonephri-tis in association with hepatitis C virus infection. *Am J Kidney Dis* 1993, 22:452–455.

81. Johnson RJ, Willson R, Yamabe H, *et al.*: Renal manifestations of hepatitis C virus infection. *Kidney Int* 1994, 46:1255.

82. Johnson RJ, Gretch DR, Couser WG, *et al.*: Hepatitis C virus associ-ated glomerulonephritis: effect of α-interferon therapy. *Kidney Int* 1994, 46:1700.

83. Misiani R, Bellavita P, Fenili D, *et al.*: Interferon-α-2a therapy in cryoglobulinemia associated with hepatitis C virus. *N Engl J Med* 1994, 330:751.

84. Poynard T, Bedossa P, Chevallier M, *et al.*: A comparison of three interferon-α-2b regimens for the long-term treatment of chronic non-A, non-B hepatitis. *N Engl J Med* 1995, 332:1457.

85. Poynard T, Leroy V, Cohard M, *et al.*: Meta-analysis of interferon randomized trials in the treatment of viral hepatitis C: effects of dose and duration. *Hepatology* 1996, 24:778.

86. Sarac E, Bastacky S, Johnson JP: Response to high-dose interferon-α after failure of standard therapy in MPGN associated with hepatitis C virus infection. *Am J Kidney Dis* 1997, 30:113.

87. Widell A, Mansson S, Persson NH, *et al.*: Hepatitis C superinfection in hepatitis C virus (HCV)-infected patients transplanted with an HCV-infected kidney. *Transplantation* 1995, 60:642–647.

88. Cockfield SM, Prieksaitis JK: Infection with hepatitis C virus increas-es the risk of *de novo* glomerulonephritis in renal transplant recipi-ents. *J Am Soc Nephrol* 1995, 6:1078.

89. Huraib S, Al Khudair W, Abu Romeh S, *et al.*: Pattern and prevalence of glomerulonephritis in renal transplant hepatitis C (HCV) patients (PTS). *J Am Soc Nephrol* 1995, 6:1093.

90. Morales JM, Fernandez-Zatarain G, Munoz MA, *et al.*: Clinical pic-ture and outcome allograft membranous glomerulonephritis in renal transplant patients with hepatitis C virus infection. *J Am Soc Nephrol* 1995, 6:1107.

91. Roth D, Cirocco R, Zucker K, *et al.*: *De novo* membranoproliferative glomerulonephritis in hepatitis C virus-infected renal allograft recipients. *Transplantation* 1995, 59:1676–1682.

92. Morales JM, Capdevila JP, Campistol JM, *et al.*: Membranous glomerulonephritis associated with hepatitis C virus infection in renal transplant patients. *Transplantation* 1997, 63:1634–1639.

93. Rao TK, Friedman EA: Outcome of severe acute renal failure in patients with acquired immunodeficiency syndrome. *Am J Kidney Dis* 1995, 25:390–398.

94. Rao TK, Filippone EJ, Nicastri AD, *et al.*: Associated focal and segmen-tal glomerulosclerosis in the acquired immunodeficiency syndrome. *N Engl J Med* 1984, 310:669–673.

95. Pardo V, Aldana M, Colton RM, *et al.*: Glomerular lesions in the acquired immunodeficiency syndrome. *Ann Intern Med* 1984, 101:429–434.

96. Gardenswartz MH, Lerner CW, Seligson GR, *et al.*: Renal disease in patients with AIDS: a clinicopathologic study. *Clin Nephrol* 1984, 21:197–204.

97. Mazbar SA, Schoenfeld PY, Humphreys MH: Renal involvement in patients infected with HIV: experience at San Francisco General Hospital. *Kidney Int* 1990, 37:1325–1332.

98. Humphreys MH: Human immunodeficiency virus–associated nephropathy. east is east and west is west? *Arch Intern Med* 1990, 150:253–255.

99. Bourgoignie JJ, Ortiz-Interian C, Green DF, *et al.*: The epidemiology of human immunodeficiency virus–associated nephropathy. In *Nephrology*, vol 1. Edited by Hatano M. Tokyo: Springer-Verlag; 1991:484–492.

100. Pardo V, Meneses R, Ossa L, *et al.*: AIDS-related glomerulopathy: occurrence in specific risk groups. *Kidney Int* 1989, 31:1167–1173.

101. Strauss J, Abitbol C, Zilleruelo G, *et al.*: Renal disease in children with the acquired immunodeficiency syndrome. *N Engl J Med* 1989, 321:625–630.

102. Nochy D, Gotz D, Dosquet P, *et al.*: Renal disease associated with HIV infection: a multicentric study of 60 patients from Paris hospi-tals. *Nephrol Dial Transplant* 1993, 8:11–19.

103. Bourgoignie JJ: Renal complications of human immunodeficiency virus type 1. *Kidney Int* 1990, 37:1571–1584.

104. Bourgoignie J: Glomerulosclerosis associated with HIV infection. *Contemp Issues Nephrol* 1996, 29:59–75.

105. D'Agati V, Appel GB: HIV infection and the kidney. *J Am Soc Nephrol* 1997, 8:138–152.

106. Humphreys MH: Human immunodeficiency virus–associated glomerulosclerosis. *Kidney Int* 1995, 48:311–320.

107. Shuka RR, Kimmel PL, Jumar A: Molecular biology of HIV-1 and kidney disease. *Contemp Issues Nephrol* 1996, 29:329–389.

108. Barisoni L, Bruggeman L, Schwartz E, *et al.*: Pathogenesis of HIV-asso-ciated nephropathy in transgenic mice. *J Am Soc Nephrol* 1997, 8:492A.

109. Ouelette DR, Kelly JW, Anders JT: Serum angiotensin converting enzyme level is elevated in patients with HIV-infection. *Arch Intern Med* 1992, 152:321–324.

110. Kimmel PL, Mishkin GJ, Umana WO: Captopril and renal survival in patients with human immunodeficiency virus nephropathy. *Am J Kidney Dis*: 1996, 28:202–208.

111. Burns G, Paul SK, Sivak SL, *et al.*: Effect of angiotensin-converting enzyme inhibition in HIV-associated nephropathy. *J Am Soc Nephrol* 1997, 8:1140–1146.

112. Bird JE, Kopp JB, Gitlitz P, *et al.*: Captopril intervention is of benefit in HIV-transgenic mice. *J Am Soc Nephrol* 1997, 8:611A.

113. Brouet JC, Clauvel JP, Danon F, *et al.*: Biological and clinical signifi-cance of cryoglobulins: a report of 86 cases. *Am J Med* 1974, 57:775–778.

114. Meltzer M, Franklin EC, Elias K, *et al.*: Cryoglobulinemia: a clinical and laboratory study. II. Cryoglobulins with rheumatoid factor activity. *Am J Med* 1966, 40:837–856.

115. Gorevic PD, Kassab HJ, Levo Y, *et al.*: Mixed cryoglobulinemia: clinical aspects and long-term follow-up of 40 patients. *Am J Med* 1980, 69:287–308.

116. D'Amico G: Cryoglobulinemic glomerulonephritis: a membranopro-liferative glomerulo-nephritis induced by hepatitis C virus. *Am J Kidney Dis* 1995, 25:361–369.

117. D'Amico G, Colasanti G, Ferrario F, Sinico RA: Renal involvement in essential mixed cryoglobulinemia. *Kidney Int* 1989, 35:1004–1014.

118. D'Amico G, Fornasieri A: Cryoglobulinemia. In *Current Therapy in Nephrology and Hypertension: A Companion to Brenner and Rector's the Kidney.* Edited by Brady HR, Wilcox CS. Philadelphia: WB Saunders Company; 1998.

119. Baylis C: Glomerular filtration and volume regulation in gravid animal models. *Clin Obstet Gynaecol* 1987, 1:789.

120. Lindheimer MD, Katz AI: The kidney and hypertension in pregnancy. In *The Kidney*, edn 4. Edited by Brenner BM, Rector FC. Philadelphia: WB Saunders Co; 1991:1551–1595.

121. August P, Mueller FB, Sealey JE, Edersheim TG: Role of renin-angiotensin system in blood pressure regulation in pregnancy. *Lancet* 1995, 345:896–897.

122. Lindheimer MD, Davison JM. Renal biopsy during pregnancy: "To b... or not to b..." *Br J Obstet Gynecol* 1987, 94:932.

123. Saltiel C, Legendre, Grunfeld JP, *et al.*: Hemolytic uremic syndrome in association with pregnancy. In *Hemolytic Uremic Syndrome and Thrombotic Thrombocytopenic Purpura.* Edited by Kaplan BS, Trompeter RS, Moake JL. New York: Marcel Dekker; 1992:241–254.

124. Watanabe-Fukunaga R, Brannan CI, Copeland NG, *et al.*: Lymphoproliferation disorder in mice explained by defects in Fas antigen that mediates apoptosis. *Nature* 1992, 356:314–317.

125. Singer GG, Carrera AC, Marshak-Rothstein A, *et al.*: Apoptosis, Fas and systemic autoimmunity: the MRL/lpr model. *Curr Opinion Immunol* 1994, 6:913–920.

126. Tax WJM, Kramers C, van Bruggen MCJ, Berden JHM: Apoptosis, nucleosomes, and nephritis in systemic lupus erythematosus. *Kidney Int* 1995, 48:666–673.

127. Berden JHM: Systemic lupus erythematosus: disturbed apoptosis? *Ned Tijdschr Geneeskd* 1997, 141:1848–1854.

128. Rumore PM, Steinman CR: Endogenous circulating DNA in systemic lupus erythematosus. Occurrence as multimeric complexes bound to histone. *J Clin Invest* 1990, 86:69–74.

129. Berden JHM: Lupus nephritis. Nephrology Forum. *Kidney Int* 1997, 52:538–558.

130. Mohan C, Adams S, Stanik V, Datta SK: Nucleosome, a major immunogen for pathogenic autoantibody-inducing T cells of lupus. *J Exp Med* 1993, 177:1367–1381.

131. Kaliyaperumal A, Mohan C, Wu W, Datta SK: Nucleosomal peptide epitopes for nephritis-inducing T helper cells of murine lupus. *J Exp Med* 1996, 183:2459–2469.

132. Burlingame RW, Rubin RL, Balderas RS, Theofilopoulos AN: Genesis and evolution of anti-chromatin autoantibodies in murine lupus implicates T-dependent immunization with self antigen. *J Clin Invest* 1993, 91:1687–1696.

133. Amoura Z, Chabre H, Koutouzov S, *et al.*: Nucleosome-restricted antibodies are detected before anti-dsDNA and/or antihistone antibodies in serum of MRL-Mp lpr/lpr and +/+ mice, and are present in kidney eluates of lupus mice with proteinuria. *Arthritis Rheumatol* 1994, 37:1684–1688.

134. Burlingame RW, Boey ML, Starkebaum G, Rubin RL: The central role of chromatin in autoimmune responses to histones and DNA in systemic lupus erythematosus. *J Clin Invest* 1994, 94:184–192.

135. Chabre H, Amoura Z, Piette JC, *et al.*: Presence of nucleosome-restricted antibodies in patients with systemic lupus erythematosus. *Arthritis Rheumatol* 1995, 38:1485–1491.

136. Appel GB, Silva FG, Pirani CL, *et al.*: Renal involvement in systemic lupus erythematosus. *Medicine* 1975, 57:371–410.

137. Sloan RP, Schwartz MM, Korbet SM, Borok RZ, and the Lupus Nephritis Collaborative Study Group: Long-term outcome in systemic lupus erythematosus membranous glomerulonephritis. *J Am Soc Nephrol* 1996, 7:299–305.

138. Bruns FJ, Adler S, Fraley DS, Segel DP: Sustained remission of membranous glomerulonephritis after cyclophosphamide and prednisone. *Ann Intern Med* 1991, 114:725–730.

139. Reichert LJM, Huysmans FTM, Assmann KJM, *et al.*: Preserving renal function in patients with membranous nephropathy: daily oral chlorambucil compared with intermittent monthly pulses of cyclophosphamide. *Ann Intern Med* 1994, 121:328–333.

140. Falk RJ, Hogan SL, Muller KE, Jenette C, and the Glomerular Disease Collaborative Network: Treatment of progressive membranous glomerulopathy. A randomized trial comparing cyclophosphamide and corticosteroids with corticosteroids alone. *Ann Intern Med* 1992, 116:438–445.

141. Appel GB, Valeri A: The course and treatment of lupus nephritis. *Ann Rev Med* 1994, 45:525–537.

142. Austin III HA, Klippel JH, Balow JE, *et al.*: Therapy of lupus nephritis. Controlled trial of prednisone and cytotoxic drugs. *N Engl J Med* 1986, 314:614–619.

143. Steinberg AD, Steinberg SC: Longterm preservation of renal function in patients with lupus nephritis receiving treatment that includes cyclophosphamide versus those treated with prednisone only. *Arthritis Rheumatol* 1991, 34:945–950.

144. Cameron JS: What is the role of long-term cytotoxic agents in the treatment of lupus nephritis? *J Nephrol* 1993, 6:172–176.

145. Esdaile JM, Levinton C, Federgreen W, *et al.*: The clinical and renal biopsy predictors of long term outcome in lupus nephritis. *Q J Med* 1989, 72:779–833.

146. Ponticelli C, Zucchelli P, Moroni G, *et al.*: Long-term prognosis of diffuse lupus nephritis. *Clin Nephrol* 1987, 28:263–271.

147. Cameron JS, Turner BR, Ogg CS, *et al.*: Systemic lupus with nephritis: a long term study. *Q J Med* 1979, 48:1–24.

148. Bansal VK, Beto JA: Treatment of lupus nephritis: a meta-analysis of clinical trials. *Am J Kidney Dis* 1997, 29:193–199.

149. Gallo G, Kumar V: Hematopoietic disorders. In *Renal Biopsy Interpretation.* Edited by Silva FG, D'Agati VD, Nadasdy T. New York: Churchill Livingstone; 1996:259–282.

150. Solomon A, Weiss DT, Kattine AA: Nephrotoxic potential of Bence Jones proteins. *N Engl J Med* 1991, 324:1845–1851.

151. Sanders PW, Booker BB: Pathobiology of cast nephropathy from human Bence Jones proteins. *J Clin Invest* 1992, 89:630–639.

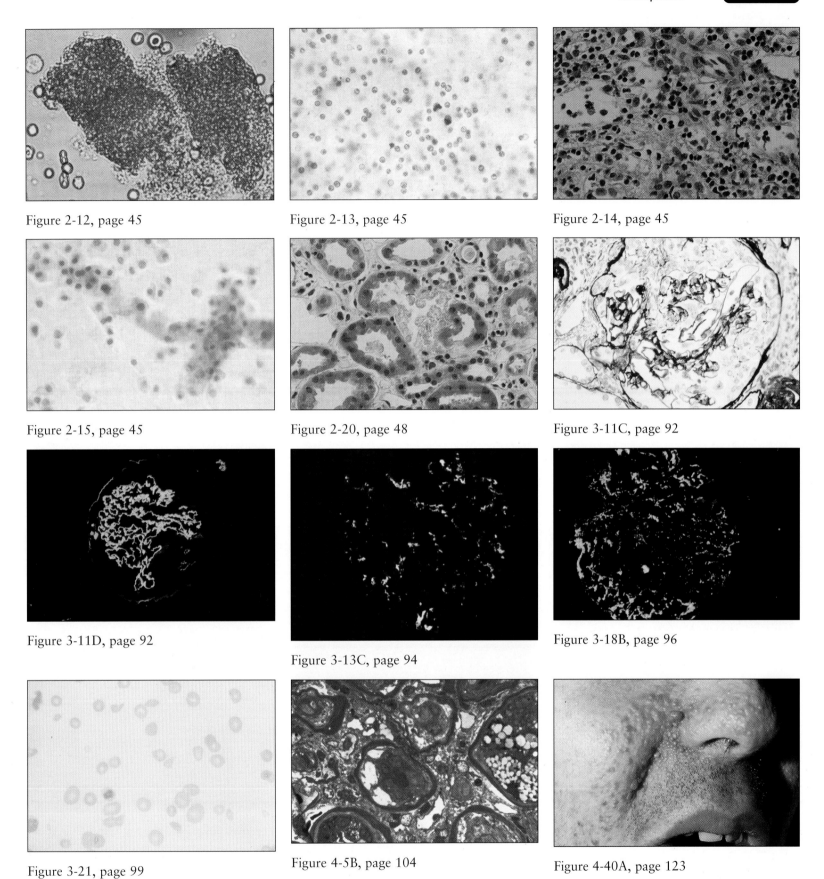

Figure 2-12, page 45

Figure 2-13, page 45

Figure 2-14, page 45

Figure 2-15, page 45

Figure 2-20, page 48

Figure 3-11C, page 92

Figure 3-11D, page 92

Figure 3-13C, page 94

Figure 3-18B, page 96

Figure 3-21, page 99

Figure 4-5B, page 104

Figure 4-40A, page 123

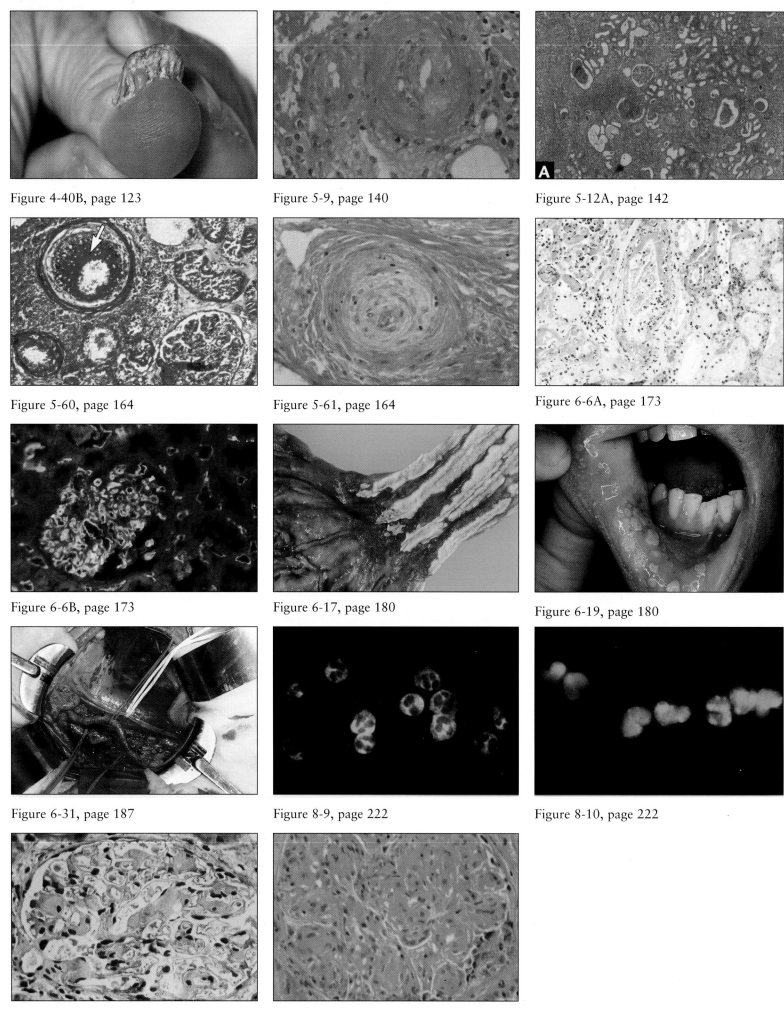

Figure 4-40B, page 123

Figure 5-9, page 140

Figure 5-12A, page 142

Figure 5-60, page 164

Figure 5-61, page 164

Figure 6-6A, page 173

Figure 6-6B, page 173

Figure 6-17, page 180

Figure 6-19, page 180

Figure 6-31, page 187

Figure 8-9, page 222

Figure 8-10, page 222

Figure 8-16, page 224

Figure 8-33b, page 234